BLUEPRINTS
NEUROLOGY

Second Edition

For every step of your medical career,
look for all the books in the *Blueprints* series

Perfect for clerkship and board review!

Blueprints Cardiology, 2nd edition
Blueprints Emergency Medicine, 2nd edition
Blueprints Family Medicine, 2nd edition
Blueprints Medicine, 3rd edition
Blueprints Neurology, 2nd edition
Blueprints Obstetrics & Gynecology, 3rd edition
Blueprints Pediatrics, 3rd edition
Blueprints Psychiatry, 3rd edition
Blueprints Radiology, 2nd edition
Blueprints Surgery, 3rd edition

Visit www.blackwellmedstudent.com to see all the great *Blueprints*:

Blueprints Notes & Cases
Blueprints Clinical Cases
Blueprints Pockets
Blueprints Step 2 Q&A
Blueprints USMLE Step 2 CS
Blueprints Step 3 Q&A
Blueprints Computer-Based Case Simulation Review: USMLE Step 3
Blueprints Clinical Procedures

BLUEPRINTS
NEUROLOGY

Second Edition

Frank W. Drislane, MD
Associate Professor of Neurology
Harvard Medical School
Comprehensive Epilepsy Center
Beth Israel Deaconess Medical Center
Boston, Massachusetts

Michael Benatar, MBChB, Dphil
Assistant Professor of Neurology
Director of the Electromyography
  Laboratory
Emory University
Atlanta, Georgia

Bernard S. Chang, MD
Assistant Professor of Neurology
Harvard Medical School
Comprehensive Epilepsy Center
Beth Israel Deaconess Medical Center
Boston, Massachusetts

Juan Acosta, MD
Clinical Research Fellow
Pain Research Unit
King's College Hospital
Denmark Hill, SE5 9RS
London, UK

John E. Croom, MD, PhD
Instructor in Neurology
Harvard Medical School
Comprehensive Epilepsy Center
Beth Israel Deaconess Medical Center
Boston, Massachusetts

Andrew Tarulli, MD
Clinical Fellow in Neurology
Harvard Medical School
Chief Resident in Neurology
Beth Israel Deaconess Medical Center
Boston, Massachusetts

Louis R. Caplan, MD
Professor of Neurology
Harvard Medical School
Chief, Cerebrovascular Service
Beth Israel Deaconess Medical Center
Boston, Massachusetts

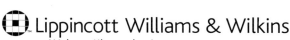 Lippincott Williams & Wilkins
a Wolters Kluwer business
Philadelphia · Baltimore · New York · London
Buenos Aires · Hong Kong · Sydney · Tokyo

Acquisitions Editor: Beverly Copland
Development Editor: Selene Steneck
Production Editor: Debra Murphy
Cover and Interior Designer: Mary McKeon
Compositor: TechBooks in New Delhi, India
Printer: Edwards Brothers in Ann Arbor, MI

351 West Camden Street
Baltimore, MD 21201

530 Walnut Street
Philadelphia, PA 19106

Printed in the United States of America

Library of Congress Cataloging-in-Publication Data

Blueprints neurology / Frank W. Drislane . . . [et al.]. 2nd ed.
  p. ; cm.
  Includes index.
  Rev. ed. of: Blueprints in neurology / by Frank W. Dislane . . . [et al.]. 2002.
  ISBN-13: 978-1-4051-0463-0 (pbk. : alk. paper)
  ISBN-10: 1-4051-0463-5 (pbk. : alk. paper) 1. Neurology—Examinations, questions, etc. 2. Physicians—Licences—United States—Examinations—Study guides.
  [DNLM: 1. Nervous System Diseases—Handbooks. 2. Neurology—Handbooks. WL 39 B658 2006] I. Drislane, Frank. II. Blueprints in neurology.

  RC336.B575 2006
  616.8'0076—dc22

                                        2005015951

To purchase additional copies of this book, call our customer service department at **(800) 638-3030** or fax orders to **(301) 824-7390**. International customers should call **(301) 714-2324.**

Visit Lippincott Williams & Wilkins on the Internet: http://www.LWW.com.
Lippincott Williams & Wilkins customer service representatives are available from 8:30 am to 6:00 pm, EST.

                                        05 06 07 08 09
                                      1 2 3 4 5 6 7 8 9 10

Table of Contents

Reviewers vii
Preface x
Acknowledgments xi
Abbreviations xii

PART ONE: Basics of Neurology 1

  1 The Neurologic Examination 2
  2 Neurologic Investigations 10

PART TWO: Common Neurologic Symptoms 19

  3 The Approach to Coma and Altered Consciousness 20
  4 Neuro-Ophthalmology 27
  5 The Approach to Weakness 38
  6 The Sensory System 46
  7 Dizziness, Vertigo, and Syncope 52
  8 Ataxia and Gait Disorders 56
  9 Urinary and Sexual Dysfunction 61
 10 Headache and Facial Pain 67

PART THREE: Neurologic Disorders 73

 11 Aphasia and Other Disorders of Higher Cortical Function 74
 12 Dementia 81
 13 Sleep Disorders 89
 14 Vascular Disease 93
 15 Seizures 102
 16 Movement Disorders 110
 17 Head Trauma 118
 18 Systemic and Metabolic Disorders 123
 19 Brain Tumors 129
 20 Demyelinating Diseases of the Central Nervous System 137
 21 Infections of the Nervous System 143

22 Disorders of the Spinal Cord 150

23 The Peripheral Nervous System 156

24 Disorders of the Neuromuscular Junction and Skeletal Muscle 166

25 Pediatric Neurology 175

Questions 183

Answers 193

Appendix: Evidence-Based Resources 201

Index 205

Reviewers

Catarina Castaneda, MD
Class of 2004
Drexel University College of Medicine
Philadelphia, Pennsylvania

Maureen Chase, MD
Resident, Emergency Medicine
Hospital of University of Pennsylvania
Jefferson Medical College
Thomas Jefferson University Hospital
Philadelphia, Pennsylvania

Suzanne Crandall
Class of 2005
Kansas City University of Medicine and Biosciences
Kansas City, Missouri

Alexis Dang, MD
Class of 2004
University of California - San Francisco
San Francisco, California

Lee S. Engel, MD, PhD
Fellow, Department of Infectious Diseases
Louisiana State University Health Sciences Center
New Orleans, Louisiana

Merritt Fajt, MD
Class of 2004
Temple University School of Medicine
Philadelphia, Pennsylvania
R1- Internal Medicine, Penn State University
Milton S. Hershey Hershey Medical Center
Hershey, Pennsylvania

Baback Gabbay, MD
Class of 2005
David Geffen School of Medicine at UCLA
Los Angeles, CA

Amir A. Ghaferi
Class of 2005
Johns Hopkins School of Medicine
Baltimore, Maryland

Hoda Ghanem, MD
Intern
UC Irvine – Internal Medicine
Irvine, California

Sarah Harper
Class of 2005
University of Pittsburgh School of Medicine
Pittsburgh, Pennsylvania

Gloria Hsu
Class of 2005
Stanford University School of Medicine
Stanford, California

Mark Lassoff, MD
Class of 2004
UMDNJ – New Jersey Medical School
Newark, New Jersey
Urology Resident
LAC+USC Medical Center
Los Angeles, California

Ryan Ley
Class of 2005
University of Nevada School of Medicine
Reno, Nevada

Meredith M. LeQuear, DO
Class of 2004
New York College of Osteopathic Medicine
Old Westbury, New York

Mark Naftanel
Class of 2005
Duke University School of Medicine
Durham, North Carolina

David J. Nusz, MD
Class of 2004
SUNY Downstate College of Medicine
Brooklyn, New York

Christi Otten
Class of 2005
University of Oklahoma Health Sciences Center – Physician Assistant program
Oklahoma City, Oklahoma

Pulak Ray
Class of 2005
University of Maryland School of Medicine
Baltimore, Maryland

Chris Reed
Class of 2005
Medical College of Wisconsin
Milwaukee, Wisconsin

Matheni Sathananthan
Class of 2006
SUNY at Buffalo School of Medicine
Buffalo, New York

Kamran Shamsa, MD
Class of 2004
University of California – San Diego
La Jolla, California

Victor Sung
Class of 2005
University of Texas Southwestern Medical Center
Dallas, Texas

Ahmet Tural, MD
Department of Infectious Diseases
Providence Physician Group
Everett, WA

Alyssa Tzoucalis
Class of 2004
Hofstra University – Physician Assistant program
Hempstead, New York

Parham Yashar, MD
Neurological Surgery PGY-1
Albert Einstein College of Medicine
Bronx, New York

Ming Zhou, MD
Class of 2004
University of Nevada School of Medicine
Las Vegas, Nevada

Preface

In 1997, the first five books in the **Blueprints** series were published as board review for medical students, interns, and residents who wanted high-yield, accurate clinical content for USMLE Steps 2 & 3. Nearly a decade later, the **Blueprints** brand has expanded into a high-quality, trusted resource covering the broad range of clinical topics studied by medical students and residents during their primary, specialty, and subspecialty rotations.

The **Blueprints** were conceived as study aids created by students, for students. In keeping with this concept, the editors of the current editions of the **Blueprints** books have recruited resident contributors to ensure that the second edition of the series continues to offer the information and approach that made the original **Blueprints** a success.

Now in their second editions, each of the five specialty **Blueprints**—**Blueprints** Emergency Medicine, **Blueprints** Family Medicine, **Blueprints** Neurology, **Blueprints** Cardiology, and **Blueprints** Radiology—has been completely revised and updated to bring you the most current treatment and management strategies. The feedback we've received from our readers has been tremendously helpful in guiding the editorial direction of the second editions; for that, we are grateful to the hundreds of medical students and residents who have responded with in-depth comments and highly detailed feedback.

Each book has been thoroughly reviewed and revised accordingly, with new features being included across the series. An evidence-based resource section has been added to provide current and classic references for each chapter, and an increased number of current board-format questions with detailed explanations for correct and incorrect answer options are included in each book. All revisions to the **Blueprints** series have been made in order to offer you the most concise, comprehensive, and cost-effective information available.

Our readers report that **Blueprints** are useful for every step of their medical career, from their clerkship rotations and subinternships to a board review for USMLE Steps 2 & 3. Residents studying for USMLE Step 3 often use the books to review areas that were not their specialty. Students from a wide variety of health care specialties, including those in physician assistant, nurse practitioner, and osteopathic programs, use **Blueprints** either as a course companion or to review for their licensure examinations.

However you use **Blueprints**, we hope that you find the books in the series informative and useful. Your feedback and suggestions are essential to our continued success.

The Publisher
Lippincott Williams & Wilkins

Acknowledgments

We thank our patients for the opportunity of working with them and learning Neurology, our colleagues and teachers in the Beth Israel Deaconess Medical Center Neurology department for teaching us more fascinating concepts about the nervous system, and our families for tolerating the many hours spent writing and revising this book.

Abbreviations

A(β)	amyloid-beta
ABP	abductor pollicis brevis
Abs	antibodies
AβPP	amyloid–beta protein precursor
ACA	anterior cerebral artery
ACE	angiotensin converting enzyme
AD	Alzheimer disease
ADEM	acute disseminated encephalomyelitis
ADHD	attention deficit–hyperactivity disorder
ADM	abductor digiti minimi
AED	antiepileptic drug
AICA	anteroinferior cerebellar artery
AIDP	acute inflammatory demyelinating polyneuropathy
AIDS	acquired immunodeficiency syndrome
AION	anterior ischemic optic neuropathy
ALS	amyotrophic lateral sclerosis
ANA	antinuclear antibody
APP	amyloid precursor protein
APS	antiphospholipid syndrome
AVM	arteriovenous malformation
AZT	zidovudine
BMD	Becker muscular dystrophy
BPPV	benign positional paroxysmal vertigo
CBC	complete blood count
cGMP	cyclic guanosine monophosphate
CIDP	chronic inflammatory demyelinating polyradiculopathy
CJD	Creutzfeldt-Jakob disease
CK	creatine kinase
CMAP	compound muscle action potential
CMT	Charcot-Marie-Tooth disease
CN	cranial nerve
CNS	central nervous system
COMT	catechol O-methyl transferase
CP	cerebral palsy
CPAP	continuous positive airway pressure
CSF	cerebrospinal fluid
CT	computed tomography
DH	detrusor hyperreflexia
DI	detrusor instability
DLB	dementia with Lewy bodies
DM	dermatomyositis
DMD	Duchenne muscular dystrophy
DSD	detrusor-sphincter dyssynergia
DTRs	deep tendon reflexes
DWI	diffusion-weighted imaging
EA	episodic ataxia
ED	erectile dysfunction
EEG	electroencephalogram
EMG	electromyography
EMG/NCS	electromyography/nerve conduction studies
ER	emergency room
ESR	erythrocyte sedimentation rate
ET	essential tremor
EWN	Edinger-Westphal nuclei
FDI	first dorsal interosseus
FEV_1	forced expiratory volume in 1 second
FLAIR	fluid-attenuated inversion recovery
FTA	fluorescent treponemal antibody
FTD	frontotemporal dementia
FVC	forced vital capacity
GAD	glutamic acid decarboxylase
GBS	Guillain-Barré syndrome
GCS	Glasgow Coma Scale
GTC	generalized tonic-clonic
HD	Huntington's disease
HIV	human immunodeficiency virus
HNPP	hereditary sensory neuropathy with liability to pressure palsy
HS	Horner's syndrome
HSAN	hereditary sensory and autonomic neuropathy
HSV	herpes simplex virus
IBM	inclusion body myositis
ICA	internal cerebral artery
ICP	intracranial pressure
ICU	intensive care unit
IIH	idiopathic intracranial hypertension
INO	internuclear ophthalmoplegia

INR	international normalized ratio	PDC	paroxysmal (nonkinesogenic) dystonic choreoathetosis
IVIg	intravenous immunoglobulin		
LEMS	Lambert-Eaton myasthenic syndrome	PEO	progressive external ophthalmoplegia
LGN	lateral geniculate nuclei	PET	positron emission tomography
LMN	lower motor neuron	PICA	posteroinferior cerebellar artery
LND	light-near dissociation	PKC	paroxysmal kinesogenic choreoathetosis
LP	lumbar puncture		
MAG	myelin-associated glycoprotein	PM	polymyositis
MCA	middle cerebral artery	PML	progressive multifocal leukoencephalopathy
MELAS	mitochondrial myopathy, encephalopathy, lactoacidosis, and stroke	PN	peripheral neuropathy
		PNS	peripheral nervous system
		POTS	postural orthostatic tachycardia syndrome
MERRF	myoclonic epilepsy with ragged red fibers		
		PP	periodic paralyses
MFS	Miller Fisher syndrome	PPD	purified protein derivative
MG	myasthenia gravis	PPRF	paramedian pontine reticular formation
MLF	medial longitudinal fasciculus		
MMN	multifocal motor neuropathy	PS1	presenilin 1
MND	motor neuron disease	PS2	presenilin 2
MRA	magnetic resonance angiography	PSP	progressive supranuclear palsy
MRC	Medical Research Council	PT	prothrombin time
MRI	magnetic resonance imaging	PTT	partial thromboplastin time
MRV	magnetic resonance venography	PVR	postvoid residual
MS	multiple sclerosis	QSART	quantitative sudomotor axon reflex test
MSA	multiple system atrophy		
MSLT	multiple sleep latency test	RAPD	relative afferent pupillary defect
MUSK	muscle-specific kinase	REM	rapid eye movement
nAChR	nicotinic acetylcholine receptor	RF	radiofrequency
NCS	nerve conduction studies	riMLF	rostral interstitial nucleus of the MLF
NCV	nerve conduction velocity		
NFTs	neurofibrillary tangles	RPR	rapid plasma reagin
NIF	negative inspiratory force	rt-PA	recombinant tissue-type plasminogen activator
NMDA	N-methyl-D-aspartate		
NMJ	neuromuscular junction	SAH	subarachnoid hemorrhage
NMS	neuroleptic malignant syndrome	SCA	spinocerebellar ataxia
NSAID	nonsteroidal anti-inflammatory drugs	SCA	superior cerebellar artery
		SE	status epilepticus
OCD	obsessive-compulsive disorder	SLE	systemic lupus erythematosus
ODS	optic disc swelling	SMA	spinal muscular atrophy
ON	optic neuritis	SNAP	sensory nerve action potential
PANDAS	pediatric autoimmune neurologic disorders associated with streptococcal infection	SPECT	single-photon emission computed tomography
		SSRI	selective serotonin reuptake inhibitor
PAS	periodic acid–Schiff		
PCA	posterior cerebral arteries	STT	spinothalamic tract
PCD	paraneoplastic cerebellar degeneration	TB	tuberculosis
		TCD	transcranial Doppler
PCNSL	primary central nervous system lymphoma	TE	time to echo
		TIA	transient ischemic attack
PCR	polymerase chain reaction	TORCH	toxoplasmosis, other agents, rubella, cytomegalovirus, herpes simplex
PD	Parkinson's disease		

TR	time to repetition	VOR	vestibulo-ocular reflex
TSC	tuberous sclerosis complex	VP	venous pulsation
UMN	upper motor neuron	VPL	ventroposterolateral
VA	visual acuity	WD	Wilson's disease
VDRL	Venereal Disease Research Laboratory		

Part One

Basics of Neurology

The Neurologic Examination

To practicing neurologists, the neurologic exam reflects the uniqueness of the specialty. In a world of technology, it remains a purely clinical tool still unmatched in its ability to identify and localize abnormalities of the nervous system. To students, however, the exam can be both mystifying and bemusing, an endless series of maneuvers designed to elicit seemingly obscure and inexplicable findings.

When its principles and elements are presented simply, though, the exam is logical and elegant, reflecting the rational diagnostic process that characterizes not just neurology but all of medicine.

■ PRINCIPLES

1. **The neurologic exam is not a standardized checklist.** Part of the intimidation of performing the exam is its sheer length; hours could be spent on examining the mental status alone. In reality, however, the exam is used in a focused and thoughtful way, depending on what hypotheses have been generated about the patient's disease from the history. A patient presenting with confusion may need quite a comprehensive mental status exam, whereas a patient presenting with a left foot drop may need detailed motor, sensory, and reflex testing of the left leg. In both cases general screening elements of the remaining parts of the exam may be sufficient.
2. **Observation is more important than confrontation.** Most abnormalities of the nervous system manifest themselves in ways visible to the observant examiner. A significant anomia becomes evident when a patient uses circumlocutions to relate his history, and proximal weakness is obvious when he has difficulty arising from a chair. It

is often more useful to describe a patient's observed activities and capabilities than to describe the findings obtained upon formal testing. Confrontation testing is subjective and variable; the grading of muscle strength depends on the examiner's effort and expectations of what the patient's "normal" strength should be. The observation of a pronator drift, for example, is less subjective.

3. **The object is to localize.** The extent and complexity of the nervous system require that any attempt to formulate a concise differential diagnosis must begin with an accurate localization of the problem to a specific region of the nervous system. Left hand weakness may stem from carpal tunnel syndrome, a brachial plexus injury, cervical spondylosis, or a right middle cerebral artery stroke, all of which have different diagnostic workups, treatments, and prognoses. The alert physician thinks, "What signs would be present in a carpal tunnel problem that would not be present in a brachial plexus problem (and vice versa)?" Those signs are then sought and the exam further refined if necessary.
4. **Not all findings have equal importance.** A common difficulty is that completion of the exam results in a long list of many minor abnormalities of questionable importance, such as a 20% decrease in temperature sensation over a patch on the left thigh. Although certainly in some cases incidental findings may be the clue to a previously unsuspected diagnosis, in most cases the highest importance must be given to findings directly related to the patient's symptoms and to "hard" findings that require definitive explanation, such as a dropped reflex or a Babinski sign.

KEY POINTS

1. The neurologic exam is not a standardized checklist.
2. Observation is more important than confrontation.
3. The object is to localize.
4. Not all findings have equal importance.

■ ELEMENTS OF THE EXAM

As discussed earlier, the specific features to include in the neurologic exam should vary with each patient; however, commonly performed elements of the exam are described in this section and listed in Table 1-1.

Mental Status

Neurologists use the mental status exam to identify cognitive deficits that help to localize a problem to a specific region of the brain. Thus the exam differs from that used by psychiatrists, whose objectives in performing the exam are different.

The first step in mental status testing is to assess the level of consciousness. This may vary from the alert wakefulness of a clinic outpatient to the coma of a patient in the intensive care unit. There is a tendency to use "medical" terminology—such as **stuporous**, **obtunded**, or **lethargic**—to describe the level of consciousness, but these have variable meanings; it is more useful to describe how well a patient stayed awake or what stimulation was required to arouse her.

■ TABLE 1-1

Commonly Performed Elements of the Neurologic Examination

Mental status	
Attention	Serial backward tasks (months of the year, digit span)
Language	Fluency of speech, repetition, comprehension of commands, naming objects, reading, writing
Memory	Three words in 5 minutes
Visuospatial function	Drawing clock, copying complex figure
Neglect	Line bisection, double simultaneous stimulation
Frontal lobe function	Generating word lists, learning a motor sequence
Cranial nerves	
II	Visual acuity, fields, pupils, funduscopic exam
III, IV, VI	Extraocular movements
V, VII	Facial sensation and movement
IX, X, XII	Palate and tongue movement
Motor	
Bulk	Palpation for atrophy
Tone	Evaluation for rigidity, spasticity
Power	Observational tests (pronator drift, arising from chair, walking on heels and toes), direct confrontation strength testing
Reflexes	
Muscle stretch reflexes	Biceps, brachioradialis, triceps, knee, ankle
Babinski sign	Stroking lateral sole of foot
Sensory	
Pinprick and temperature	Pin, cold tuning fork
Vibration and joint position sense	Tuning fork and moving digits
Coordination	
Accuracy of targeting	Finger-to-nose, heel-to-shin
Rhythm of movements	Rapid alternating movements, rhythmic finger or heel tapping
Gait	
Stance	Narrow or wide base
Romberg's sign	Steadiness with feet together and eyes closed
Stride and arm swing	Assessment for shuffling, decreased arm swing
Ataxia	Ability to tandem walk

Next, assuming the level of consciousness allows for further testing of cognitive functions, attention is tested, typically with serial forward and backward tasks. These include digit span, reciting the months of the year, or spelling the word **"world,"** all forward and backward. Attention is usually tested early, because significant inattention compromises the ability to perform subsequent cognitive tests and may render their interpretation difficult.

Next, language is assessed. As noted previously, listening to the patient tell his history may be all that is necessary to gauge language ability. Formal testing, however, includes assessing the fluency of spontaneous speech, the ability to repeat, the ability to comprehend commands, the ability to name both common and less common objects, and the ability to read and write.

For memory testing, most commonly the patient is given three words and asked to recall them several minutes later, with the aid of hints if necessary. More information can be gained by giving longer lists of words and charting the patient's learning (and forgetting) curve. Visual memory can be tested with three simple shapes for the patient to draw from memory in several minutes.

Visuospatial function can be tested in a variety of ways. Patients can be asked to draw a clock, a cube, or another simple figure; alternatively, they can be asked to copy a complex figure drawn by the examiner (Figure 1-2).

Neglect is a mental status finding typically not sought by nonneurologists, yet its presence can be a very important sign. Patients with dense neglect may fail to describe items on one side of a picture or of their surroundings, or may fail to bisect a line prop-

erly. Subtle neglect may manifest as extinction to double simultaneous stimulation, in which a patient can sense a single stimulus on either side but when bilateral stimuli are presented simultaneously will sense only the one on the nonneglected side.

Tests of frontal lobe function include learning a simple motor sequence of hand postures, inhibiting inappropriate responses when following a "go/no-go" paradigm, or generating lists of words beginning with a particular letter or belonging to a particular category.

KEY POINTS
1. The mental status exam should begin with assessment of level of consciousness and attention, because these can affect the interpretation of subsequent tests.
2. Language, memory, visuospatial function, neglect, and tests of frontal lobe function are other key elements of the mental status exam that can suggest focal brain lesions.

Cranial Nerves

It is usually easiest to test the cranial nerves (or at least to record the results) in approximate numerical order (Table 1-2).

Olfaction (cranial nerve I) is rarely tested, but when this is important, each nostril should be tested separately with a nonnoxious stimulus, such as coffee or vanilla.

Tests of optic nerve (II) function include visual acuity (using a near card), visual fields (tested by confrontation with wiggling fingers or with a small red object, which is more sensitive), and the pupillary light reflex, the afferent limb of which is mediated by this nerve. Funduscopic examination is the only means by which a part of the central nervous system (the retina) can be directly visualized.

Extraocular movements (III, IV, and VI) are tested in three ways: by having the patient pursue a moving target that is a drawing of the letter "H" in front of his face (pursuit), by directing his gaze rapidly to various stationary targets (saccades), and by fixating on an object while his head is being turned passively (vestibulo-ocular movements). The presence of nystagmus should be noted.

Muscles of mastication (V) are tested by assessing strength of jaw opening and palpating over the masseters bilaterally while the jaw is clenched. Facial sensation can be tested to all modalities over the

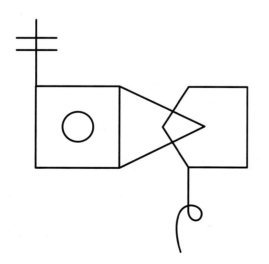

Figure 1-1 • Example of a complex figure to be copied by the patient as test of visuospatial function.

TABLE 1-2

The Cranial Nerves

Nerve	English Name	Exit Through Skull	Function
I	Olfactory	Cribriform plate	Olfaction (test using nonnoxious substance)
II	Optic	Optic canal	Vision (acuity, fields, color), afferent limb of pupillary reflex
III	Oculomotor	Superior orbital fissure	Superior rectus, inferior rectus, medial rectus, inferior oblique, levator palpebrae, efferent limb of pupillary reflex
IV	Trochlear	Superior orbital fissure	Superior oblique (of contralateral eye)
V	Trigeminal	Superior orbital fissure (V_1), foramen rotundum (V_2), foramen ovale (V_3)	Muscles of mastication, tensor tympani, tensor veli palatini, facial sensation, afferent limb of corneal reflex
VI	Abducens	Superior orbital fissure	Lateral rectus
VII	Facial	Internal auditory meatus	Muscles of facial expression, stapedius, taste on anterior two-thirds of tongue, efferent limb of corneal reflex
VIII	Vestibulocochlear	Internal auditory meatus	Hearing, vestibular function
IX	Glossopharyngeal	Jugular foramen	Movement of palate, sensation over palate and pharynx, taste over posterior one-third of tongue, afferent limb of gag reflex
X	Vagus	Jugular foramen	Movement of palate, sensation over pharynx, larynx and epiglottis, efferent limb of gag reflex, parasympathetic function of viscera
XI	Accessory	Jugular foramen	Sternocleidomastoid and trapezius movement
XII	Hypoglossal	Hypoglossal foramen	Tongue movement

forehead (V_1), cheek (V_2), and jaw (V_3). The afferent limb of the corneal reflex is mediated by this nerve.

Muscles of facial expression (VII) are tested by having the patient raise her eyebrows, squeeze her eyes shut, or show her teeth. Though uncommonly tested, taste over the anterior two-thirds of the tongue is mediated by this nerve and can be evaluated with sugar or another nonnoxious stimulus.

Hearing (VIII) may be evaluated in each ear simply by whispering or rubbing fingers; more detailed assessment of hearing loss may be accomplished with the Weber or Rinne tuning fork (512 Hz) test. Vestibular function can be tested in many ways, including evaluation of eye fixation while the patient's head is rapidly turned or by observation for drift in one direction while the patient is walking in place with the eyes closed.

Palatal elevation should be symmetric, and the voice should not be hoarse or nasal (IX and X). Failure of the right palate to elevate implies pathology of the right glossopharyngeal nerve. The gag reflex is also mediated by these nerves.

Sternocleidomastoid strength is tested by having the patient turn the head against resistance; weakness on turning to the left implies a right accessory nerve (XI) problem. The trapezius muscle is tested by having the patient shrug his shoulders.

Tongue protrusion should be in the midline. If the tongue deviates toward the right, the problem lies with the right hypoglossal nerve (XII).

KEY POINTS

1. Cranial nerve testing is most easily performed and recorded in approximate numerical order.
2. Key elements of the cranial nerve exam include assessment of vision and eye movements, facial movement and sensation, and movements of the palate and tongue.

Motor Exam

The motor exam includes more than just strength testing—in fact, strength should usually be the portion of the exam performed last.

First, bulk is assessed by observing and palpating the muscles and comparing each side to the other and the patient's overall muscle bulk to that expected for age. The presence of fasciculations or of adventitious movements such as tremor or myoclonus should also be noted.

Tone is one of the most important parts of the motor exam. In the upper extremities, tone is checked by moving the patient's arm at the elbow in both flex-ion-extension and circular movements, by moving the wrist in a circular fashion, and by rapidly pronating and supinating the forearm using a handshake grip. Abnormalities of tone such as spasticity and rigidity are discussed in subsequent chapters. Tone in the lower extremities can be tested well only with the patient supine. The examiner lifts the leg up suddenly under the knee; only in the presence of increased tone will the heel come off the bed.

Finally, strength or power is assessed, by both functional observation and direct confrontation (Figure 1-2). A pronator drift may be observed in an arm held

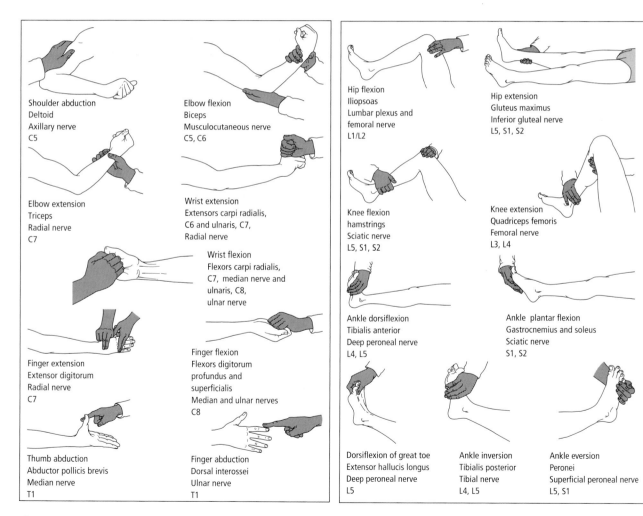

Figure 1-2 • Power testing of individual movements. For each movement, the predominant muscle, peripheral nerve, and nerve root are given.
(Reproduced with permission from Ginsberg L. Lecture Notes Neurology. 8th ed. Oxford: Blackwell Publishing, 2005:40–41.)

TABLE 1-3	
Medical Research Council Grading of Muscle Power	
0	No contraction of muscle visible
1	Flicker or trace of contraction visible
2	Active movement at joint, with gravity eliminated
3	Active movement against gravity
4	Active movement against gravity and some resistance
5	Normal power

KEY POINTS

1. The motor exam begins with assessment of bulk and tone.
2. Abnormalities of increased tone include both spasticity and rigidity.
3. Strength testing involves both functional observation as well as confrontation testing of individual muscles' power.
4. Strength is graded on the MRC scale from 0 to 5.

supinated and extended in front of the body. The patient may be asked to rise from a chair without using her arms or to walk on her heels or toes. The power of individual muscles assessed by direct confrontation testing is graded according to the Medical Research Council (MRC) scale (Table 1-3), although refinements of the scale (such as the use of 4−, 4, and 4+) or the use of a 10-point scale will increase precision.

Reflexes

Muscle stretch (or "deep tendon") reflexes can be useful aids in localizing or diagnosing both central and peripheral nervous system problems (Figure 1-3).

In the upper extremities, the biceps, brachioradialis, and triceps reflexes are the ones commonly tested. Pectoral and finger flexor reflexes can also be

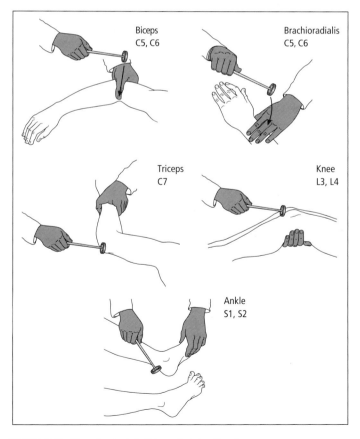

Figure 1-3 • Muscle stretch ("deep tendon") reflexes.
(Reproduced with permission from Ginsberg L. Lecture Notes Neurology. 8th ed. Oxford: Blackwell Publishing, 2005:44.)

tested. Hoffmann's sign is sought by flicking the distal phalanx of the middle finger while observing for flexion of the thumb.

In the lower extremities, patellar (knee jerk) and ankle reflexes are the ones commonly tested. The adductor reflex can also be tested. The Babinski sign is sought by stroking the lateral sole of the foot while observing for extension of the great toe. Clonus, if present, can be elicited by forcibly dorsiflexing the ankle when it is relaxed.

Sensory Exam

The sensory exam can be frustrating to perform because of the tedium of potentially examining the entire body surface (see dermatome map in Chapter 6) as well as the inherent subjectivity and all-too-frequent inconsistencies in patients' responses.

In general, sensation should be tested in detail in areas relevant to a patient's complaints, especially if the complaints are sensory in nature. Otherwise, screening elements of the sensory exam that are targeted at the distal lower extremities, where most asymptomatic sensory abnormalities are likely to be found, may be sufficient.

Pinprick sensation is tested with a safety pin, the sharp edge of a broken-off cotton swab, or special pins designed for the neurologic exam.

Temperature sensation, mediated by the same pathway, is most easily tested with the side of a tuning fork, which, if freshly retrieved from an instrument bag, will be quite cold on the skin.

Vibration is tested by striking the 128-Hz tuning fork and placing its stem against the joint being tested, typically beginning at the toes.

Joint position sense, or proprioception, is tested beginning most distally by holding the patient's great toe by its sides and moving it slightly upward or downward.

Light touch is the least useful modality to test, because it is carried by a combination of pathways and is unlikely to provide clues to localization or diagnosis.

KEY POINTS

1. The sensory exam is usually the most subjective portion of the neurologic exam.
2. In a patient without sensory complaints, screening elements of the sensory exam that are targeted at the distal extremities may be sufficient.
3. Pinprick and temperature are carried in one pathway; vibration and joint position sense in another.

Coordination

This portion of the exam, often incorrectly referred to as "cerebellar" testing, in fact serves to test coordinated movements whose successful completion requires the interaction of multiple components of the motor system, not just the cerebellum.

Finger-to-nose testing can identify the presence of dysmetria (inaccuracy of targeting) or intention tremor.

Heel-to-shin testing can elicit incoordination in the lower extremities.

Rapid alternating movements, rhythmic finger tapping, and heel tapping are particularly sensitive to coordination problems. Patients may have trouble with the timing or cadence of these movements. *Dysdiadochokinesis* is the term used to describe difficulty with rapid alternating movements.

Gait

Aside from orthopedic surgeons, neurologists are among the only doctors to routinely test a patient's gait, yet the "normal" function of walking requires the proper functioning of so many different aspects of the nervous system that it is frequently a sensitive way to detect an abnormality. In addition, certain diseases, such as Parkinson disease, have quite distinctive gaits associated with them.

The patient with a normal stance maintains the feet at an appropriately narrow distance apart; a wide-based stance is abnormal.

The Romberg sign is present when the patient maintains a steady stance with feet together and eyes open but sways and falls with feet together and eyes closed. Its presence usually implies a deficit of joint position sense, not cerebellar function, as is commonly believed.

Stride length should be full. Short-stepped or shuffling gaits are characterized by a decrease in stride length and clearance off the ground.

Ataxia of gait results in an inability to walk in a straight line; patients may stagger from one side to the other or consistently list toward one side. Ataxia is typically associated with a wide-based stance. Ataxia can be brought out most obviously by having the patient attempt tandem gait, walking heel to toe.

The arms normally swing in the opposite direction from their respective legs during ambulation. Decreased arm swing is a feature of extrapyramidal disorders.

Finally, difficulty initiating ambulation or understanding the appropriate motor program for walking, leaving the feet "stuck to the floor" despite intact motor and sensory function, characterizes the gait of frontal lobe dysfunction, sometimes referred to as *gait apraxia*. Hydrocephalus is one etiology of such a gait disorder.

KEY POINTS

1. Gait is one of the most important elements of the neurologic exam because it is sensitive for many deficits, and certain diseases have characteristic gait disorders.
2. Stance, stride length, arm swing, ability to tandem walk, and initiation of walking should all be assessed in the gait exam.
3. The Romberg sign suggests a deficit in joint position sense.

Neurologic Investigations

■ CEREBROSPINAL FLUID ANALYSIS

Cerebrospinal fluid (CSF) bathes the internal and external surface of the brain and spinal cord. It is produced by the choroid plexus of the ventricles and absorbed through the villi of the arachnoid granulations that project into the dural venous sinuses. CSF is produced continually at a rate of about 0.5 mL per minute; the total volume is approximately 150 mL. The entire CSF volume is thus replaced about every 5 hours. Lumbar puncture (LP) via the L3-4 interspace is the most commonly used means of obtaining CSF for analysis. LP is contraindicated by the presence of a space-occupying lesion that is causing mass effect, raised intracranial pressure, or local infection or inflammation at the planned puncture site.

Technique

LP is best performed with the patient in the lateral recumbent position with the legs flexed up over the abdomen. Optimal positioning is the key to a successful and atraumatic LP. Ideally, a pillow should be placed between the legs, and the patient should lie on the edge of the bed where there is better support to keep the back straight. The anterosuperior iliac spine is at the level of the L3-4 vertebral interspace. The LP may be performed at this level, one interspace higher, or one to two interspaces lower. Remember that the spinal cord ends at the level of L1-2. The needle is inserted with the bevel facing upward, so that it will enter parallel to the ligaments and dura that it pierces rather than cutting them transversely. The needle is directed slightly rostrally to coincide with the downward angulation of the spinous processes. The needle is advanced gently until CSF is obtained. To measure the opening pressure reliably, the patient's legs should

be extended slightly and note should be made of fluctuation of the CSF meniscus within the manometer with respiration.

Interpretation of Results

CSF is a clear, colorless fluid. The glucose content is about two-thirds that of blood, and it contains up to 40 to 50 mg/dL protein. Fewer than five cells are present, and these are lymphocytes. Measured by LP in the lateral recumbent position, the opening pressure is about 60 to 150 mm H_2O.

Xanthochromia refers to the yellow discoloration of the supernatant of a spun CSF sample. Its presence helps to distinguish an in vivo intrathecal hemorrhage from a traumatic tap [in which red blood cells (RBCs) have not lysed and the supernatant is still colorless].

The implications of various CSF findings are summarized in Table 2-1. The CSF findings in a variety of common conditions are summarized in Table 2-2. Special tests may be performed as indicated. Some examples include cytology for suspected malignancy, oligoclonal banding for suspected immune-mediated processes such as multiple sclerosis, 14,3,3-protein for Creutzfeldt-Jakob disease, and a variety of polymerase chain reactions and serologic tests for various infections.

Safety, Tolerability, and Complications

Cerebral or cerebellar herniation may occur when lumbar puncture is performed in the presence of either a supratentorial or infratentorial mass lesion. A computed tomography (CT) scan should be performed prior to an LP except in cases of suspected meningitis and when a CT scan cannot be performed. Radiologic contraindications to LP include closure of the fourth ventricle and quadrigeminal cistern. Low-

■ TABLE 2-1

Interpretation of CSF Findings

Red blood cells	
No xanthochromia	Traumatic tap
Xanthochromia	Subarachnoid hemorrhage; hemorrhagic encephalitis
White blood cells	
Polymorphs	Bacterial or early viral infection
Lymphocytes	Infection (viral, fungal, mycobacterial); demyelination (MS, ADEM); CNS lymphoma
Elevated protein	Infection; demyelination; tumor (e.g., meningioma); age
Low glucose	Bacterial infection; mycobacterial infection
Oligoclonal bands	Demyelination (MS); CNS infections (e.g., Lyme disease); noninfectious inflammatory processes (e.g., SLE)
Positive EBV PCR	Highly suggestive of CNS lymphoma in patients with AIDS or other immunosuppressed states

MS, multiple sclerosis; ADEM, acute disseminated encephalomyelitis; CNS, central nervous system; SLE, systemic lupus erythematosus; EBV PCR, Epstein-Barr virus polymerase chain reaction; AIDS, acquired immunodeficiency syndrome.

pressure headache is the most common complication of lumbar puncture and is most effectively treated by having the patient lie flat and increase her intake of liquids and caffeine. Rarely, it may be necessary to administer an epidural blood patch (see Chapter 10).

KEY POINTS

1. A CT scan should be performed prior to lumbar puncture except when bacterial meningitis is suspected.
2. Lumbar puncture is performed at or below the L2-3 interspace.
3. Xanthochromia indicates recent intrathecal hemorrhage.

■ COMPUTED TOMOGRAPHY AND MAGNETIC RESONANCE IMAGING

Technical Considerations

CT measures the degree of x-ray attenuation by tissue. Attenuation is defined simply as the removal (by absorption or scatter) of x-ray photons and is quantified on an arbitrary scale (in Hounsfield units) that is represented in shades of gray. Differences in the shades directly reflect the differences in the x-ray attenuation of different tissues, a property that depends on their atomic number and physical density. Images are usually obtained in either an axial or a coronal plane. Three-dimensional

■ TABLE 2-2

CSF Findings in Common Neurologic Diseases

Disease	Cells (pleocytosis)	Protein	Glucose	Other
Bacterial meningitis	Polymorphs	High	Low	Culture and Gram stain may be positive
Viral meningitis/encephalitis	Lymphocytes	High	Normal	Viral PCR may be positive
Tuberculous meningitis	Lymphocytes	High	Very low	Positive for acid-fast bacilli
Guillain-Barré syndrome	None	High (degree depends on interval from symptom onset)	Normal	—
MS	Few lymphocytes	Slightly high	Normal	OCBs usually present
ADEM	Lymphocytes or polymorphs	Usually high	Normal	OCBs usually absent
Subarachnoid hemorrhage	Lymphocytes and many red blood cells	May be high	Normal	Xanthochromia

reconstruction and angiography are possible with new-generation spiral CT scanners.

Magnetic resonance imaging (MRI) is similar to CT in that radiant energy is directed at the patient and detected as it emerges from the patient. MRI differs, however, in its use of radiofrequency (RF) pulses rather than x-rays. The images in MRI result from the varying intensity of radio-wave signals emanating from tissue in which hydrogen ions have been excited by an RF pulse. A detailed understanding of magnetic resonance physics is not necessary for the interpretation of routinely used MRI sequences. It is sufficient to understand that the patient is placed in a magnet and that an RF pulse is administered. Signal intensity is measured at a time interval, known as **time to echo** (TE), following RF administration. The RF pulse is administered many times in generating an image; the **time to repetition** (TR) is the time between these RF pulses.

Two basic MRI sequences in common usage are T1- (short TE and TR) and T2- (long TE and long TR) weighted images. Fat is bright on a T1-weighted image, which imparts a brighter signal to the myelin-containing white matter. Water (including CSF) is dark on T1 and bright on T2. T2 images are most useful in evaluating the spinal cord (Figure 2-1). Gadolinium is the contrast agent used in MRI, and gadolinium-enhanced images are usually acquired with a T1-weighted sequence. Contrast-enhanced images are invaluable in determining the presence of brain tumors, abscesses, other areas of inflammation, and new multiple sclerosis lesions (see Figure 19-3).

Other commonly used MRI sequences are fluid-attenuated inversion recovery (FLAIR) and susceptibility- and diffusion-weighted imaging (DWI). FLAIR is a strong T2-weighted image, but one in which the signal from CSF has been inverted and is thus of low rather than high intensity. FLAIR is the single best screening image sequence for most pathologic processes of the central nervous system (CNS). It is very useful in assessing the chronic lesion burden in multiple sclerosis (see Figure 20-2). A susceptibility-weighted sequence is one that is sensitive to the disruptive effect of a substance on the local magnetic field. Examples of substances that exert such a susceptibility effect are calcium, bone, and the blood breakdown products ferritin and hemosiderin. Areas of increased susceptibility appear black on these images.

DWI demonstrates cellular toxicity with high sensitivity and is most commonly employed in the diagnosis of acute stroke, where it can be positive within half an hour of symptom onset. Areas of restricted diffusion appear bright on DWI. Figure 2-2 provides examples of T1, T2, FLAIR, and DWI images.

Clinical Utility

Head CT is often the initial investigation used in a variety of neurologic disorders, including headache, trauma, seizures, subarachnoid hemorrhage, and stroke. The sensitivity of a CT scan for detecting lesions depends on many factors, including the nature and duration of the underlying disease process. The sensitivity for detecting areas of inflammation, infection, or tumor may be increased by the administration of intravenous contrast. Contrast enhancement indicates local disruption of the blood-brain barrier. CT is the investigation of choice for demonstrating fresh blood.

Apart from providing better anatomic definition, MRI is particularly useful for imaging the contents of the posterior fossa and craniocervical junction, which are seen poorly on CT because of artifact from surrounding bone. DWI is the most sensitive technique available for demonstrating early tissue ischemia and is therefore extremely useful in the evaluation of patients with suspected stroke.

Safety, Tolerability, and Complications

CT scanning employs x-rays and is thus relatively contraindicated during pregnancy. The use of RF waves in MRI makes this the imaging modality of choice in pregnant women. There is no cross-reactivity between the iodinated contrast agents used in CT and the gadolinium used as a contrast agent in MRI. When contrasted imaging is required, MRI may therefore be preferable when there is a history of allergy to intravenous contrast. Similarly, gadolinium does not have the nephrotoxicity of iodinated contrast. MRI may be

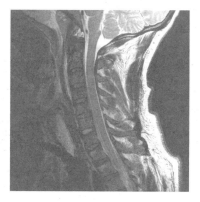

Figure 2-1 • T2-weighted MRI of the cervical spine.

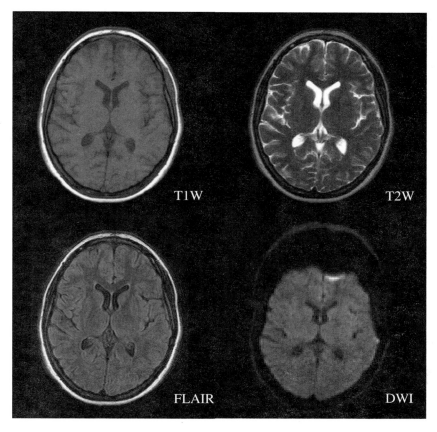

Figure 2-2 • Normal T1, T2, FLAIR, and DWI images of the brain.

used safely only in the absence of metal objects (foreign bodies, plates, and screws) and pacemaker and defibrillator devices. Some people with claustrophobia cannot tolerate MRI; under these circumstances, CT is preferred.

This is the most sensitive and specific imaging study of the intracranial and extracranial circulation. Risks of the procedure include contrast dye reaction, stroke due to dislodged plaque from the catheter, and bleeding from the cannulation site. Although the risks of

KEY POINTS

1. CT is the imaging modality of choice for demonstrating acute intracranial bleeding.
2. MRI is required for adequate imaging of the posterior fossa and craniocervical junction.
3. DWI is the most sensitive MRI sequence for demonstrating early cerebral ischemia or infarction.

■ VASCULAR IMAGING STUDIES

Conventional angiography involves cannulation of the great vessels and injection of contrast dye to obtain an image of the vascular anatomy (Figure 2-3).

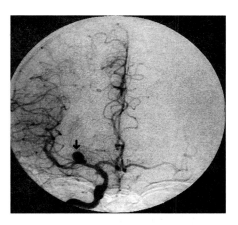

Figure 2-3 • Conventional cerebral angiogram demonstrating aneurysm of the right middle cerebral artery (arrow). (Reproduced with permission from Patel PR. Lecture Notes Radiology. 2nd ed. Oxford: Blackwell Publishing, 2005:278.)

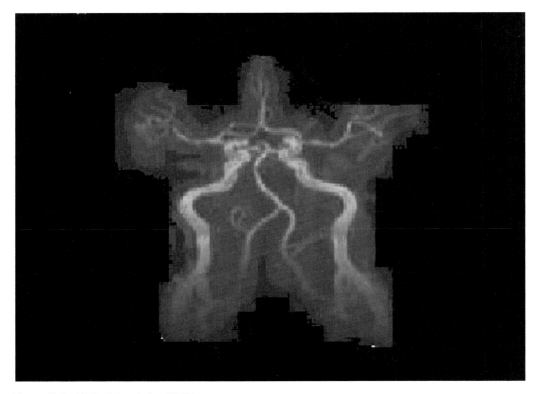

Figure 2-4 • MRA of the circle of Willis.

the procedure, and developments in magnetic resonance angiography (MRA) (below), have decreased
the number of conventional angiograms performed, it
remains the "gold standard" in vascular imaging.

MRA uses blood flow as a contrast agent and MR
technique to define vascular anatomy (Figure 2-4).
Compared with conventional angiograpy, MRA is less
invasive and can be performed more quickly and less
expensively, but it is not as sensitive or specific for
cerebrovascular disease. MRA is performed commonly on the intracranial circulation of stroke patients
to look for evidence of vascular narrowing or occlusion. "Fat-suppressed" MRA of the neck is useful for
determining the presence of vertebral or carotid
artery dissections. Magnetic resonance venography
(MRV) can be used to demonstrate venous sinus
thrombosis and other venous disease.

Extracranial Doppler sonography measures blood
flow by determining the difference between emitted
and received ultrasound frequencies. It is used commonly to detect stenosis or occlusion of the extracranial carotid circulation, especially in the planning
stages for carotid endarterectomy. Transcranial
Doppler (TCD) detects intracranial stenosis and

emboli. Most of the intracranial circulation, however,
is inaccessible to TCD. Although somewhat less accurate than MRA or conventional angiography, Doppler
studies are noninvasive and virtually without contraindication.

KEY POINTS

1. Conventional angiography is the gold standard for
   evaluating cerebrovascular anatomy.
2. MRA is less invasive but also less accurate than
   conventional angiography.
3. MRV is useful for assessing the presence of venous
   sinus thrombosis.

■ OTHER IMAGING STUDIES

Positron emission tomography (PET) scans measure
regional brain metabolism. Hypermetabolism can be
demonstrated during seizures (though it is rare to
get the scan during a seizure), while hypometabolic
regions may be evident interictally. Such a finding

can be very useful in planning epilepsy surgery, especially in the temporal areas. Single-photon emission computed tomography (SPECT) uses a radioactive isotope to demonstrate increased blood flow during seizures. Both PET and SPECT scans have been studied in the evaluation of dementia. While regional patterns of abnormality help study disease processes, they are not specific enough for diagnosis in individual patients. Magnetic resonance spectroscopy is primarily a research tool used to demonstrate areas of neuronal damage or dysfunction and has been studied in the assessment of brain tumors, demyelinating disease, and infections of the CNS.

ELECTROENCEPHALOGRAPHY

The electroencephalogram (EEG) provides a record of the electrical activity of the cerebral cortex. Normal EEG patterns are characterized by the frequency and amplitude of the recorded electrical activity, and the patterns of activity correlate with the degree of wakefulness or sleep. The normally observed frequency patterns are divided into four groups: alpha (8 to 13 Hz), beta (14 to 30 Hz), theta (4 to 7 Hz), and delta (0.5 to 3.0 Hz) (Figure 2-5). Under normal circumstances, alpha waves are observed over the posterior head regions in the relaxed awake state with the eyes closed. Lower-amplitude beta activity is more prominent over the frontal regions. Theta and delta activity is normal during drowsiness and sleep, and the different stages of sleep are defined by the relative proportions and amplitudes of theta and delta activity (see Chapter 13).

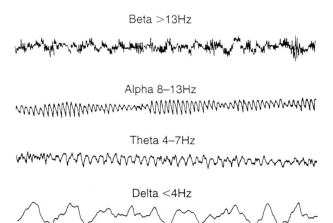

Beta >13Hz

Alpha 8–13Hz

Theta 4–7Hz

Delta <4Hz

Figure 2-5 • Electroencephalographic frequencies.

Technique

The standard EEG is recorded from electrodes attached to the scalp in a symmetric array. The pattern in which these electrodes are connected to each other is referred to as the *montage*, of which there are essentially two types: bipolar and referential. In a bipolar montage, all electrodes are active and a recording is made of the difference in electrical activity between two adjacent electrodes. In a referential montage, the electrical activity is recorded beneath the active electrode relative to a distant electrode or common average signal. The signal recorded by an EEG is a sum of excitatory and inhibitory postsynaptic potentials of cortical neurons.

Clinical Utility

To appreciate the utility of the EEG, it is important to understand its limitations. First, the patterns of electrical activity recorded by the EEG are rarely (if ever) specific to their cause. For example, the presence of diffuse theta or delta activity during the awake state suggests an encephalopathy but does not indicate the etiology. Second, the EEG records the electrical activity of cortical neurons. Although subcortical structures influence cortical activity, the surface EEG may be insensitive to dysfunction of deep structures. For example, seizures originating in the medial frontal or temporal lobes may not be readily apparent on the surface EEG. Furthermore, the EEG provides a measure of the electrical activity of the cortex at the time of the recording and is therefore frequently normal in paroxysmal conditions such as seizures. The interictal EEG, for example, may be abnormal in only about 50% of adults with epilepsy. The frequency of interictal EEG abnormalities may be higher in certain forms of epilepsy.

Several common patterns of abnormal activity are recognized. Focal arrhythmic or polymorphic slow activity in the theta or delta range suggests local dysfunction in the underlying brain. Vascular disease is a common cause of such findings, but the slowing cannot specify the etiology. Generalized arrhythmic slow activity often indicates a diffuse encephalopathy. Interictal epileptiform findings include sharp- and spike-wave discharges, with or without an accompanying slow wave. Electrographic seizures may take various forms. The most common are rhythmic spike- or sharp- and slow-wave discharges or rhythmic slow waves. They may be focal or generalized. Activation procedures can be used to enhance the likelihood of finding abnormal EEG patterns: hyperventilation is useful for provoking EEG changes in patients with absence seizures, while photic stimulation can induce EEG changes in patients with myoclonic seizures.

KEY POINTS

1. Alpha frequency (8 to 13 Hz) is the dominant posterior rhythm in the awake restful state with the eyes closed.
2. Epilepsy is a clinical diagnosis; interictal epileptiform EEG findings are demonstrable only in the minority of patients with epilepsy.

■ NERVE CONDUCTION STUDIES AND ELECTROMYOGRAPHY

Nerve conduction studies (NCS) and electromyography (EMG) are appropriately used as an extension of the clinical examination.

Technique

In performing NCS, an electrical stimulus is applied over a nerve and recordings are made from surface skin electrodes. For motor studies, the recording electrodes are placed over the endplate of a muscle innervated by the nerve being stimulated. The nerve is stimulated in at least two locations (distal and proximal), and the distance between the two sites of stimulation is measured carefully. The distal latency, compound muscle action potential (CMAP), and conduction velocity are recorded. The CMAP is a recording of the contraction of the underlying muscle. The distal latency is the time interval between stimulation over the distal portion of the nerve and the initiation of the CMAP. Conduction velocity is calculated by measuring the difference in latency to CMAP initiation between proximal and distal sites of stimulation. For sensory studies, the nerve is stimulated at one site and the sensory nerve action potential (SNAP) is recorded either at a more proximal site (orthodromic study) or at a more distal site (antidromic study). Repetitive nerve-stimulation studies are used to demonstrate either decremental or incremental CMAP responses in disorders of the neuromuscular junction.

Electromyography involves the insertion of a needle into individual muscles. Recordings are made of the muscle electrical activity upon insertion (insertional activity), while the muscle is at rest (spontaneous activity), and during contraction (volitional motor unit potentials). To increase the strength of muscular contraction, motor units can fire more quickly (activation) or more motor units can be added (recruitment). Reduced activation is seen in CNS disease. Reduced recruitment suggests a neurogenic lesion, while early recruitment can be seen in early myopathic disease. For routine EMG studies, activity is recorded from a group of muscle fibers simultaneously. Single-fiber EMG is the technique used in the investigation of disorders of the neuromuscular junction.

Clinical Utility

NCS and EMG are used primarily to assist in the localization of dysfunction within the peripheral nervous system and to define pathophysiology more clearly. For example, NCS and EMG may help to differentiate a C8–T1 radiculopathy from a lower brachial plexopathy or an ulnar neuropathy in the patient who presents with numbness of the fourth and fifth fingers with weakness of the hand. Similarly, the combination of motor NCS, repetitive nerve stimulation, and EMG may help to localize motor dysfunction (i.e., weakness) to the peripheral nerve, the neuromuscular junction, or the muscle (Table 2-3). In

---

■ TABLE 2-3

Electromyography in Neurogenic and Myopathic Disorders

	Neurogenic	Myopathic
Insertional activity	↑ (active denervation)	Usually normal ↑ (necrotizing myopathies)
Spontaneous activity	↑ (active denervation)	Usually normal ↑ (necrotizing myopathies)
Volitional motor unit potentials Recruitment	Large amplitude; polyphasic Reduced	Small amplitude; polyphasic Usually normal early

TABLE 2-4

Nerve Conduction Studies in Demyelinating and Axonal Neuropathies

	Demyelinating	Axonal
Distal latency	Prolonged	Normal
Conduction velocity	Markedly reduced	Normal; may be slightly reduced
CMAP amplitude	Normal or mildly reduced	Reduced

CMAP, compound muscle action potential.

a patient with a polyneuropathy, NCS may help to define the relative degree of motor and sensory involvement and to distinguish primary demyelinating from axonal disease (Table 2-4).

KEY POINTS

1. The goal of NCS and EMG is to localize the neurologic dysfunction within the peripheral nervous system.
2. Repetitive nerve stimulation and single-fiber EMG are useful in the diagnosis of disorders of the neuromuscular junction.

Part Two

Common Neurologic Symptoms

The Approach to Coma and Altered Consciousness

The neurologic evaluation and management of a patient with coma or altered consciousness can be intimidating for the student, because such patients are usually critically ill and may require prompt intervention. The fundamental principles behind the evaluation of a neurologic problem, however, should not be discarded. On the contrary, an orderly and hypothesis-based approach may be even more important in a comatose patient than in others, given the need for timely diagnosis and the relative limitations on history and examination.

Definition

Coma is defined as a state of unarousable unresponsiveness. Typically the patient lies with eyes closed and does not open them even to vigorous stimulation, such as sternal rub, nasal tickle, or nailbed pressure. Alterations in consciousness short of coma are often described using terms such as **drowsiness**, **lethargy**, **obtundation**, and **stupor**, but these terms tend to be used imprecisely and it is generally best to describe simply how the patient responded to various degrees of stimulation. The Glasgow Coma Scale assigns a numerical score to a patient's level of responsiveness and is commonly used by neurosurgeons in cases of head trauma (see Table 17-1). Its utility lies in its ease of use by nurses and paramedics, its interrater reproducibility, and its prognostic value following head injury.

KEY POINTS

1. Coma is a state of unarousable unresponsiveness.
2. It is important to describe a patient's responses to various degrees of stimulation.
3. The Glasgow Coma Scale, which has prognostic value in patients with head trauma, is reproducible and easy to use.

Clinical Approach

An algorithm for approaching patients with coma or altered consciousness is presented in Figure 3-1. The initial steps of stabilization and evaluation culminate

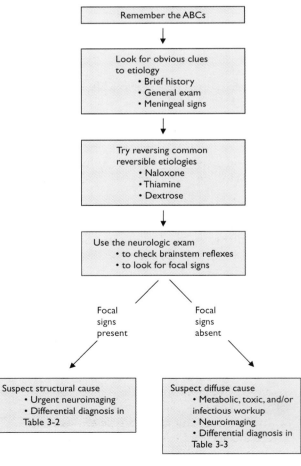

Figure 3-1 • The approach to coma and altered consciousness.

in the neurologic exam, which is performed with two goals in mind: to assess brainstem function and to look for focal signs. The differential diagnosis and further investigations stem from this clinical assessment.

1. **Remember the ABCs.** In any patient with altered consciousness, the airway, breathing, and circulation should be checked and maintained according to usual protocols, including intubation and mechanical ventilation if required.
2. **Look for obvious clues to etiology.** A brief history and general exam should be performed to search for obvious clues. A history of medical problems such as diabetes, hepatic failure, alcoholism, or a seizure disorder may be provided by the family, noted on a medical alert bracelet, or deduced from prescription labels. The circumstances in which the patient was found can offer clues to the onset or etiology of depressed consciousness. The general exam may yield telling signs, such as an odor on the breath, needle tracks on the skin, or a tongue laceration. It is important to check for meningeal signs in any unconscious patient because both bacterial meningitis and subarachnoid hemorrhage may lead to depressed consciousness.
3. **Try reversing common reversible etiologies.** Most emergency rooms (ERs) make it standard practice to administer naloxone, thiamine, and dextrose to any patient with depressed consciousness and no obvious etiology. Note that thiamine should always be given before glucose, because the latter can precipitate Wernicke encephalopathy if given alone.
4. **Check brainstem reflexes and look for focal signs.** These are the two primary goals of the neurologic exam in this setting, because the subsequent diagnostic and therapeutic steps will depend on these clinical findings.

KEY POINTS

1. The clinical approach to the patient with altered consciousness begins with the ABCs: airway, breathing, and circulation.
2. Look for obvious clues to etiology.
3. Try reversing common reversible etiologies.
4. Use the neurologic exam to check brainstem reflexes and look for focal signs.

Examination

It is important to proceed with the neurologic exam of a comatose patient in an orderly fashion—it is easy to be intimidated or distracted by the array of attached tubes and lines or by the intensity and anxiety of other clinicians. An appropriate way to begin is to progress systematically through the sequence of the usual neurologic exam, making adjustments as necessary for the patient's altered level of responsiveness.

Mental status testing in these patients begins with assessing the level of consciousness. An increasing gradient of stimulation should be applied and the patient's responses recorded. For example, does he lie with his eyes closed but open them slowly when spoken to in a loud voice? Does he groan but not open his eyes when sternal rub is applied? For many patients, further cognitive testing may not be possible. For those who can be aroused even briefly, however, a short evaluation of attention, language, visuospatial function, and neglect is in order, because this may reveal a gross focal finding such as an aphasia or dense neglect of the left side.

Cranial nerves should be examined in detail, because this is the portion of the exam most relevant to the assessment of brainstem function. In an arousable patient, most cranial nerves can be tested in the usual manner. In a patient who is not arousable enough to follow commands, several important brainstem reflexes should be tested (Table 3-1), including the pupillary, corneal, oculocephalic, and gag reflexes. In addition, a funduscopic examination should always be performed. For many patients with altered consciousness, testing for a blink to visual threat may be the only way to judge visual fields. If the patient cannot move her face to command, the examiner may be restricted to looking for an asymmetry at rest, such as a flattened nasolabial fold on one side. The presence of an endotracheal tube may make such observation difficult.

Motor tone should be checked in all extremities. If the patient can cooperate with some testing, a gross hemiparesis can be ruled out by having the patient hold her arms extended or legs elevated and observing for downward drift. Otherwise, the examiner may be restricted to observing for asymmetry of spontaneous movements (or to asking caretakers whether all extremities have been seen to move equally). Failing that, noxious stimuli such as nailbed pressure or a pinch on a flexor surface can be applied to each limb and the speed and strength of withdrawal noted, although abnormalities here may result from sensory loss as well as motor dysfunction. Decorticate and

TABLE 3-1

Brainstem Reflexes

Reflex	Cranial Nerves Involved	How to Test
Pupillary	II (afferent); III (efferent)	Shine light in each pupil and observe for direct (same side) and consensual (contralateral side) constriction
Oculocephalic (doll's eyes)	VIII (afferent); III, IV, VI (efferent)	Forcibly turn head horizontally and vertically and observe for conjugate eye movement in opposite direction (contraindicated if cervical spine injury has not been ruled out)
Caloric testing (if necessary)*	Same	Inject 50 mL ice water into each ear and observe for conjugate eye deviation toward the ear injected
Corneal	V_1 (afferent); VII (efferent)	Touch lateral cornea with cotton tip and observe for direct and consensual blink
Gag	IX (afferent); X/XI (efferent)	Stimulate posterior pharynx with cotton tip and observe for gag

* Caloric testing should be performed if turning the head is contraindicated or does not result in eye movement. Never assume the eyes are immobile unless caloric testing has been done.

decerebrate posturing, signs of brainstem dysfunction, may be seen either spontaneously or in response to noxious stimuli (Figure 3-2).

Muscle stretch reflexes can be tested in the usual manner, and a Babinski sign should be sought.

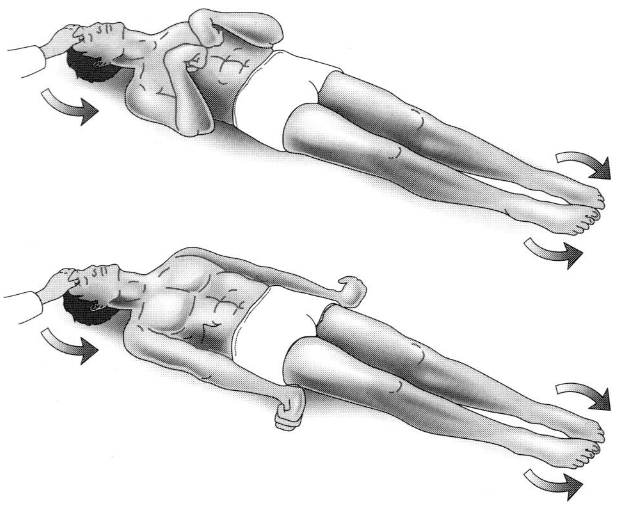

Figure 3-2 • Decorticate (above) and decerebrate (below) posturing in response to noxious stimuli. Both indicate brainstem dysfunction, although decorticate posturing suggests dysfunction slightly more superior than decerebrate posturing. (Reproduced with permission from Kandel ER, Schwatz JH, Jessell TM. Principles of Neural Science. 4th ed. New York: McGraw-Hill, 2000:903.)

Sensory testing in most patients with altered consciousness is limited to testing of light touch or pain sensation. Noxious stimulation to each limb, as described previously, may be useful in looking for gross sensory abnormalities.

Coordination and gait may be tested in patients who are arousable enough.

KEY POINTS

1. The mental status exam in patients with altered consciousness primarily assesses the level of responsiveness.
2. The cranial nerve exam includes the testing of important brainstem reflexes, including the pupillary, corneal, and oculocephalic reflexes.
3. The remainder of the examination should be dedicated to looking for focal abnormalities.

Differential Diagnosis

In theory, there are two main ways in which consciousness can be depressed: the brainstem can be dysfunctional or both cerebral hemispheres can be dysfunctional simultaneously. In fact, acute disease in the brainstem (e.g., pontine hemorrhage) can lead to coma, as can processes affecting both cerebral hemispheres at once (e.g., hypoglycemia). Unilateral cerebral hemispheric lesions, however, can also lead to coma if they are large or severe enough to cause swelling and compression of the opposite hemisphere or downward pressure on the brainstem.

Therefore most neurologists interpret the information obtained from the exam of the comatose patient using the following principle: the presence or absence of brainstem reflexes suggests how deep the coma is, while the presence or absence of focal signs narrows the differential diagnosis and guides the workup.

Thus, in milder cases of depressed consciousness, the pupillary, corneal, and gag reflexes may all be preserved. In more severe cases, some or all of these brainstem reflexes may be lost, no matter what the etiology. (Note that if a brainstem reflex is abnormal in an asymmetric fashion, such as a unilateral unreactive pupil, this would be interpreted as a focal sign and suggests compression of or primary disease in the brainstem.)

The presence of focal signs either on cranial nerve testing or in the remainder of the examination—including such findings as hemiparesis, aphasia, reflex asymmetry, facial droop, or a unilateral Babinski sign—suggests a structural cause of depressed consciousness (Box 3-1). Examples include a large unilateral stroke or intracranial hemorrhage. The absence of focal signs suggests a diffuse cause of depressed consciousness, including metabolic, toxic, or hypoxic-ischemic etiologies (Box 3-2). Examples include coma from fulminant hepatic failure, barbiturate overdose, or anoxia following prolonged cardiac arrest.

BOX 3-1	STRUCTURAL CAUSES OF DEPRESSED CONSCIOUSNESS

Acute ischemic stroke
   Brainstem
   Unilateral cerebral hemisphere (with edema)
Acute intracranial hemorrhage
   Intraparenchymal
   Subdural
   Epidural
Brain tumor (with edema or hemorrhage)
   Primary
   Metastatic
Brain abscess

KEY POINTS

1. In theory, consciousness can be depressed either by dysfunction of the brainstem or dysfunction of both cerebral hemispheres simultaneously; in reality, large unilateral hemispheric lesions (with pressure on the other side) qualify as well.
2. The presence or absence of brainstem reflexes suggests how deep the coma is.
3. The presence of focal signs suggests a structural cause of coma.
4. The absence of focal signs suggests a diffuse cause of coma, such as metabolic, toxic, infectious or hypoxic-ischemic etiologies.

Laboratory and Radiographic Studies

The distinction between structural and diffuse causes of depressed consciousness, arrived at by interpreting the findings on exam, suggests different pathways of diagnostic workup.

The presence of focal findings on examination, suggesting a structural cause, demands urgent head imaging, almost always a noncontrast CT scan. One should be looking for signs of a large acute stroke, an intracranial hemorrhage, or a mass lesion that may have enlarged rapidly or had hemorrhage within it. (Contrast-enhanced CT should be avoided if acute hemorrhage is possible.) Even in cases where focal brainstem signs are found, the initial choice of head imaging may have to be a CT scan rather than MRI, despite the poor quality of the former in evaluating the brainstem, because of the possibility of a large cerebral hemispheric lesion compressing the brainstem as well as because of the more immediate availability of CT.

The absence of focal findings on examination, suggesting a diffuse cause, warrants an extensive workup for causes of metabolic, toxic, or infectious etiologies. Blood testing—including complete blood count (CBC), electrolytes, glucose, liver function tests, and toxicologic screen—may be necessary. If infection is suspected, a chest x-ray, urinalysis, and blood or urine cultures may be called for. There should be a low threshold for obtaining an LP. If a basic workup is unrevealing, one should search for more unusual causes (such as myxedema coma by checking thyroid function tests). Head imaging is usually needed even in these cases of suspected diffuse cause because it may demonstrate signs of global hypoxic-ischemic injury, diffuse cerebral edema, or bilateral lesions mimicking a diffuse process, although the urgency is

BOX 3-2	DIFFUSE CAUSES OF DEPRESSED CONSCIOUSNESS

Metabolic
  Electrolyte abnormality
    Hyponatremia, hypernatremia, hypocalcemia, hypercalcemia, hypomagnesemia, hypermagnesemia, hypophosphatemia
  Glucose abnormality
    Hypoglycemia, nonketotic hyperosmolar coma, diabetic ketoacidosis
  Hepatic failure
  Uremia
  Thyroid dysfunction
  Myxedema coma, thyrotoxicosis
  Adrenal insufficiency
Toxic
  Alcohol
  Sedatives
  Narcotics
  Psychotropic drugs
  Other exogenous toxins (carbon monoxide, heavy metals)
Infectious
  Meningitis (bacterial, viral, fungal)
  Diffuse encephalitis
Hypoxic-ischemic
  Respiratory failure
  Cardiac arrest
Other
  Subarachnoid hemorrhage
  Carcinomatous meningitis
  Seizures or postictal state

particular diagnosis, such as hepatic encephalopathy or anoxic brain injury. Finally, the EEG can rule out nonconvulsive status epilepticus as a cause of coma in cases in which this is (or is not) clinically suspected.

KEY POINTS

1. If a structural cause of coma is suspected, urgent head imaging, usually with a noncontrast head CT, should be performed.
2. If a diffuse cause is suspected, an extensive workup for metabolic, toxic, or infectious causes should be undertaken.
3. Head imaging in suspected diffuse cases may demonstrate cerebral edema, signs of global hypoxic-ischemic injury, or bilateral lesions mimicking a diffuse process.
4. Almost without exception, head CT should be performed before LP.
5. EEG can assess the depth of coma and can occasionally suggest a specific diagnosis.

Treatment and Prognosis

The treatment of coma and altered consciousness rests on the specific diagnosis. Metabolic, infectious, or toxic etiologies require mostly medical management, while some structural causes of coma may require neurosurgical intervention. Specific treatments for particular conditions are detailed in later chapters, in particular Chapter 14 for strokes and hemorrhages, Chapter 17 for head trauma, Chapter 18 for systemic and metabolic disorders, Chapter 19 for brain tumors, and Chapter 21 for CNS infections.

When increased intracranial pressure (ICP) is suspected clinically or radiographically, treatments aimed at lowering ICP should be applied. These include raising the head of the bed, hyperventilation, and the use of an osmotic diuretic such as mannitol. Corticosteroids tend to be useful only in cases of edema associated with brain tumors. The lowering of ICP may be a neurologic or neurosurgical emergency if the patient shows signs of brain herniation, which is discussed in more detail in Chapter 17.

The prognosis of depressed consciousness is mostly dependent on etiology—the patient with a barbiturate overdose may recover completely, whereas one with a severe anoxic injury likely will not. Age is an important prognostic factor as well. One of the most frequent reasons for admission to an intensive care

not as high as for patients with focal findings. Of course, a head CT should be performed before obtaining an LP almost without exception in the evaluation of a patient with depressed consciousness, given the risk of precipitating brain herniation if a large intracranial mass (particularly in the posterior fossa) is present. (If bacterial meningitis is suspected, empiric antibiotic treatment can be started if CT scanning is delayed.)

Frequently, an EEG is ordered in patients with coma or altered consciousness. Although many of its findings may be nonspecific, the EEG can help to assess how deep a coma is based on the degree of background slowing. In addition, there are occasionally more specific patterns on EEG that suggest a unit (ICU) or neurologic consultation is to estimate the prognosis of a patient in coma following cardiopulmonary arrest. In these cases the circumstances and duration of the arrest are important, and published studies have correlated outcome with findings on neurologic examination performed at least 24 hours after the arrest.

KEY POINTS

1. The treatment of coma or altered consciousness depends on etiology.
2. The lowering of intracranial pressure may be a neurologic emergency if the patient shows signs of brain herniation.
3. Prognostic factors for coma or altered consciousness include both etiology and patient age.

SPECIAL TOPICS

■ PERSISTENT VEGETATIVE STATE

Persistent vegetative state is a state in which patients have lost all awareness and cognitive function but may remain with their eyes open, exhibit sleep-wake cycles, and maintain respiration and other autonomic functions. Patients may progress into this state after being in coma for a prolonged period if their vital functions have been supported.

■ LOCKED-IN SYNDROME

Although a locked-in syndrome can be confused with coma at first glance, a patient with locked-in syndrome is awake and may be intact cognitively, with no abnormality of consciousness. Usually a consequence of large lesions in the base of the pons, the locked-in syndrome leaves patients unable to move the extremities and most of the face. If all other motor function is lost, they may be limited to communicating by vertical eye movements or blinks.

■ BRAIN DEATH

Death can be declared either when there has been irreversible cessation of cardiopulmonary function or there has been irreversible cessation of all functions of the entire brain, including the brainstem. A declaration of death based on the latter criterion is commonly referred to as **brain death**. Many institutions have specific guidelines for how brain death must be determined, but in general the patient must be comatose, have absent brainstem reflexes, and have no spontaneous respirations even when the P_{CO_2} has been allowed to rise (the apnea test). Confounding factors such as hypothermia or drug overdose must not be present. Confirmatory tests most commonly include an EEG, which can demonstrate electrocerebral silence ("flat line"), or cerebral angiography, which can demonstrate absence of blood flow to the brain. Local institutional guidelines for declaration of brain death should always be consulted.

KEY POINTS

1. A persistent vegetative state may follow prolonged coma and is characterized by preserved sleep-wake cycles and maintenance of autonomic functions, with absence of awareness and cognition.
2. Locked-in syndrome, in which awareness and cognitive function are preserved but almost complete paralysis occurs, is often caused by large lesions in the base of the pons.
3. Brain death is a declaration of death based on irreversible cessation of all brain functions.

■ ACUTE CONFUSIONAL STATE

Definition

The terms **confusion, delirium,** and **encephalopathy** are often used nonspecifically to indicate a disturbance of mental status in which the patient is unable to carry out a coherent plan of thought or action. Most neurologists employ the terms **confusion** or **encephalopathy,** while **delirium** (commonly used by psychiatrists) often implies a state of encephalopathy characterized by a waxing and waning level of alertness.

At its core, an acute confusional state results from a problem of attention. Thus, a patient's failure to answer questions in a coherent manner or to carry out an intended series of actions in an expected way derives from an inability to maintain attention for long enough to proceed through the cognitive or motor steps required for the task. On formal mental status testing, therefore, patients with confusion typically do poorly on standard tests of attention, such as spelling the word "world" in reverse, reciting the months of the year backward, or completing serial subtractions. Such inattention may be significant enough to make impossible the performance of more detailed mental status testing. Depending on the underlying etiology of the acute confusional state, other associated features may be present on neurologic or general physical examination as well.

Differential Diagnosis

The differential diagnosis of acute confusion includes a number of different disorders, among them aphasia (particularly Wernicke), psychosis, and complex partial seizures. Patients with Wernicke aphasia may appear "confused" but in fact are attentive and able to carry out coherent series of actions; their deficit lies solely in their ability to communicate. Although patients with psychosis may also behave as if they were acutely confused, pure confusional states do not result in frank psychotic symptoms like hallucinations or delusions. Complex partial seizures can be characterized by behavior that appears "confused," but seizures are typically self-limited in duration and may be associated with clonic motor movements or automatisms such as lip-smacking.

Diagnostic Evaluation

An acute confusional state is most commonly caused by an underlying systemic or neurologic disorder, including infection, metabolic disturbance, inflammatory condition, or hypoxic-ischemic state, among many possibilities. Focal brain disorders, particularly acute right hemispheric lesions, can also lead to confusion. The appropriate diagnostic workup in a patient with confusion is therefore potentially quite extensive. Blood work and urinalysis to search for infectious or metabolic disturbances are often warranted. If there is clinical suspicion for a CNS infection, CSF analysis should be performed. Neuroimaging should be obtained if the neurologic history or examination suggests the possibility of an acute focal lesion. An EEG can help to determine whether there is a widespread dysfunction (encephalopathy) or focal abnormalities. It is unlikely to demonstrate the precise cause of an acute confusional state but can help to confirm a diagnosis, since characteristic findings of an encephalopathy may be present.

Treatment and Prognosis

The treatment and prognosis of acute confusional states depend largely on the underlying etiology. Most cases of confusion arise from a reversible underlying cause and will resolve if the underlying disorder is treated appropriately. Confusional states arising from structural neurologic lesions or more chronic underlying disturbances may be less likely to improve spontaneously.

KEY POINTS

1. An acute confusional state, also sometimes called delirium, is characterized by an inability to carry out a coherent plan of thought or action.
2. Acute confusion is primarily the result of a core problem with attention.
3. Systemic infections and metabolic disturbances are common causes of an acute confusional state, although many possible etiologies exist.

4 Neuro-Ophthalmology

An understanding of visual impairment, pupillary disturbances, and oculomotor control is essential in the diagnosis of neurologic disorders. Maximal interpretation of our environment is accomplished through the integration of visual, somatosensory, motor, and auditory information.

A systematic approach to evaluating patients with "visual" problems includes the analysis of: vision, eye movements, and integration of visual information. This chapter covers the first two; the third constitutes part of higher cortical function, discussed elsewhere (see Chapter 11).

■ ANATOMY

Light enters the cornea and stimulates the rods and cones in the retina, where the visual stimuli are converted into electrical signals that are sent through the optic nerve to centers in the brain for further processing and visual perception. The visual pathway (with various field defects) is shown in Figure 4-1.

The more posterior parts of the cerebral hemispheres are involved in seeing and analyzing visual information, including written language, and the more anterior parts control looking at and exploring visual space.

Ninety percent of retinal axons terminate in a retinotopic fashion in the lateral geniculate nucleus, the principal subcortical structure that carries visual information to the cerebral cortex through the optic radiations. The primary visual cortex is visual area 1 (V1), corresponding to Brodmann's area 17, or striate cortex, which receives information from the contralateral visual hemifield. This information is then transferred to associative visual cortex, including areas 18 and 19, and to many higher-order centers in the posterior parietal and inferior temporal cortices, where the perception of motion, depth, color, location, and form takes place.

SYMPTOMS APPROACH TO NEURO-OPHTHALMOLOGIC DISTURBANCES

The most common neuro-ophthalmologic symptoms are loss of vision and diplopia. Other symptoms include eye pain, visual hallucinations, and oscillopsia. Two important signs discussed in this chapter are the abnormal optic disc and anisocoria (unequal pupils).

■ VISUAL LOSS

Visual disturbances can be described as positive or negative phenomena. Positive visual phenomena include brightness, shimmering, sparkling, hallucinations, shining, flickering, or colors, often suggesting migraine or seizures. Negative visual phenomena can be described as blackness, grayness, dimness, or shade-obscuring vision, as seen in patients with strokes or transient ischemic attacks.

When the complaint is loss of vision, ask the following questions:

1. Is this a monocular or binocular problem? Does the problem go away when one eye is closed?
2. Does it affect a portion or the entire visual field?
3. Is it transient or persistent?
4. Are there associated symptoms, such as headache, visual auras, motor or sensory disturbances, changes in mentation, seizures, or eye pain (e.g., with optic neuritis)?

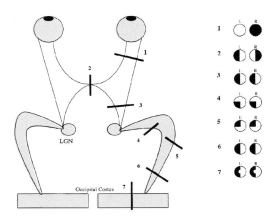

Localization	Visual field defect
1. Optic nerve	1. Right eye blindness
2. Chiasm	2. Bitemporal visual field defect
3. Optic tract	3. Left homonymous hemianopia
4. Optic radiations (parietal)	4. Left inferior homonymous quadrantonopia
5. Optic radiations (temporal or Meyer's loop)	5. Left superior homonymous quadrantonopia
6. Optic radiations (both)	6. Left homonymous hemianopia
7. Occipital cortex	7. Left homonymous hemianopia with macular sparing

Figure 4-1 • The visual pathway, with lesions and resultant visual field defects.

Diagnostic Evaluation

The evaluation of acquired visual loss (Box 4-1) begins with determining whether the problem is at the level of the eye, optic nerve, chiasm, optic tract, lateral geniculate nuclei (LGN), optic radiation, or occipital cortex. Once the site of dysfunction is determined, the workup is targeted to the specific cause.

The diagnostic evaluation includes assessment of visual acuity and color vision, test for afferent pupillary defects, testing of visual fields, and ophthalmoscopic evaluation. The ophthalmoscopic evaluation looks for damage to the retinal nerve fiber layer, optic atrophy, swollen disc, abnormal optic disc (hypoplastic, tilted, etc.), vascular lesions, and retinal emboli.

To test visual acuity (VA), use a distance chart with good illumination. At the bedside, the near chart (handheld Snellen chart) is often enough. If the VA is poor, try using a pinhole (you can create one by making small holes in a blank card). If the pinhole test improves the VA, the problem is in refraction. If the patient is unable to read letters, try counting fingers, followed by perception of movement and finally perception of a bright light. Impairment of VA is usually a problem in the refractive apparatus of the eye or the optic nerve, or both. Rarely, chiasmal or retrochiasmal lesions cause changes in VA.

Color vision is tested by using Ishihara plates. Another method is looking for red desaturation (decreased perception of red color), which can be seen early in optic nerve problems (particularly optic neuritis).

When testing pupils, report their size and reaction to light, both consensually and in accommodation. Use a bright light. Look for a relative afferent pupillary defect (RAPD), also known as a Marcus-Gunn pupil. To perform this test, place the patient in a dimly illuminated room and ask for fixation in the distance. A bright light is flashed alternately for 2 to 3 seconds in each eye. If the light is directed toward one eye and the ipsilateral pupil appears to dilate, an RAPD is present (i.e., the dilating pupil is "deafferented": it does not constrict to direct light but constricts consensually to light shone in the other eye).

Visual field testing at the bedside is done by confrontation. Cover one eye at a time. Move your fingers or a small white or red object over the different quadrants and compare the patient's visual field to yours. Table 4-1 compares the clinical characteristics of visual loss according to localization.

KEY POINTS

1. Organize your exam when examining vision. Remember to use a bright light.
2. Examine one eye at a time.
3. Monocular visual loss implies problems in the eye, optic nerve, or chiasm. Binocular visual loss implies a chiasmal or retrochiasmal lesion.
4. The pattern of visual field loss helps in the localization of the site of the lesion (see Figure 4-1).

BOX 4-1   CAUSES OF VISUAL LOSS

Retina
  Detachment
  Infectious: CMV, toxoplasmosis
  Toxic: ethambutol
  Degenerative: macular degeneration, retinitis
    pigmentosa
  Ischemic: embolic
Optic disc
  AION: vasculitic and nonvasculitic
  Optic neuritis
  Glaucoma
  Papilledema (late)
  Sarcoidosis
  Tumor
Optic nerve
  Demyelination
  Tumor, including meningioma, glioma, etc.
  Thyroid ophthalmopathy
  Trauma
Chiasm
  Tumor: pituitary tumors such as adenoma,
    craniopharyngioma, and glioma
  Sphenoid mucocele
  Internal carotid artery aneurysm
  Trauma
  Demyelination
  Vascular
  Toxic
Retrochiasmal
  Tumor: glioma, meningioma, metastasis
  Stroke involving the visual pathway
  Demyelination
  Degenerative diseases

CMV, cytomegalovirus; AION, anterior ischemic optic neuropathy.

■ DISORDERS OF THE PUPIL

Unequal pupil size (anisocoria) is common. The challenge is to distinguish a physiologic from a pathologic anisocoria.

Anatomy

Light activates retinal ganglion cells, which send their axons through the optic nerve, chiasm, and optic tract to synapse in the pretectal midbrain nuclei, also known as **Edinger-Westphal nuclei** (EWN) in the rostral portion of the third nerve nucleus. Efferent parasympathetic fibers from the EWN travel with the third cranial nerve (CN). In the cavernous sinus, they run with the inferior division of the third nerve and ultimately synapse in the ciliary ganglion. The iris contains two muscles that regulate pupil size. The sphincter is a pupilloconstrictor innervated by parasympathetic fibers of the third nerve. The dilator (pupillodilator) is innervated by the cervical sympathetic system. The sympathetic system starts in the ipsilateral posterolateral hypothalamus (first-order neuron) and projects down the brainstem to the intermediolateral cell column at the C8–T1 spinal level. The second-order neurons synapse in the superior cervical ganglion and represent the preganglionic neurons. Third-order neurons (postganglionic) travel along the internal carotid artery into the cavernous sinus and from there into the orbit to the pupillodilator muscles.

Diagnostic Evaluation

Document pupil reactivity and size in bright and dim illumination. Remember that up to 25% of normal people have asymmetric pupils without pathologic significance. In physiologic anisocoria, the amount of anisocoria does not change with different illumination. Pupils should respond normally to light and near stimulation. If the anisocoria is not physiologic, the next question to be answered is which pupil is abnormal, the dilated or the constricted one.

First, examine the pupils in the dark (turn the lights off and look at the pupils during the first 5 to 10 seconds). A dilation lag in the small pupil and anisocoria greater in darkness means a sympathetic defect in that pupil. Horner's syndrome (HS) is characterized by unilateral miosis, ptosis, and (sometimes) ipsilateral facial anhidrosis as a result of impaired sympathetic innervation. There are many different causes of HS, but in all of them cocaine eyedrops fail

■ TABLE 4-1

Comparison of Visual Loss According to Localization

Lesion Level	Causes	Symptoms/Signs	Visual Field Defect
Eye	Usually refractive error; central retinal artery occlusion; retinal detachment; central retinal vein occlusion	RAPD present; usually unilateral; vision improves with pinhole	Depends on the cause; only one eye affected
Optic nerve	Usually inflammatory lesions (MS and sarcoid); ischemic (vasculitis, atherosclerosis), such as AION; infiltrative (neoplasia)	Monocular visual loss; ipsilateral RAPD; disc swelling	Central, centrocecal, arcuate, or wedge field defect in the affected eye
Chiasm	Parasellar mass, including pituitary adenoma, craniopharyngioma, meningioma, aneurysm, etc.	Ipsilateral RAPD; binocular visual loss	Bitemporal hemianopia; central scotoma and centrocecal scotoma; important to evaluate contralateral superior temporal visual field
Lateral geniculate nucleus	Infarction, neoplasia, AVM	Binocular visual loss; no RAPD	Incongruous contralateral hemianopia
Optic radiation	Infarction, inflammatory, neoplasia, AVM	Binocular visual loss; ipsilateral smooth pursuit abnormalities; spasticity of conjugate gaze; no RAPD	
Temporal lobe			Superior contralateral quadrantanopia
Parietal lobe			Inferior contralateral quadrantanopia
Occipital lobe	Infarction (PCA strokes), inflammatory, neoplasia, AVM	Binocular visual loss; no RAPD	Congruous contralateral hemianopia with macular sparing

AION, anterior ischemic optic neuropathy; PCA, posterior cerebral artery; RAPD, relative afferent pupillary defect; AVM, arteriovenous malformation.

to dilate the abnormal pupil. If the cocaine test is negative, hydroxyamphetamine eyedrops will help to distinguish a preganglionic from a postganglionic HS (the pupil with a postganglionic HS fails to dilate with hydroxyamphetamine). The different causes of HS are summarized in Box 4-2.

Once you have established that the abnormal pupil is the larger one (mydriatic), localization of the problem starts by following the course of the third nerve from the midbrain or third nerve nucleus to the iris muscle. If the problem is at the level of the midbrain, other neurologic signs are usually present (hemiparesis, nystagmus, loss of consciousness, tremor, etc.).

Third nerve palsy is characterized by ptosis, dilated pupil, and ophthalmoplegia. Because the parasympathetic fibers run in the outer part of the third nerve and the motor fibers are more internal, compression of the nerve initially produces a dilated pupil without compromising eye movements. On the other hand, vascular problems producing third nerve ischemia (e.g., diabetes) will produce a pupil-sparing third nerve lesion in which the pupil is normal and reactive but there is palsy of the ocular muscles innervated by the third nerve.

A tonic (Adie's) pupil results from interruption of the parasympathetic supply from the ciliary ganglion (cell bodies or postganglionic fibers). Symptoms include anisocoria, photophobia, and blurred near vision (because of some accommodation paresis). The exam shows a dilated pupil, poor light reaction (with the typical segmental contraction), and light-near dissociation. It can be confirmed by demonstrating supersensitivity of the affected pupil to 0.1%

BOX 4-2	ETIOLOGY OF HORNER'S SYNDROME

First-order Horner's, or central Horner's:
    Hypothalamic infarcts, tumor
    Mesencephalic stroke
    Brainstem: ischemia (Wallenberg's syndrome),
        tumor, hemorrhage
    Spinal cord: syringomyelia, trauma
Second-order Horner's, or preganglionic:
    Cervicothoracic cord/spinal root trauma
    Cervical spondylosis
    Pulmonary apical tumor: Pancoast tumor
Third-order Horner's, or postganglionic:
    Superior cervical ganglion (tumor, iatrogenic, etc.)
    Internal carotid artery: dissection, trauma,
        thrombosis, tumor, etc.
    Base of skull: tumor, trauma
    Middle ear problems
    Cavernous sinus: tumor, inflammation (Tolosa-Hunt
        syndrome), aneurysm, thrombosis, fistula

pilocarpine, which will produce more contraction in the affected pupil than in the normal pupil.

An Argyll Robertson pupil is classically associated with syphilis. Usually both pupils are small and irregular, with impaired light reaction and intact near response (light-near dissociation); pupils also dilate poorly to mydriatic agents.

KEY POINTS

1. Horner's syndrome (HS) is characterized by ipsilateral miosis, ptosis, and facial anhidrosis.
2. A complete third nerve palsy presents with mydriasis, ptosis, and ophthalmoplegia.
3. An Adie's pupil is dilated, with segmental contraction and light-near dissociation.
4. Argyll Robertson pupils are small and poorly reactive to light but have preserved near response; they are typically associated with syphilis.
5. Light-near dissociation (LND): Normally the pupillary constriction to light is greater than to a near stimulus. The opposite is called LND. It implies a defect in light response, as in optic neuropathy, or the presence of aberrant regeneration, as in the Adie pupil. Other causes of LND include dorsal midbrain lesions and severe bilateral visual loss.

ABNORMAL OPTIC DISC

The term **papilledema** implies optic disc swelling resulting from increased ICP. Other forms of optic disc swelling due to local or systemic causes should just be called **optic disc swelling** (ODS).

The etiology of papilledema is a blockage of axoplasmic transport in the optic nerve. The clinical symptoms depend on the underlying cause [pain on eye movements with demyelinating optic neuritis, sudden visual loss in anterior ischemic optic neuropathy (AION), morning headache with space-occupying lesions, etc.]. The most common symptom of ODS is transient visual obscurations, described as a dimming or "blacking out" of vision and usually lasting just a few seconds. They are usually precipitated by changes in posture (bending or straightening) and can occur many times per day.

The most common causes of unilateral optic disc edema are optic neuritis, AION, and orbital compressive lesions. As a rule, optic nerve function is abnormal in each. The appearance of the optic disc may be indistinguishable in these entities, but certain features of it may suggest a specific diagnosis. Disc hemorrhages, for example, are much more common in AION than in optic neuritis or compressive lesions. The term **Foster-Kennedy syndrome** refers to ipsilateral optic disc atrophy due to compression by a space-occupying lesion in the frontal lobe and papilledema in the contralateral optic disc due to increased ICP.

Table 4-2 summarizes abnormalities of the optic disc and describes the most relevant clinical characteristics.

KEY POINTS

1. Always remember to carry your ophthalmoscope.
2. An abnormal optic disc has many possible causes (see Table 4-2).
3. LP determines intracranial pressure.

DIPLOPIA

Double vision usually arises from a misalignment of the eyes, which may occur from decompensation of a previous strabismus but in most cases is a symptom

■ TABLE 4-2

Assessment of Abnormal Optic Disc

Abnormality	Etiology	Clinical Manifestation and Fundoscopy	Diagnosis/Therapy
Increased	Space-occupying lesion (tumor, AVM, aneurysm, edema, etc.) Idiopathic intracoanial hypertension (IIH), also known as pseudotumor cerebri	Symptoms: morning headache, ataxia, and transient visual obscuration No RAPD, central acuity spared No color loss enlarged blind spot Fundi show bilateral disc hyperemia	Clinical MRI/CT LP with opening pressure **Therapy:** specific to the cause **IIH:** acetazolamide, nerve decompression, shunt
Drusen (calcified hyaline bodies) or pseudopapilledema	Small hyaline concretions (familial, autosomal dominant)	Asymptomatic Enlarged blind spot with normal visual acuity (initially) Fundi: glistening hyaline bodies + VP No disc hyperemia or exudates	Clinical CT and orbital ultrasound to see calcified hyaline bodies
Optic neuritis	Usually indicates demyelination (MS, SLE, adrenoleukodystrophy, sarcoidosis, tumor) Others: viral, meningitis, Behçet's, Whipple's, and Crohn's diseases	Painful visual loss Uhthoff's phenomenon (worsening visual function during exercise, hot baths, etc.) RAPD Retro-orbital pain Loss of color discrimination Central scotoma is classic Fundi: variable: from normal optic disc to optic atrophy or papillitis.	Clinical MRI looking for demyelination LP Visual evoked potentials **Therapy:** IV methylpred-nisolone is indicated. If MRI of the head shows more than three demyelinating lesions, the probability of developing MS is up to 50% in 5 years
Ischemia (AION)	Vascular: carotid occlusion, embolic TIAs Inflammatory: temporal arteritis	Sudden painless visual loss Patients usually over age 50 Associated hypertension diabetes Hypotensive episodes Variable visual field abnormalities and common RAPD Fundi: usually unilateral segmental disc edema	Medical workup for diabetes, hypertension, vasculitis MRA or ultrasound of the carotid artery TIA workup **Therapy:** specific to the cause

AION, anterior ischemic optic neuropathy; VP, venous pulsation; RAPD, relative afferent pupillary defect; MS, multiple sclerosis.

of neurologic disease. Abnormal eye movements can result from lesions in individual extraocular muscles, abnormalities of the neuromuscular junction, or dysfunction of the oculomotor nerves, their central nuclei, or central connections. Some useful concepts for understanding eye movements are summarized in Table 4-3.

Anatomy of Eye Movements

The three CNs involved in eye movements are the oculomotor (III), the trochlear (IV), and the abducens (VI). CN III innervates the superior rectus, medial rectus, inferior rectus, levator palpebrae, pupil constrictor, and inferior oblique muscles. Its dysfunction

TABLE 4-3

Some Terms Used to Define Eye Misalignment

Strabismus	Misalignment of the eyes
Comitant	Misalignment is constant in all directions of gaze, and each eye has full range of movement (usually an ophthalmologic problem)
Noncomitant	The degree of misalignment varies with the direction of gaze (usually a neurologic problem)
Phoria	Misalignment of the eyes when binocular vision is absent
Tropia	Misalignment of the eyes when both eyes are opened and binocular vision is possible

produces ptosis, mydriasis, and ophthalmoparesis with the eye deviated down and out (when all parts of CN III are involved). In addition, depending on the site of the lesion, there may be one of the following patterns:

- **Nucleus of CN III:** Bilateral ptosis and weakness of contralateral superior rectus; failure of eye elevation
- **Subarachnoid space:** Meningismus, constitutional symptoms, and other CN defects
- **Tentorial edge compression:** Depressed level of consciousness, hemiparesis, and history of trauma or supratentorial mass lesion

CN IV innervates the superior oblique muscle that intorts and depresses the adducted eye. Fourth nerve lesions produce oblique diplopia, worse on downgaze when the affected eye is adducted. The patient usually complains of diplopia when reading or going down stairs. Patients compensate with a contralateral head tilt (in other words, the diplopia improves with head tilt away from the side of the lesion).

CN VI innervates the lateral rectus muscle. Lesions produce esotropia, especially on ipsilateral gaze. Sixth nerve palsy can be a nonlocalizing sign of increased ICP.

The most common causes of oculomotor nerve dysfunction in older adults include microvascular occlusion and ischemia, commonly associated with hypertension, diabetes mellitus, and atherosclerosis.

Destruction of the abducens nucleus in the brainstem leads to complete (binocular) ipsilateral conjugate gaze palsy because of simultaneous damage to the interneurons connected to the contralateral third nerve through the medial longitudinal fasciculus (MLF) (Figure 4-2).

Clinical Manifestations

Is it monocular or binocular? If binocular, is it horizontal or vertical? Is it worse at near or at far? And finally, is the problem localized to an extraocular muscle (paresis or fatigue), brainstem MLF (internuclear ophthalmoplegia), or the orbit itself?

The MLF connects the abducens nucleus with the contralateral third nerve nucleus. Lesions of the MLF produce an internuclear ophthalmoplegia (INO). The clinical characteristics of a right INO include inability to adduct the right eye in left lateral gaze plus nystagmus of the abducting left eye. Adduction during convergence is preserved because this action does not depend on the MLF. Bilateral INOs can be seen in Wernicke encephalopathy (along with gait ataxia or confusional state), botulism, myasthenia gravis, brainstem strokes, and demyelination.

"One-and-a-half syndrome" occurs as a consequence of a lesion involving the paramedian pontine reticular formation (PPRF), or sixth nerve nucleus and the adjacent ipsilateral MLF. These produce an ipsilateral gaze palsy and INO on the contralateral side (the only eye movement present in the lateral plane is abduction of the contralateral eye) (Figure 4-2).

Vertical eye movements are controlled by the rostral interstitial nucleus of the MLF (riMLF) located in the pretectal midbrain area, near the CN III nucleus. Fibers controlling upgaze from the riMLF cross to the contralateral side using the posterior commissure to communicate with the inferior oblique and superior rectus subnuclei of the CN III complex. The downgaze pathway is less well understood but does not travel in the posterior commissure. Abnormal vertical gaze movements can be found in dorsal midbrain syndromes. Parinaud syndrome is characterized by upgaze disturbance, convergence-retraction nystagmus on attempted upgaze, and light-near dissociation of the pupils. It is generally produced by a pineal tumor compressing the dorsal midbrain.

Finally, skew deviation is a vertical tropia, generally caused by brainstem or cerebellar lesions. The

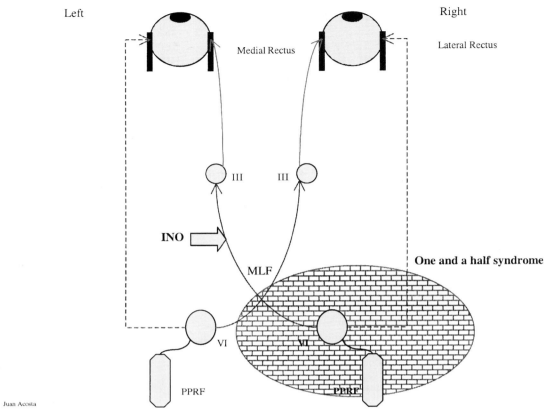

Figure 4-2 • Damage to the paramedian pontine reticular formation (PPRF), sixth nerve nucleus, and both medial longitudinal fasciculi (MLF) produces the "one-and-a-half syndrome syndrome" (patterned oval). The only eye movement present in the horizontal plane in this case is the abduction of the left eye. Internuclear ophthalmoplegia (INO) occurs after damage of the MLF. In this graphic, damage to the left MLF alone would produce inability to adduct the left eye and nystagmus in the right eye with right lateral gaze.

hypotropic (lower) eye is often on the side of the lesion.

Diagnostic Evaluation

The evaluation includes a careful history and a detailed neurologic exam. Some tests done to evaluate diplopia include the following:

- **Cover test:** Ask the patient to fixate on a small target. Cover one eye and watch the other eye. If the eye makes a refixation movement, this means that it was not aligned on the target. If the eye moves nasally, the patient has an exotropia; if it moves temporally, an esotropia. For example, a third nerve palsy produces exotropia and hypotropia of the paretic eye. Abducens palsy produces esotropia of the affected eye.

- **Alternate cover test:** Detects phoria (esophoria or exophoria). Phorias do not cause diplopia because the eyes are aligned when both are open simultaneously.

- **Park's three-step test:** Detects a fourth-nerve palsy:

1. Hypertropia (relative upward deviation) of the paretic eye.
2. Hypertropia increases when the patient looks to the opposite side.
3. Hypertropia increases when the patient tilts the head to the same side.

- **Oculocephalic maneuver (doll's-eye test):** Useful in unconscious patients to evaluate the integrity of the vestibular and oculomotor apparatus. It is done by rapid horizontal and vertical movement of the head. The vestibulo-ocular reflex rotates

the eyes in the direction opposite to head movement.
- **Saccades:** Rapid, conjugate movement of the eyes between objects (e.g., fingertips). In general, disorders of eye movement will produce slowness of saccades in the direction of the paretic muscle.
- **Pupillary size and reflexes**
- **Periocular signs or proptosis**

KEY POINTS

1. The PPRF acts as the horizontal gaze center, activating the abducens nucleus in response to supranuclear gaze commands.
2. The abducens nucleus contains motor neurons and internuclear neurons that travel with the MLF to the contralateral oculomotor nuclei in the midbrain.
3. Lesions of the MLF produce an INO.
4. Lesions of the PPRF and ipsilateral MLF produce the one-and-a-half syndrome (gaze palsy to the ipsilateral side and INO in contralateral gaze).
5. The riMLF is the vertical gaze center, analogous to the PPRF for horizontal gaze.
6. A gaze palsy may indicate a supranuclear or nuclear dysfunction. The doll's-eye maneuver or caloric testing will distinguish them. If doll's-eye movements are normal, the dysfunction is supranuclear.

◼ SUPRANUCLEAR EYE MOVEMENTS

Saccades are rapid eye movements to redirect the eyes to a new fixation object. In general, voluntary saccades originate in the frontal eye field and superior colliculus contralateral to the direction of gaze. These areas have a direct connection with the contralateral PPRF and participate in saccadic movements. Other areas that contribute to saccadic control include the dorsolateral prefrontal cortex, supplementary eye field, and parietal lobe. Vertical saccades may also originate in frontal eye fields or superior colliculi and connect to the contralateral riMLF. Inability to produce saccades is called **oculomotor apraxia.**

Abnormal saccades include those that overshoot (hypermetric) or undershoot (hypometric) and unwanted saccades or saccadic intrusions (square wave jerks, ocular flutter, and opsoclonus).

Pursuit movements permit the eyes to conjugately track a moving visual target to keep it in focus. The control is hemispheric and ipsilateral. Visual cortex inputs reach the temporo-occipital region. The occipitoparietotemporal junction is responsible for integrating the movement data. The fibers course into the deep parietal lobe and continue to the ipsilateral dorsolateral pontine nucleus. Then they travel sequentially to the cerebellar vermis, nucleus prepositus hypoglossi, medial vestibular nuclei, and finally to the abducens nuclei for horizontal pursuit. Vertical pursuits are mediated by the interstitial nucleus of Cajal rather than the riMLF (as for vertical saccades).

Pursuit disorders may be difficult to identify. Neurologic diseases such as Parkinson disease, progressive supranuclear palsy, drugs, and aging can slow down pursuits. Deep parietal lobe lesions produce pursuit abnormalities as well. Because of the long pathway involved in this type of movement, its value in localizing a lesion is limited.

The vestibulo-ocular reflex (VOR) coordinates eye movements with head movement, preventing the visual image from slipping during movements of the head. Slow, passive head movements can elicit it. The pathway involves the semicircular canals (rotation) and otoliths (linear acceleration) and travels to the vestibular nuclei. From there, it proceeds to the abducens nuclei and then to CNs III and IV through the MLF. Abnormalities of the VOR result in nystagmus (see following section).

◼ NYSTAGMUS

Nystagmus is a rhythmic to-and-fro movement of the eyes that can be congenital, physiologic, or a sign of CNS dysfunction, peripheral vestibular loss, or visual loss. It can be either pendular or jerking. In jerk nystagmus, the eye drifts away from fixation in a pursuit-like movement and returns with a fast, saccadic movement. The direction of the nystagmus is named by the direction of this fast component. Table 4-4 gives a brief description of physiologic and acquired nystagmus and possible causes.

Special attention needs to be paid to vestibular nystagmus. It is very common to be called to the ER

■ TABLE 4-4

Types of Nystagmus

Type	Characteristics
Physiologic or nonpathologic:	
Optokinetic nystagmus	Normal response to a continuously moving object.
Vestibulo-ocular	By rotations of the subject's head. Also irrigation of the ear (caloric test).
Endpoint nystagmus	Few beats of nystagmus in eccentric gaze.
Congenital nystagmus	Jerk or pendular, present after birth and remains throughout life.
Pathologic or acquired nystagmus:	
Periodic alternating nystagmus	Horizontal jerk nystagmus that changes direction every 2–3 minutes. Acquired forms are associated with craniocervical junction abnormalities, multiple sclerosis, bilateral blindness, and toxicity from anticonvulsants.
Downbeat nystagmus	Present in primary position. Also seen in disorders of the craniocervical junction (Chiari malformation), spinocerebellar degeneration, multiple sclerosis, familial periodic ataxia, and drug intoxication.
Upbeating nystagmus	In primary position is associated with lesions of the anterior cerebellar vermis and lower brainstem. Also occurs with drug intoxication and Wernicke's encephalopathy.
See-saw nystagmus	One eye elevates and intorts while the other depresses and extorts. Associated with third ventricle tumors and bitemporal hemianopsia, trauma, and brainstem vascular disease.
Gaze-evoked nystagmus	Similar to endpoint nystagmus but amplitude is greater and it occurs in a less eccentric position of the eyes. Most common cause is drug intoxication. Also seen in cerebellar disease and brainstem or hemisphere pathology.
Rebound nystagmus	Seen as a transient, rapid, horizontal jerk when eyes are moving to or from eccentric position. Usually associated with cerebellar or posterior fossa lesions.
Vestibular nystagmus	Usually horizontal with a rotatory component. Associated with peripheral inner ear disorders, Ménière's disease, vascular disorder, and drug toxicity.

■ TABLE 4-5

Tips for Differentiating Central from Peripheral Nystagmus

	Peripheral (vestibular)	Central (brainstem)
Direction	Unidirectional, fast phase away from the lesion	Bidirectional or unidirectional
Purely horizontal without rotatory component	Uncommon	Common
Vertical nystagmus	Never present	May be present
Visual fixation	Inhibits nystagmus and vertigo	No changes
Tinnitus or deafness	Often present	Rarely present
Romberg sign	Toward the slow phase	Variable
Vertigo	Severe	Mild
Duration	Short but recurrent	May be chronic
Causes	Vascular disorders, trauma, toxicity, Ménière's disease, vestibular neuronitis	Vascular, demyelination, and neoplastic/paraneoplastic disorders

to evaluate a patient with the acute onset of vertigo; the ER doctor immediately becomes concerned when the patient has nystagmus. Table 4-5 describes a few characteristics to help differentiate central from peripheral nystagmus.

KEY POINTS

1. Peripheral nystagmus is often unidirectional, with the fast phase away from the lesion; it combines horizontal and torsional movements and is inhibited by fixation.
2. Central nystagmus is normally bidirectional; often purely horizontal, vertical, or torsional; and not inhibited by fixation.
3. Saccades are fast eye movements that redirect the fovea to a new target. Horizontal saccades are initiated in the contralateral frontal eye field or superior colliculus.
4. Vertical saccades originate from bilateral frontal eye fields or the superior colliculus.
5. Conjugate gaze deviation is observed in lesions of the frontal lobe with destruction of the frontal eye field; the eyes deviate toward the side of the lesion. During a seizure, the eyes often turn away from the frontal focus.

5 The Approach to Weakness

Weakness is one of the most common presenting neurologic complaints. Many patients may tolerate some degree of numbness, tingling, or even pain, but often it is when weakness sets in that medical attention is finally sought. Similarly, friends or family members will not notice a patient's sensory problems, but significant weakness will be obvious to all.

At the same time, weakness can be one of the most difficult neurologic problems to sort out, because the pathways that control motor function span the entire axis of the nervous system. Left leg weakness can arise from a peripheral nerve lesion, a lumbosacral plexus problem, or a stroke in the right cerebral hemisphere. Each of these has a different workup, prognosis, and treatment, and it is the job of the physician to use the history and examination to distinguish among them.

PRINCIPLES

Figure 5-1 presents a flowchart to aid in the diagnosis of weakness. The key steps in the clinical approach are outlined below.

1. **Make sure that true weakness is the complaint.** Sometimes patients will use the term *weak* to mean a general sense of fatigue; others will say a limb is "weak" when it is clumsy or numb. Having the patient confirm that decreased strength is the symptom may be useful. Likewise, a limb that is painful to move may seem "weak"; whether there is true underlying weakness may be difficult to discern.
2. **Identify which muscles are weak.** This seems like an obvious point but must be emphasized. It is not sufficient to know that a patient has left leg weakness. Testing must be done in enough detail to know which muscles in the left leg are weak or, if they are all diffusely weak, which are weaker than others.
3. **Determine the pattern of weakness.** This is frequently the crux of the entire diagnosis. It is the pattern of weakness that will reveal when left leg weakness is due to a peroneal nerve problem and not a right hemispheric stroke. Needless to say, one must be familiar with the different patterns of weakness and their implications.
4. **Look for associated signs and symptoms.** If a leg is weak, determine whether it is also numb, tingling, or painful. Check the reflexes carefully. Often the motor deficit overshadows other problems, whose presence may be helpful in supporting or excluding certain diagnoses.
5. **Use laboratory and electrophysiologic tests wisely.** Blood tests or neuroimaging studies can be useful in the appropriate settings, and electromyography/ nerve conduction studies (EMG/NCS) can act as an extension of the clinical exam in localizing the problem to a particular segment of the peripheral nervous system. Tests are most useful in the setting of a complete clinical evaluation and formed diagnostic hypothesis, however.

KEY POINTS

1. Weakness can be caused by lesions along the entire neuraxis, from brain to muscle.
2. The diagnosis rests on determining what the pattern of weakness is, searching for associated signs and symptoms, and using laboratory tests and EMG/NCS to confirm clinical hypotheses.

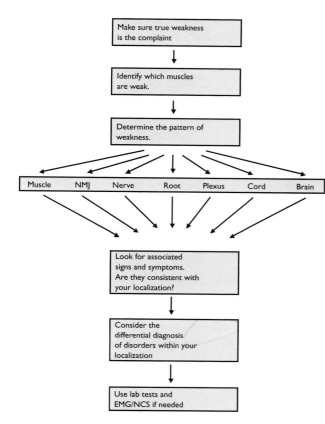

Figure 5-1 • The approach to weakness.

DIFFERENTIAL DIAGNOSIS

It is useful to consider the disorders that cause weakness in an anatomic order, from most distal in the nervous system (primary muscle disorders) to most proximal (disorders of the cerebral hemisphere). Below, each anatomic category is presented with the clues that might lead a clinician to suspect a disorder in that location. Individual diseases in each category are discussed in the later chapters covering specific neurologic disorders.

■ PRIMARY MUSCLE DISORDERS

Pattern of Weakness

Primary muscle problems tend to cause weakness predominantly in proximal muscles, in a symmetric fashion. Distal muscles are affected later or not as severely. In addition, neck flexors and extensors, which are not affected in most nerve or brain lesions, may be weak in a muscle disorder.

Associated Signs and Symptoms

Associated signs and symptoms may occasionally include muscle pain if the muscle disorder is inflammatory, such as polymyositis. By their nature, primary disorders of muscle should not cause sensory signs or other symptoms. Reflexes are characteristically preserved unless the process is so severe that the muscles are nearly paralyzed.

Laboratory Studies

Some disorders of muscle are characterized by an elevated serum creatine kinase (CK) level. The demonstration of characteristic "myopathic" changes on an EMG can help confirm a primary muscle disorder.

Differential Diagnosis

Primary muscle disorders, discussed in Chapter 24, include both acquired problems (myopathies), which can result from inflammatory or toxic etiologies among other causes, and congenital problems (muscular dystrophies).

KEY POINTS

1. Primary muscle disorders typically cause symmetric proximal weakness and can affect neck muscles.
2. Sensory signs and symptoms are not present.
3. Serum CK level is elevated in some muscle disorders, and EMG may show a characteristic "myopathic" pattern.

■ NEUROMUSCULAR JUNCTION DISORDERS

Pattern of Weakness

Neuromuscular junction (NMJ) problems can vary in the pattern of weakness they cause, though most affect proximal extremity muscles. Some NMJ disorders can lead to ptosis as well as weakness of extraocular, bulbar, and neck muscles. The characteristic feature of NMJ disorders is not the pattern of weakness, however, but the fluctuation. The degree of weakness may change from hour to hour. Depending on the specific disease, strength may be worse after using the muscles or toward the end of the day; it may improve after resting or in the morning (fatigability). Alternatively, strength may paradoxically improve after exercise in other conditions.

Associated Signs and Symptoms

By their nature, NMJ problems, which affect only the junction between the motor axon terminal and the muscle, should not lead to sensory signs or symptoms. Some NMJ disorders may have associated autonomic features.

Laboratory Studies

EMG/NCS can demonstrate nearly pathognomonic findings for certain NMJ disorders on specialized testing. Some of the diseases in this category have specific serum markers, such as antiacetylcholine receptor antibodies in myasthenia gravis.

Differential Diagnosis

NMJ disorders are discussed in Chapter 24; they include myasthenia gravis and Lambert-Eaton myasthenic syndrome, among others.

KEY POINTS

1. NMJ disorders can cause weakness of proximal muscles; some characteristically affect extraocular and bulbar muscles.
2. The key to diagnosing NMJ disorders is fluctuation in the degree of weakness.
3. Sensory signs and symptoms are not present.
4. EMG/NCS can be nearly pathognomonic in some cases.

■ PERIPHERAL NERVE DISORDERS

Pattern of Weakness

Each muscle in the upper or lower extremity is innervated by an individual peripheral nerve (Table 5-1). A lesion involving a particular peripheral nerve will lead to weakness in the muscles innervated by that nerve while sparing other, often neighboring muscles.

Disorders affecting a single peripheral nerve are known as **mononeuropathies**. Certain systemic

■ TABLE 5-1

Commonly Tested Movements

Movement	Muscle	Nerve	Root
Shoulder abduction	Deltoid	Axillary	C5
Elbow flexion	Biceps	Musculocutaneous	C5/C6
Elbow extension	Triceps	Radial	C7
Wrist extension	Wrist extensors	Radial	C7
Finger flexion	Finger flexors	Median, ulnar	C8/T1
Finger extension	Finger extensors	Radial	C7
Finger abduction	Interossei	Ulnar	C8/T1
Hip flexion	Iliopsoas	Nerve to iliopsoas	L1/L2/L3
Hip abduction	Gluteus medius, minimus	Superior gluteal	L5
Hip adduction	Hip adductors	Obturator	L3
Hip extension	Gluteus maximus	Sciatic	S1
Knee flexion	Hamstrings	Sciatic	L5/S1
Knee extension	Quadriceps	Femoral	L3/L4
Plantar flexion	Gastrocnemius, soleus	Tibial	S1
Dorsiflexion	Tibialis anterior	Peroneal	L5
Foot eversion	Peroneus muscles	Peroneal	S1
Foot inversion	Tibialis posterior	Tibial	L5
Great toe extension	Extensor hallucis longus	Peroneal	L5

conditions can lead to dysfunction of multiple peripheral nerves in succession, a disorder known as **mononeuropathy multiplex**. Finally, when peripheral nerves are all affected diffusely, in a **polyneuropathy**, dysfunction typically occurs in the longest nerves first. Thus, weakness from a polyneuropathy usually appears first in the distal muscles, symmetrically.

Associated Signs and Symptoms

Mononeuropathies may cause sensory symptoms—such as numbness, tingling, or pain—in the distribution of the relevant peripheral nerve. Mononeuropathy multiplex is characteristically associated with pain. Polyneuropathies, depending on etiology, usually have associated sensory loss and depressed or absent reflexes, particularly in the distal extremities.

Laboratory Studies

EMG/NCS can confirm the clinical suspicion of a problem localized to the peripheral nerves. NCS can identify whether the pathologic process affects primarily the axons or the myelin of the nerve, an essential step in formulating a differential diagnosis. EMG may yield insight as to the relative acuity or chronicity of a nerve disorder.

Differential Diagnosis

Mononeuropathies most commonly occur as a result of entrapment (as in carpal tunnel syndrome). Mononeuropathy multiplex is associated with systemic vasculitis and other metabolic or rheumatologic diseases. Demyelinating polyneuropathies can be hereditary (such as Charcot-Marie-Tooth disease) or acquired (as in Guillain-Barré syndrome), while axonal polyneuropathies have many potential underlying causes. Peripheral nerve disorders are discussed in Chapter 23.

KEY POINTS

1. Mononeuropathies lead to weakness in muscles innervated by a single peripheral nerve.
2. Polyneuropathies first affect the muscles of the distal extremities symmetrically.
3. EMG/NCS can confirm peripheral nerve involvement, identify axonal or demyelinating features, and evaluate the relative chronicity of a nerve disorder.

■ NERVE ROOT DISORDERS

Pattern of Weakness

Each nerve root relevant to the upper or lower extremity exits the spinal cord and eventually traverses a plexus (either brachial or lumbosacral) in which its fibers separate and become part of multiple different peripheral nerves, which then go on to innervate multiple different muscles. The result is that most muscles are innervated by fibers that originate from more than one nerve root, although some muscles are predominantly innervated by fibers from one nerve root (see Table 5-1). In any case, a lesion of a single nerve root will cause weakness in the muscles innervated predominantly by fibers from that root, while leaving other, often neighboring muscles unaffected.

A problem involving a single nerve root is termed a **radiculopathy.** Some processes lead to dysfunction of multiple nerve roots at once (**polyradiculopathy**), leaving a pattern of weakness that may be more diffuse and difficult to sort out because multiple muscles related to multiple nerve roots can be weak bilaterally.

Associated Signs and Symptoms

Radiculopathies often have associated tingling or pain, frequently radiating out from the neck or back. Objective sensory loss is rare in disorders affecting a single nerve root because there is overlap from neighboring roots. If the nerve root is one that subserves a particular muscle stretch reflex (Table 5-2), that reflex may be depressed or absent.

■ TABLE 5-2

Commonly Tested Muscle Stretch Reflexes

Reflex	Root
Biceps	C5
Brachioradialis	C6
Triceps	C7
Finger flexor	C8/T1
Patellar (knee jerk)	L4
Hip adductor	L3
Ankle jerk	S1

Laboratory Studies

EMG/NCS can confirm that nerve roots are the culprit in a weak patient and can be particularly useful for cases where clinical differentiation between a root problem and a peripheral nerve problem is murky. Single radiculopathies usually require MRI of the spine to rule out structural causes, whereas polyradiculopathies usually require lumbar puncture (LP) to look for infectious or inflammatory conditions.

Differential Diagnosis

Single radiculopathies can be caused by herniated discs or by reactivation of varicella zoster virus (shingles), for example. Polyradiculopathies are often inflammatory or infectious. These disorders are discussed in Chapter 23.

KEY POINTS

1. A radiculopathy causes weakness in the muscles innervated predominantly by fibers from one nerve root.
2. Radiating pain and tingling are common symptoms.
3. If the nerve root subserves a particular muscle stretch reflex, that reflex may be depressed or absent.
4. A polyradiculopathy may lead to weakness of multiple muscles related to multiple nerve roots bilaterally.

■ PLEXUS DISORDERS

Pattern of Weakness

The intricacies of brachial and lumbosacral plexus anatomy (Figure 5-2) are often quite intimidating for students, but it need not be, because—ironically—it is their complex anatomy that makes localizing lesions to a plexus more straightforward than expected. Put simply, if multiple muscles in a limb are weak and do not conform to the pattern of a particular nerve root or peripheral nerve, a plexus problem should be suspected.

In the leg, for example, weakness in both hip flexors and hip adductors would have to involve the L1, L2, and L3 roots or both the nerve to the iliopsoas and the obturator nerve (see Table 5-1); a much more likely explanation is a lesion in the upper part of the lumbosacral plexus.

Associated Signs and Symptoms

Because the plexus is where multiple nerve roots intermingle their fibers to form multiple peripheral nerves, it is unsurprising that plexus disorders can have associated sensory findings (in the distribution of one or more roots or nerves) or dropped reflexes (subserved by one or more roots).

Laboratory Studies

EMG/NCS is frequently ordered in cases of clinically suspected plexopathies to help confirm the localization to the plexus, given the less than straightforward

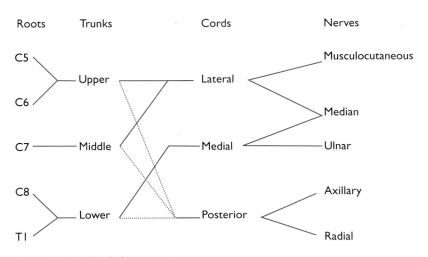

Figure 5-2 • Brachial plexus anatomy.

anatomy. MRI of the brachial plexus or pelvis (or lumbosacral plexus) may be necessary to rule out mass lesions.

Differential Diagnosis

Plexopathies can be caused by idiopathic inflammation, radiation, infiltration by metastases, hemorrhage, or trauma. They are discussed in Chapter 23. Diabetic patients are prone to develop a characteristic lumbosacral plexopathy known as **diabetic amyotrophy.**

KEY POINTS

1. A plexus problem should be suspected when multiple muscles in a limb are weak and do not conform to a particular nerve root or peripheral nerve pattern.
2. There may be associated sensory signs or reflex loss.
3. Plexopathies can be confirmed by EMG/NCS and have many potential causes.

■ SPINAL CORD DISORDERS

Pattern of Weakness

Spinal cord disorders cause weakness in two ways. First, the anterior horn cells located at the level of the lesion are affected, leading to weakness of the muscles innervated by the nerve root at that level. This mimics a radiculopathy, with weakness in a particular nerve root pattern. Second, there is weakness below the level of the lesion due to interruption of the descending corticospinal tracts. This weakness occurs in an upper motor neuron (UMN) pattern (Figure 5-3).

Associated Signs and Symptoms

Depending on the extent of the lesion, there may be sensory findings due to interruption of the ascending tracts. There may be a sensory level (loss of sensation below a particular dermatomal level) on the torso. Typically, reflexes below the level of a spinal cord lesion are increased, and there may be Babinski signs. Bladder and bowel incontinence may occur.

Laboratory Studies

MRI of the spine can rule out structural etiologies or demonstrate intrinsic inflammation within the cord. LP may be needed to evaluate infectious or inflammatory possibilities.

Differential Diagnosis

Spinal cord disorders are discussed in Chapter 22; they may stem from inflammation (transverse myelitis), infarction, compression, or other causes. Amyotrophic lateral sclerosis causes degeneration of both the corticospinal tracts and anterior horn cells.

KEY POINTS

1. Spinal cord disorders lead to weakness in a UMN pattern below the lesion and weakness in a nerve root pattern at the level of the lesion.
2. There may be sensory loss below the level of the lesion due to interruption of ascending tracts.
3. Reflexes below the level of the lesion are typically increased, and Babinski signs may be present.
4. Bladder and bowel incontinence may occur.

■ DISORDERS OF THE CEREBRAL HEMISPHERES AND BRAINSTEM

Pattern of Weakness

Lesions in the cerebral hemispheres lead to weakness of the contralateral body in an UMN pattern (see Figure 5-3). Knowledge of the homunculus of the motor strip (Figure 5-4) explains why lesions in the parasagittal part of the cerebral hemisphere cause weakness primarily in the leg, whereas lesions more laterally in the hemisphere cause weakness primarily in the face and arm. Deep hemispheric lesions, as in the internal capsule, may lead to weakness of all three parts of the contralateral body (face, arm, and leg), because motor fibers from all areas of the motor strip join together as they travel toward the brainstem.

Lesions in the base of the pons may lead to weakness of the ipsilateral face and contralateral arm and leg (crossed signs), because descending motor fibers to the face have crossed at that level but those to the body have not.

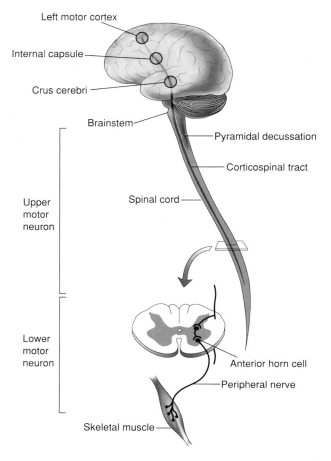

Left motor cortex

Internal capsule

Crus cerebri

Brainstem

Pyramidal decussation

Corticospinal tract

Spinal cord

Upper
motor
neuron

Lower
motor
neuron

Anterior horn cell

Peripheral nerve

Skeletal muscle

The descending motor pathway is divided into two parts.

The Upper Motor Neuron	The Lower Motor Neuron
Constitutes the neuron in the motor strip of the cerebral hemisphere and its descending axon all the way through the pyramidal decussation into the spinal cord	Constitutes the anterior horn cell and its projecting axon all the way through the root and nerve to the neuromuscular junction of the innervated muscle
Disorders of the UMN lead to a particular pattern of weakness: In the upper extremity, extensors and abductors become weaker than flexors and adductors. In the lower extremity, muscles that shorten the leg become weaker than muscles that extend the leg. In addition, UMN lesions lead to associated signs such as spasticity, hyperactive reflexes, and Babinski signs.	Disorders of the LMN lead to associated signs such as wasting and fasciculations.
In the face, lesions in the UMN (motor strip in cerebral hemisphere down to decussation in the pons) lead to weakness of the lower face but not the upper face, and weakness with volitional movements but not with emotional smile.	In the face, lesions in the LMN (peripheral facial nerve, as in Bell's palsy), lead to weakness of the upper and lower face, seen with all movements.

Figure 5-3 • Upper motor neuron (UMN) versus lower motor neuron (LMN).

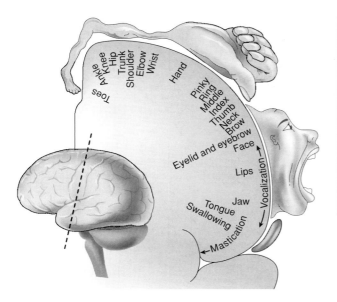

Figure 5-4 • The homunculus of the motor strip.

KEY POINTS

1. Cerebral hemispheric lesions lead to weakness of the contralateral side in a UMN pattern.
2. Parasagittal lesions lead primarily to leg weakness, more lateral lesions lead primarily to face and arm weakness, and deep lesions may lead to weakness of all three parts.
3. Cerebral hemispheric lesions may have accompanying cognitive signs, such as aphasia or neglect.
4. Brainstem lesions may have accompanying CN findings.

Associated Signs and Symptoms

Lesions of the cerebral hemispheres frequently have associated cognitive signs, such as those described in Chapter 11. Left hemispheric lesions may cause aphasia or apraxia, while right hemispheric lesions may cause neglect or visuospatial dysfunction. Lesions of the brainstem may cause cranial nerve problems, such as extraocular movement disorders.

Laboratory Studies

Imaging of the brain is important to evaluate almost all of the potential etiologies in this category. The choice of MRI or CT depends on the suspected etiology and relative acuity.

Differential Diagnosis

The differential diagnosis includes such diverse etiologies as stroke (Chapter 14), demyelinating disease (Chapter 20), traumatic injury (Chapter 17), brain tumor (Chapter 19), and infection (Chapter 21).

6

The Sensory System

The sensory system includes somatosensory and special senses: smell, vision, taste, hearing, and vestibular sensation. The common characteristic in all is the presence of a receptor, an afferent nerve, and a dorsal root or cranial nerve ganglion that carries the information to the CNS.

Somatosensory abnormalities may be characterized by increase, alteration, impairment, or loss of feeling. The diagnosis of these problems includes analysis of the nature, location, characteristics, and distribution of symptoms.

■ ANATOMY OF THE SENSORY PATHWAYS

Each sensory modality has a receptor. Information from the receptor is then carried to the CNS by individual fibers in the nerve (peripheral or cranial) known as first-order neurons. Pain and temperature are carried by thinly myelinated and unmyelinated slowly conducting fibers (A-delta and C fibers, respectively) that synapse at the level of the dorsal horn of the spinal cord. From here, the axons from the second-order neurons cross and travel contralaterally in the spinothalamic tract (STT), also called the anterolateral system (Figure 6-1). Proprioception, vibration, and light touch run ipsilaterally in heavily myelinated fibers (A-alpha and A-beta fibers) in the dorsal column system, reaching the second-order neuron at the level of the medulla in the nuclei gracilis and cuneatus. Axons from these nuclei cross at the lower medulla to form the medial lemniscus (Figure 6-2).

There is a somatotopic arrangement of fibers in these tracts.

- **Spinothalamic tract:** At the level of the spinal cord, sacral segments are located laterally, lumbar fibers more medially, and cervical segments in the most medial locations.
- **The dorsal columns:** The medial fibers are from the legs and lateral fibers from the arms. At the level of the medial lemniscus, the upper body fibers become medial and those of the lower body lateral.

Facial sensation is carried to the brainstem by the trigeminal nerve. The STT and the trigeminal tract terminate in the thalamus (ventroposterolateral and ventroposteromedial, respectively), with further cortical projections through the third-order neurons to the postcentral cortex in a somatotopic arrangement similar to that in the motor cortex, with the face in the lowest area and the leg in the parasagittal area. Fine sensory discrimination and localization of pain, temperature, touch, and pressure require normal functioning of the sensory cortex.

■ EXAMINATION OF THE SENSORY SYSTEM

This is a difficult part of the neurologic exam and requires the patient's cooperation. The evaluation of different primary sensory modalities [temperature, pain (pinprick), light touch, vibration, and propioception] is necessary to characterize sensory loss and its extent. In some instances, it is difficult to demonstrate sensory abnormalities in a patient with sensory symptoms; in others, the exam shows sensory findings in an asymptomatic patient. Whatever the situation, the sensory examination must be organized and methodical.

Touch sensation is tested with a wisp of cotton, using a very soft stimulus. Pain sensation is tested with a pin. Thermal modalities are tested using

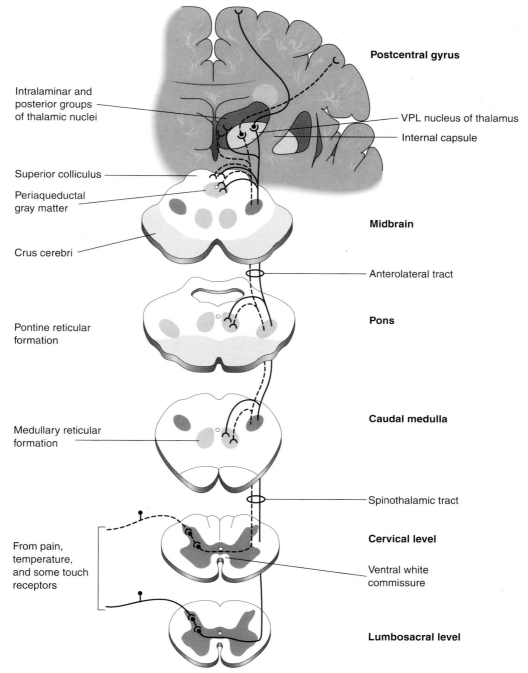

Figure 6-1 • Anterolateral system.

objects with a temperature range between 10 and 50°C, because beyond those limits the stimulus becomes painful. Moving the great toe up and down and asking the patient to indicate the direction of movement test joint position sense. Proprioception can also be tested by moving an object up or down on the skin and asking the patient the direction of the movement. The testing of vibration sense requires a tuning fork (128 Hz) to be applied to toes and other bony prominences.

The next step is to record the sensory abnormalities using accepted definitions.

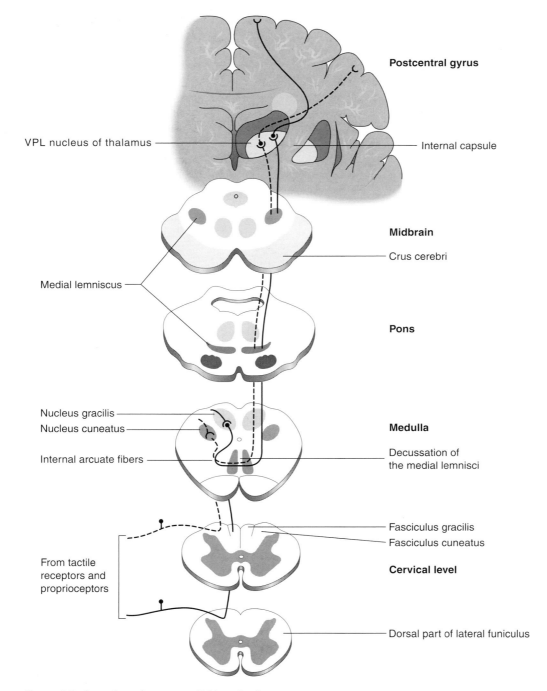

Figure 6-2 • Posterior column—medial lemniscal system.

It is important to register the patient's own words rather than using the terms below. Not only the presence or absence of sensation but also slight differences and gradations should be recorded. The following list defines some of the terminology used to describe sensory abnormalities:

- **Paresthesias** are abnormal sensations described by the patient as tingling, prickling, pins and needles, etc.
- **Dysesthesias** are unpleasant sensations triggered by painless stimuli.
- **Hyperesthesia** is increased sensitivity to sensory stimuli. The opposite is **hypesthesia.**

- **Allodynia** is pain provoked by normally innocuous stimuli.
- **Dissociated sensory loss** refers to the loss of one of the sensory systems with preservation of another. For example, in a syrinx, the STT is compromised early, with loss of pain and temperature in the dermatomes involved but preservation of posterior column function and therefore a normal response to light touch and normal proprioception. This occurs frequently with central cord syndromes (see Chapter 22).

■ APPROACH TO THE PATIENT WITH SENSORY LOSS

Sensory dysfunction becomes manifest through two types of symptoms: **negative**, such as numbness, loss of cold or warm sensation, blindness, and deafness; or **positive**, such as pain, paresthesias (tingling, pins and needles), visual sparkles, and tinnitus. The former usually means disruption of nerve excitation; the latter in general means excitation or disinhibition.

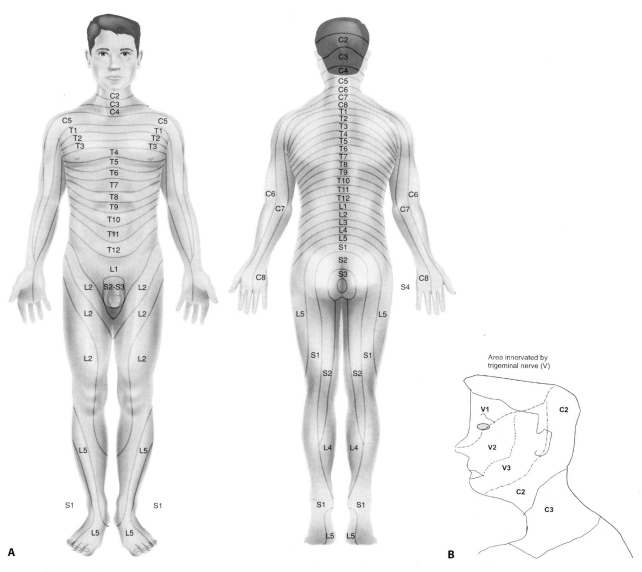

Figure 6-3 • Dermatome map.

In a patient complaining of sensory disturbances, the first goal is to establish the presence or absence of a neurologic lesion and then, if present, to establish its location. Sometimes the sensory problems accompany other symptoms—such as weakness, neglect, visual field cuts, behavioral problems, or seizures—that may help to determine the lesion's location.

The goal is to recognize sensory abnormalities by modality and to judge the level at which they are produced. Although in theory it is easy to distinguish peripheral nerve from segmental nerve or root, spinal cord, or other CNS locations, this is in fact often not possible or at best imprecise. In general, compression of a peripheral nerve has a distribution of sensory loss in the territory of that specific nerve. Root problems give a dermatomal pattern of loss (Figure 6-3). Spinal cord disease leads to a characteristic loss of sensation below a certain level. In brainstem lesions, the sensory

■ TABLE 6-1

Patterns of Sensory Loss According to Localization

Site of the Lesion	Sensory Findings	Other Neurologic Abnormalities	Examples
Peripheral nerve	Loss of LT, T, PP, and proprioception in the influenced area; associated weakness in muscles innervated by that nerve	Distal muscle weakness, atrophy, areflexia	Peroneal neuropathy; median and ulnar neuropathies
Root	Loss of all sensory modalities in a dermatomal distribution	Weakness in a myotomal distribution, atrophy, segmental hyporeflexia	L5 radiculopathy; cervical radiculopathy
Plexus	Sensory loss in the distribution of two or more peripheral nerves	Muscle weakness that cannot be localized to a single nerve or root	Brachial plexopathy due to trauma, inflammation, infiltration, etc.
Spinal cord	Sensory level: bilateral loss of all sensory modalities Sensory dissociation Contralateral hypesthesia and ipsilateral loss of proprioception (Brown-Séquard syndrome) Proprioceptive loss and corticospinal tract involvement Saddle anesthesia	Paraplegia, tetraplegia; initially areflexia, then hyperreflexia below the lesion; Babinski sign	Myelopathy; central cord syndromes; Brown-Séquard syndrome; subacute combined degeneration
Brainstem	Ipsilateral facial numbness and contralateral body numbness	Alternating hemiplegia; cranial nerve findings; INO, ataxia	Posterior circulation strokes; tumor
Thalamus	Hemibody anesthesia	May have motor findings	Lacunar stroke; hemorrhage
Posterior limb of internal capsule	Hemibody anesthesia	Hemiplegia	Lacunar stroke; hemorrhage; tumor
Cortex	All modalities affected on the contralateral side	Sensory neglect; agraphesthesia	Parietal stroke; hemorrhage; AVM
Psychogenic	Hyperesthesia for one modality in one area with anesthesia for another modality in the same area; changing sensory findings Nonphysiologic sensory level changes (abrupt midline changes, vibration asymmetry over the forehead, etc.)	Any	Psychogenic (This is a rule-out diagnosis; therefore, all other explanations need to be excluded before reaching this conclusion.)

LT, light touch; T, temperature; PP, pinprick; INO, internuclear ophthalmoplegia; AVM, arteriovenous malformation.

abnormalities may occur on the ipsilateral side of the face and contralateral side of the body. Central sensory loss involving the thalamus or sensory cortex will generally affect the contralateral face, arm, and leg.

Once the location of sensory loss has been characterized, it is important to determine what sensory modality is involved, because different pathologic processes can affect different sensory systems.

The last step in evaluating these sensory abnormalities is to establish the cause. There are many primary neurologic diseases as well as systemic diseases that can present with sensory symptoms. They are explored in more detail in Chapter 23 on peripheral neuropathies.

The different patterns of sensory loss and the location of the respective neurologic problem are represented in Table 6-1. This table provides a guide to the process of diagnosis based on clinical symptoms and the physical exam, without the need for further technologic resources.

KEY POINTS

1. It is important to obtain a good history of the sensory abnormalities and direct the exam according to it.
2. Nerve damage produces sensory problems in the distribution of the damaged nerve; root damage produces sensory problems in a dermatome; and plexus damage produces sensory problems in a group of nerves in the same limb.
3. Spinal cord lesions produce a sensory level; brainstem lesions cause a crossed sensory loss; and thalamus and cortex lesions produce sensory loss in the contralateral face, arm, and leg.

Dizziness, Vertigo, and Syncope

Because "dizziness" means different things to different people, it is not a useful term in describing one's symptoms. Broadly speaking, the possibilities include vertigo, light-headedness, dysequilibrium, and a fourth category of ill-defined dizziness. Vertigo is an illusion or hallucination of movement that is usually rotatory but may be linear. Light-headedness may also be described as feeling faint and may refer to a presyncopal state. This chapter focuses on these two categories.

Dysequilibrium is a sensation of imbalance or unsteadiness that is usually referable to the legs rather than to a feeling inside the head. The neurologic abnormalities responsible for this symptom are outlined in detail in Chapter 8. Finally, there are people who simply cannot define their symptoms accurately as well as those with anxiety.

■ VERTIGO

Most vertigo is caused by an acute asymmetry or imbalance of neural activity between the left and right vestibular systems. Vertigo does not result from symmetric bilateral loss of vestibular function (as with ototoxic drugs) or from a slow unilateral loss of vestibular function (e.g., with an acoustic neuroma); the brain appears to habituate to slow changes. A useful approach (Box 7-1) to sorting out the etiology is to determine the periodicity and duration of the symptoms and whether they are positional or spontaneous. A determination should also be made as to whether the vertigo is of peripheral or central origin; the most helpful features in this regard are the presence and nature of the associated symptoms and signs. Tinnitus or hearing loss suggests a peripheral cause, whereas diplopia, dysarthria, dysphagia, or other symptoms of brainstem dysfunction indicate a

central process. Accompanying nausea and vomiting is often more prominent with peripheral causes of vertigo, and the ability to walk or maintain posture may be more impaired with central disease. Neither of these latter features, however, is very reliable. Finally, the nature of the nystagmus may suggest the source of the vertigo. Vertical and direction-changing gaze-evoked nystagmus indicates a central process. Unidirectional nystagmus may arise from either central or peripheral dysfunction.

Vestibular neuronitis presents as an acute unilateral (complete or incomplete) peripheral vestibulopathy. The designation **neuronitis** is inaccurate because there is no evidence of inflammation, but the term is retained here because of its common usage. Patients develop a sudden and spontaneous onset of vertigo, nausea, and vomiting. The onset is usually over minutes to hours; symptoms peak within 24 hours and then improve gradually over several days or weeks. Complete recovery may not occur for months. Nystagmus is strictly unilateral and may be suppressed by visual fixation. Recovery represents central compensation for the loss of peripheral vestibular function.

Labyrinthine concussion may result from head injury irrespective of whether there is an associated skull fracture. Vertigo is sometimes accompanied by hearing loss and tinnitus.

Infarction of the labyrinth, brainstem, or cerebellum. The blood supply to the central and peripheral vestibular apparatus and the cerebellum is via the vertebrobasilar system (posterior and anterior inferior cerebellar arteries and the superior cerebellar artery). Blood supply to the inner ear is via the internal auditory artery, a branch of the anteroinferior cerebellar artery. Infarction of the inner ear presents with a sudden onset of deafness, vertigo, or both.

BOX 7-1	APPROACH TO THE PATIENT WITH VERTIGO

Spontaneous vertigo
   Single prolonged episode
      Vestibular neuronitis
      Labyrinthine concussion
      Lateral medullary or cerebellar infarction
   Recurrent episodes
      Ménière's disease
      Perilymph fistula
      Migraine
      Posterior circulation ischemia
Positional vertigo
   Peripheral
      Benign positional paroxysmal vertigo (BPPV)
   Central

Brainstem or cerebellar stroke is the most important differential diagnosis in patients with suspected acute vestibular neuronitis. The type of nystagmus and the presence of associated neurologic signs are the main distinguishing factors. A central-type nystagmus results from cerebellar or brainstem infarction, and almost invariably there are associated cranial nerve signs, weakness, ataxia, or sensory changes that clearly indicate a central process.

Ménière disease is characterized by episodic vertigo with nausea and vomiting; fluctuating, but progressive hearing loss; tinnitus; and a sensation of fullness or pressure in the ear. It is caused by an intermittent increase in endolymphatic volume.

A **perilymph fistula** results from disruption of the lining of the endolymphatic system. Typically, the patient reports hearing a "pop" at the time of a sudden increase in middle ear pressure, with sneezing, nose-blowing, coughing, or straining. This is followed by the abrupt onset of vertigo.

Patients with **benign positional paroxysmal vertigo** (BPPV) have episodes of vertigo that are precipitated by changes in position, such as turning over in bed or looking upward. The attacks are brief, usually lasting seconds to minutes, and symptoms typically begin after a few seconds' latency following the change in position. Attacks occur most frequently when the individual is reclining in bed at night or upon awakening in the morning. There may be associated severe nausea and vomiting. Attacks may occur in clusters, with patients remaining asymptomatic for months or years in between.

BPPV results from freely moving crystals of calcium carbonate within one of the semicircular canals. When the head is stationary, these crystals settle in the most dependent part of the canal (usually posterior). With head movements, the crystals move more slowly than the endolymph within which they lie; once the head comes to rest, their inertia causes ongoing stimulation of the hair cells, resulting in the illusion of movement (vertigo). Diagnosis is established by demonstrating the characteristic downbeating and torsional nystagmus with the Dix-Hallpike test (Figure 7-1, upper). The offending ear is the one that is toward the ground when vertigo occurs during the test. A positioning (Epley) maneuver (Figure 7-1, lower) can be used to remove the crystals from the posterior semicircular canal. The head is turned in the direction of the offending ear. The illustration demonstrates treatment for BPPV originating from the left ear.

KEY POINTS

1. Vertigo is a hallucination of movement that results from acute unilateral vestibular dysfunction.
2. Tinnitus and hearing loss often accompany peripheral vertigo; diplopia, dysarthria, or other symptoms of brainstem dysfunction indicate a central cause.
3. Isolated vertigo is almost never caused by brainstem ischemia.
4. Recurrent episodes of vertigo lasting seconds to minutes triggered by a change in head position are typical of benign positional paroxysmal vertigo.

■ SYNCOPE

Syncope is a transient loss of consciousness and postural tone that results from brain hypoperfusion. Prior to losing consciousness, patients often report light-headedness and a variety of visual symptoms (blurred or tunnel vision, graying or blacking out). The term **presyncope** is used when patients experience this prodrome of symptoms but do not subsequently lose consciousness. Observers may note that the patient appears pale or is sweating. Syncope is most commonly a manifestation of hypotension due to cardiac causes, low intravascular volume, or excessive vasodilation. Cardiac causes include asystole, third-degree heart block, tachyarrhythmias, outflow

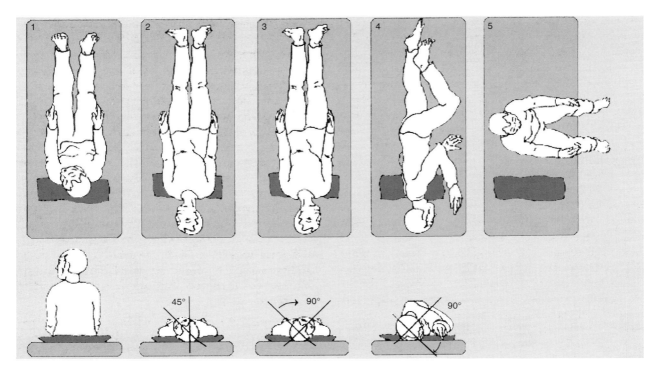

Figure 7-1 • The Dix-Hallpike maneuver is illustrated in the first two frames of the figure. The patient's head is rotated 45 degrees to one side and then extended 30 degrees over the edge of the bed. The examiner looks for a rotatory and down-beating nystagmus. The Epley positioning maneuver begins with the positioning used for the Dix-Hallpike maneuver and continues with a series of other positions, as illustrated.
(Reproduced with permission of the Department of Neurology, Charité, Humbolt University, Berlin.)

obstruction, valvular disease, or myocardial infarction. Low intravascular volume can result from dehydration, blood loss, or Addison's disease and can result in either syncope or orthostatic hypotension. Excessive vasodilation usually has a neurologic cause. There are essentially two neurologic varieties of syncope, both involving some dysfunction of the autonomic nervous system that results in excessive vasodilation. The more common is neurogenic syncope, in which acute hypotension results from a sudden reflex change in autonomic cardiovascular control. Less commonly, orthostatic hypotension and syncope may result from autonomic failure.

Neurogenic syncope is an acute hemodynamic reaction produced by a sudden change in the activity of the autonomic nervous system. Its pathophysiology involves a reflex triggered by excessive afferent discharges from arterial (including cardiac or great vessel) or visceral mechanoreceptors. Afferent impulses via the vagus nerve lead to cardioinhibition and vasodepression, resulting in hypotension and bradycardia. Different terms are used to describe this reflex, depending on the trigger (Table 7-1).

Autonomic failure is characterized by an inability to activate efferent sympathetic fibers appropriately, particularly on assumption of the upright posture. This usually leads to orthostatic hypotension, but syncope can also result. The underlying pathologic process can be either central (e.g., spinal cord injury or degenerative neurologic conditions that affect the autonomic nervous system, such as multiple system

■ TABLE 7-1

Reflex Syncope

Type of Syncope	Pathophysiologic Trigger
Micturition syncope	Rapid emptying of a distended bladder
Carotid sinus hypersensitivity	Compression of the carotid sinus
Neurocardiogenic syncope	Vigorous contraction of an underfilled ventricle
Vasovagal syncope	Strong emotions or acute pain

atrophy and Parkinson's disease) or peripheral (e.g., diabetes resulting in autonomic neuropathy), but the hallmark of both is the failure to release norepinephrine on standing. Patients usually complain of light-headedness and presyncopal symptoms in response to a sudden change in posture or prolonged standing. There may be associated weakness, fatigue, cognitive slowing, headache, neck pain, or buckling of the legs.

In evaluating patients with syncope or orthostatic hypotension, a thorough history and medical and neurologic examinations are warranted. The history is critical in detailing the precipitating circumstances of the event and excluding other conditions, such as seizures, that can be confused with syncope. If a cardiac cause is suspected, an electocardiogram or more prolonged cardiac monitoring with a Holter monitor may be indicated in order to exclude an underlying arrhythmia. An echocardiogram is indicated if a structural cardiac lesion (e.g., valvular) is suspected. In addition, clinical findings, orthostatic signs, and blood work (hemoglobin, hematocrit, blood urea nitrogen, and creatinine) can indicate intravascular volume depletion and its causes, such as blood loss or dehydration. If a neurologic cause for syncope is suspected, the exam can demonstrate a degenerative neurologic condition or a peripheral neuropathy. If no clear cause for syncope can be identified, tilt-table testing may be helpful in documenting autonomic dysfunction and diagnosing neurogenic syncope, particularly when the clinical history is unclear.

In managing patients with symptomatic orthostatic hypotension or syncope, it is important to recognize the potential contribution of drugs such as diuretics, antihypertensives, vasodilators, and antidepressants. Raising the head of the bed will reduce nocturnal diuresis, and patients should be advised to move gradually from the supine to standing position. A variety of drugs are available to ameliorate the symptoms of orthostatic hypotension, with midodrine and fludrocortisone being most commonly used. Beta blockers can be used to treat neurogenic syncope by suppressing overactive cardiac mechanoreceptors.

KEY POINTS

1. Presyncopal symptoms include light-headedness, headache, neck pain, blurring of vision, cognitive slowing, and buckling of the knees.
2. Syncope results from cerebral hypoperfusion.
3. The two main neurologic causes of syncope are neurogenic syncope and autonomic failure (central or peripheral).
4. Neurogenic syncope results from inappropriate activation of a cardioinhibitory and vasodepressor reflex, which may be triggered by micturition, deglutition, carotid sinus compression, sudden underfilling of the ventricle, or heightened vagal tone.
5. The hallmark of autonomic failure is the failure to release norepinephrine on standing.
6. Orthostatic hypotension may result from intravascular volume depletion, autonomic failure, or medications.

Ataxia and Gait Disorders

Ataxia is a term derived from Greek meaning "irregularity" or "disorderliness"; it is a general term often used to describe the manifestations of diseases of the cerebellum or its connections. It is important, however, to recognize that not all ataxia is cerebellar in origin. For example, the deafferentation due to the loss of position sense also results in an ataxia. Hence it is appropriate to distinguish cerebellar ataxia from sensory ataxia.

The cerebellum controls the force, direction, range, rate, and rhythm of movements; a disturbance of these elements results in the signs and symptoms characteristic of cerebellar disease (Box 8-1). Ataxia is not the only process that may underlie a gait disorder; these other causes are described separately below.

ATAXIA

Diagnostic Approach

The spectrum of disorders characterized by prominent ataxia is diverse. A limited differential diagnosis can often be generated by considering the acuity with which symptoms begin and whether the disorder is temporary, episodic, or progressive. It is also helpful to consider the age of onset, family history, and mode of inheritance. A classification based on this approach is outlined in Box 8-2. The details of a few of these disorders are specified below. Associated symptoms and signs may also provide useful diagnostic information; some of these are summarized in Table 8-1. Finally, at a clinical level, a distinction can often be made between lesions of the vermis and those of the cerebellar hemispheres. Vermal lesions typically produce prominent truncal and gait ataxia. Hemispheric lesions, however, typically manifest with ipsilateral limb ataxia.

■ CEREBELLAR HEMORRHAGE OR INFARCTION

Cerebellar hemorrhage or infarction typically presents with the abrupt onset of vertigo, vomiting, and inability to walk. Level of arousal may be depressed if there is compression of the fourth ventricle with hydrocephalus or if there is pressure on the brainstem. Cerebellar stroke should be considered a medical emergency because neurosurgical intervention may be required for decompression if there is brainstem compression or risk of herniation.

BOX 8-1	SIGNS AND SYMPTOMS OF CEREBELLAR DISEASE

Dysmetria: Abnormality of the range and force of a movement; manifests as erratic, jerky movements with over- and undershooting the target (hence limb or ocular dysmetria)

Intention tremor: Rhythmic side-to-side oscillations of the limb as it approaches the target

Dysdiadochokinesia: Abnormality of the rate and rhythm of a movement demonstrated by asking the patient to perform a rapid alternating movement

Gait ataxia: Broad-based and unsteady, with an inability to walk in a straight line and a tendency to lurch from side to side

Truncal ataxia: Impaired control of truncal posture; when severe, unable to even sit unsupported

Dysarthria: Slow scanning and monotonous speech

Nystagmus

BOX 8-2	CLASSIFICATION OF THE ATAXIAS

Acute or subacute onset with resolution or episodic course
  Postinfectious and infectious cerebellitis
  Cerebellar hemorrhage or infarction
  Drugs (e.g., phenytoin, barbiturates, antineoplastic agents)
  Multiple sclerosis
  Hydrocephalus*
  Posterior fossa mass*
  Foramen magnum compression*
  Dominantly inherited episodic ataxias
  Childhood metabolic disorders (e.g., aminoacidurias, disorders of pyruvate and lactate metabolism)
Acute or subacute onset with progressive course
  Paraneoplastic cerebellar degeneration
  Alcoholic or nutritional cerebellar degeneration
Chronic onset and progressive course
  Autosomal dominant spinocerebellar degenerations
  Autosomal recessive cerebellar degenerative disorders
  Infectious (e.g., Creutzfeldt-Jakob disease)
  Vitamin E deficiency
  Hypothyroidism
  Childhood metabolic disorders (e.g., mitochondrial encephalomyelopathies, Wilson's disease, ataxia-telangiectasia)

* May also cause insidious onset and chronically progressive ataxia.

ALCOHOLIC CEREBELLAR DEGENERATION

Alcoholic cerebellar degeneration is a consequence of long-standing alcohol abuse and is usually accompanied by an alcoholic polyneuropathy. Alcohol is the most common cause of acquired cerebellar degeneration. The vermis bears the brunt of the damage; the presentation, therefore, is usually with progressive gait and truncal ataxia that evolves over a period of weeks or months. Cessation of drinking and supplementation of nutrition offer the best (although limited) chance of improvement.

POSTINFECTIOUS CEREBELLITIS

Postinfectious cerebellitis typically affects children between the ages of 2 and 7 and usually follows a varicella or other viral infection. Children present with acute onset of limb and gait ataxia as well as dysarthria. Severity ranges from mild unsteadiness to complete inability to walk. The diagnosis is one of exclusion; this usually requires a careful search for underlying drug intoxication and for a mass lesion in the posterior fossa. The illness lasts a few weeks and recovery is usually complete.

PARANEOPLASTIC CEREBELLAR DEGENERATION

Paraneoplastic cerebellar degeneration (PCD) typically presents with the acute or subacute onset of a

TABLE 8-1

Associated Symptoms and Signs in Cerebellar Ataxia

Associated Symptom or Sign	Diagnostic Possibilities
Vomiting	Cerebellar stroke, posterior fossa mass
Fever	Viral cerebellitis, infection, or abscess
Malnutrition	Alcoholic cerebellar degeneration or vitamin E deficiency
Depressed consciousness	Cerebellar stroke, childhood metabolic disorders
Dementia	Creutzfeldt-Jakob disease, inherited spinocerebellar ataxia
Optic neuritis or atrophy	Multiple sclerosis
Ophthalmoplegia	Wernicke's encephalopathy, Miller-Fisher syndrome, multiple sclerosis, cerebellar stroke, posterior fossa mass
Extrapyramidal signs	Wilson's disease, Creutzfeldt-Jakob disease, olivopontocerebellar atrophy
Hyporeflexia or areflexia	Miller-Fisher syndrome, Friedreich's ataxia, alcoholic cerebellar degeneration, hypothyroidism
Downbeat nystagmus	Foramen magnum lesion, posterior fossa mass

pancerebellar syndrome with truncal, gait, and limb ataxia; dysarthria; and disturbances of ocular motility (ocular dysmetria, nystagmus). The disease usually evolves to its maximal extent over a period of weeks and then stabilizes, leaving the patient with profound disability. PCD is typically associated with an underlying gynecologic or small cell lung cancer and may become manifest prior to diagnosis of the tumor. MRI is usually normal. The CSF may have an elevated protein or a lymphocytic pleocytosis but is frequently normal. A variety of autoantibodies (e.g., anti-Yo, anti-Hu) have been described in this condition.

FRIEDREICH'S ATAXIA

Friedreich's ataxia is an autosomal recessive disorder characterized by a progressive ataxia that usually affects the arms more than the legs as well as by severe dysarthria. Onset is usually in childhood. Classic associated findings are loss of reflexes, spasticity and extensor plantar responses, and impaired vibration and position sense.

INHERITED EPISODIC ATAXIA

The episodic ataxia (EA) syndromes are characterized by brief episodes of ataxia, vertigo, nausea, and vomiting. EA-1 is caused by mutations in a voltage-gated potassium channel. Episodes are brief, and an interattack skeletal muscle myokymia is associated. EA-2 is caused by mutations in the pore-forming α_1 subunit of the P/Q-type voltage-gated calcium channel. Attacks are longer, lasting several minutes; there is interictal nystagmus; and a progressive irreversible ataxia may develop late in the disease.

AUTOSOMAL DOMINANT SPINOCEREBELLAR DEGENERATIONS

The clinical diagnosis is based on the occurrence of cerebellar ataxia, with or without additional neurologic signs, and a family history consistent with autosomal dominant inheritance. The typical presentation is the insidious onset of progressive impairment of gait and dysarthria in early adult life. Associated neurologic abnormalities (e.g., oculomotor, pyramidal, or extrapyramidal signs) may suggest the underlying genotype. Mild to moderate cognitive decline is a late feature in most of the spinocerebellar ataxias (SCAs). Many SCAs for which the genetic defect has been

identified have been shown to be caused by trinucleotide (CAG) expansions. SCA6 is allelic to EA-2, with the mutated gene being the pore-forming α_1 subunit of the P/Q-type voltage-gated calcium channel. The normal function of the other SCA genes is presently unknown.

MILLER FISHER SYNDROME

The Miller Fisher syndrome (MFS) is a disorder characterized by the triad of ataxia, areflexia, and ophthalmoplegia. The ataxia is due to proprioceptive loss rather than to cerebellar dysfunction. MFS is thought to be a variant of the Guillain-Barré syndrome; as such, it is most likely mediated by a postinfectious immune process. IgG anti-GQ_{1b} antibodies are detectable in the serum of over 90% of patients with this syndrome. It is usually a self-limiting disorder with a relatively good prognosis for full recovery.

KEY POINTS

1. Sudden onset of cerebellar ataxia with associated vomiting and depressed level of consciousness suggests a cerebellar stroke.
2. Alcoholic cerebellar degeneration typically affects the vermis and manifests itself with gait and truncal ataxia.
3. Postinfectious cerebellitis is a relatively common cause of ataxia in children.
4. Paraneoplastic cerebellar degeneration is a pancerebellar syndrome and is most often associated with small cell lung cancer or a gynecologic malignancy.
5. The inherited episodic ataxias are caused by mutations in calcium and potassium channel genes.
6. The autosomal dominant SCAs are a group of degenerative disorders caused by trinucleotide expansions.

OTHER GAIT DISORDERS

Abnormalities of gait are common and frequently multifactorial. This is especially true in the elderly, in whom falls often result. Not all gait disorders are the result of disease of the nervous system. For example, local mechanical factors such as pain and arthritis may impair ambulation. These factors are not discussed further here.

Clues to the etiology of the gait disorder may be derived from the presence of other neurologic abnormalities, such as weakness, spasticity, rigidity, bradykinesia, ataxia, or frontal lobe dysfunction. Sometimes, however, an abnormal gait is sufficiently characteristic to permit identification of the underlying disorder based solely on the features of the gait. The following sections are devoted to descriptions of the different types of gait disorders. The differential diagnosis of each type of gait is presented in Table 8-2.

■ HEMIPARETIC GAIT

The affected leg is stiff and does not flex at the hip, knee, or ankle. The leg is circumducted, with a tendency to scrape the floor with the toes. The arm is held in flexion and adduction and does not swing freely. A spastic (paraparetic) gait is essentially that of a bilateral hemiparesis. The adductor tone is increased, and the legs tend to cross during walking (scissoring gait).

■ AKINETIC-RIGID GAIT

Posture is stooped, with flexion of the shoulders, neck, and trunk. Gait is narrow-based, slow, and shuffling with small steps and reduced arm swing. Instead, the arms are carried flexed and slightly ahead of the body. There is often difficulty with gait initiation. Postural reflexes are impaired, and the patient may take a series of rapid small steps (festination) forward (propulsion) or backward (retropulsion) in an effort to preserve equilibrium. The foregoing description is typical of patients with idiopathic Parkinson's disease, but these features may also be seen in other extrapyramidal disorders. One difference in progressive supranuclear palsy is that posture tends toward extension rather than flexion.

■ FRONTAL GAIT

Posture is flexed, and the feet may be slightly apart. Gait initiation is impaired; the word "magnetic" is used to describe the patient's difficulty in lifting the feet off the ground. The patient advances with small, shuffling, and hesitant steps. With increasing severity, the patient may make abortive stepping movements in one place without being able to move forward.

■ WADDLING GAIT

A waddling gait is characteristic of hip-girdle weakness. During normal walking, the hip abductors contract to fix the weight-bearing leg and thus allow the opposite leg to rise and the trunk to tilt toward the fixed leg. Weakness of the abductors and consequent failure to stabilize the weight-bearing hip cause the pelvis and trunk to tilt toward the opposite side during walking.

■ TABLE 8-2

Etiology of Various Abnormal Gaits

Gait Disorder	Anatomical Location	Pathology
Hemiplegic	Brainstem, cerebral hemisphere	Stroke, tumor, trauma
Paraplegic	Spinal cord	Demyelination (e.g., multiple sclerosis), transverse myelitis, compressive myelopathy
	Bihemispheral	Diffuse anoxic injury
Akinetic-rigid	Basal ganglia	Parkinson's disease; other parkinsonian syndromes
Frontal	Frontal lobes	Hydrocephalus, tumor, stroke, neurodegenerative disorder
	Subcortical	Binswanger's disease
Waddling	Hip-girdle weakness	Muscular dystrophy, spinal muscular atrophy, acquired proximal myopathy
Slapping	Large-fiber neuropathy Dorsal columns	Vitamin B_{12} deficiency Tabes dorsalis

SENSORY ATAXIA

Loss of proprioceptive input from the feet impairs the patient's ability to determine his position in space. Gait, therefore, becomes cautious. It is wide-based, and steps are slow. Contact with the ground is made by the heel, and the forefoot then strikes the floor with a slapping sound (hence **slapping gait**). Walking on uneven surfaces or in the dark is particularly difficult for such a patient.

PSYCHOGENIC GAIT

There is no single typical characteristic to this gait. Instead, a range of abnormalities may be seen. With psychogenic leg weakness, for example, the patient tends to drag her leg behind or push it ahead of her. The circumduction characteristic of the genuine hemigait (described above) is absent. Another feature is that the patient may adopt extreme postures and lurch wildly in all directions but without falling, thus demonstrating good strength and more than adequate postural reflexes. The term **astasia-abasia** is used to describe this sort of acrobatic psychogenic gait.

KEY POINTS

1. Hemiparetic gait suggests hemispheric dysfunction, most often stroke.
2. Paraparetic gait typically suggests spinal cord disease.
3. Akinetic-rigid gait is a feature of parkinsonian syndromes.
4. Frontal gait suggests hydrocephalus (including normal-pressure hydrocephalus), neurodegenerative process, or bifrontal or diffuse subcortical disease.
5. Waddling gait suggests proximal muscle (hip girdle) weakness.
6. Slapping gait indicates large-fiber sensory or dorsal column dysfunction.

Urinary and Sexual Dysfunction

Urinary bladder dysfunction is associated with a wide variety of neurologic diseases including stroke, dementia, Parkinson's disease, multiple sclerosis, and diabetes. An understanding of how these diseases cause incontinence is important in both diagnosis and management.

■ BLADDER INCONTINENCE

Anatomy and Physiology

Neural circuits in the brain and spinal cord coordinate the activity of visceral smooth muscle (bladder and urethra) and striated muscle (external urethral sphincter) to control micturition (voiding). These circuits act as on-off switches to shift the lower urinary tract between storage (sympathetic) and elimination (parasympathetic) modes (Figure 9-1).

Bradley has defined the different neuroanatomic connections important for bladder control as "circuits." The first circuit connects the dorsomedial frontal lobe to the medial (M) region in the pons, providing the volitional control of micturition. The second, or spinobulbospinal circuit, is a reflex arc that starts in the urinary bladder and projects to the M region of the pons, with outflow connections to the parasympathetic sacral spinal motor nuclei. The third circuit is a spinal segmental reflex arc with afferent fibers from the detrusor muscle to the pudendal nucleus in the sacral spinal cord and efferent fibers to the striated sphincter muscles (see Figure 9-1).

M-region stimulation produces a decrease in urethral pressure, followed by a rise in detrusor muscle pressure and voiding. The M region projects to the intermediolateral columns of the sacral cord. The lateral (L) region is at the same level of the pons; its stimulation produces a powerful contraction of the urethral sphincter (storage). Damage at the level of the pontine micturition center will produce a loss of inhibitory control over spinal reflexes. As the bladder becomes distended, the micturition reflex is automatically activated without the patient's awareness or control, and detrusor hyperreflexia and incontinence occur.

Diagnostic Evaluation

The first objective in the evaluation of bladder incontinence is to determine if the problem is neurogenic or not. A detailed history is essential. It is important to obtain information about initiation; voiding problems such as frequency, stream characteristics, urine volume, fullness, and urgency; effects of posture, cough, Valsalva maneuver, and medications; and associated bowel and sexual dysfunction.

Thorough physical and neurologic examinations are necessary. The examiner seeks signs of frontal lobe dysfunction, parkinsonian features, sensory level, myelopathy, and so forth. Laboratory evaluation includes basic urinalysis to rule out infection. Measurement of the postvoid residual (PVR) by bladder ultrasound or catheterization is important in the characterization of bladder dysfunction. The PVR represents the residual volume in the bladder after voiding. A normal PVR is less than 50 mL. Urodynamic studies can clarify the characteristics of the incontinence, determine the underlying neurologic abnormality, categorize the vesicourethral dysfunction, and provide a basis for appropriate therapy.

Some urodynamic studies include the following:

- **Cystometry:** Provides information about bladder compliance, capacity, and volume at first sensation

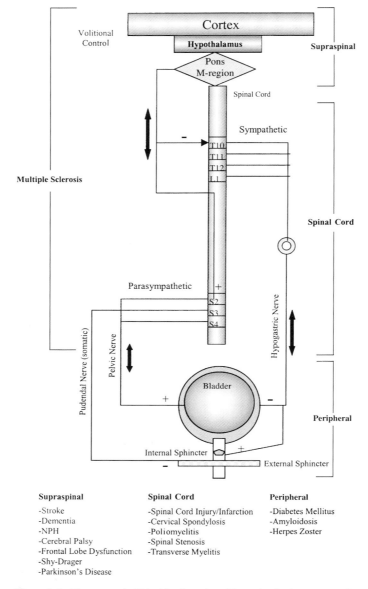

Figure 9-1 • The control of bladder function. (Figure by Dr. Juan Acosta.)

and at urge to void; voiding pressure; and the presence of uninhibited detrusor contractions.

- **Cystourethroscopy:** Assesses the integrity of the lower urinary system and identifies important urethral and bladder lesions.
- **Retrograde urethrography**
- **Neurophysiologic studies:** These include EMG of the sphincter and pelvic floor.

Urodynamic findings in various types of neurogenic bladder dysfunctions are listed in Table 9-1.

KEY POINTS

1. The M region in the pons is the site of activation of micturition.
2. History and a complete neurologic exam are important in the evaluation of bladder incontinence.
3. PVR should be less than 50 mL. Increased PVR implies poor bladder emptying. Sphincter dyssynergia and atonic bladder are common neurogenic causes of elevated PVR.

TABLE 9-1

Urodynamic Findings in Neurogenic Bladder

Type	Capacity	Compliance	Others
Spastic bladder	Decreased	Reduced	Uninhibited detrusor contractions
Atonic bladder	Increased	Increased	Low voiding pressure and flow rate

Classification

This classification is based on symptoms:

Urge incontinence is an involuntary loss of urine associated with a strong desire to void (urgency), usually associated with detrusor instability (DI). When the DI is the result of a neurologic problem, the term **detrusor hyperreflexia** (DH) is used; its clinical expression is a spastic bladder. DH is common in patients with strokes, suprasacral spinal cord lesions, and multiple sclerosis. It is usually accompanied by detrusor-sphincter dyssynergia (DSD), which is inappropriate contraction of the external sphincter with detrusor contraction. This can result in urinary retention, vesicoureteral reflux, and subsequent renal damage.

Stress incontinence is an involuntary loss of urine during coughing, sneezing, laughing, or other physical activities that increase intra-abdominal pressure (in the absence of detrusor contraction or an overdistended bladder). This is common in multiparous women who have cystoceles or weakened muscles of the pelvic floor. Other causes include urethral hypermobility; significant displacement of the urethra and bladder neck; and intrinsic urethral sphincter deficiency due to congenital weakness in patients with myelomeningocele or epispadias or who have had prostatectomy, trauma, or radiation.

Mixed incontinence is a combination of urge and stress incontinence.

Overflow incontinence is an involuntary loss of urine associated with overdistention of the bladder, reflecting a lower motor neuron problem. Patients report constant dribbling or urge or stress incontinence symptoms. The resultant atonic bladder can be produced by an underactive or acontractile detrusor (due to drugs, diabetic neuropathy, lower spinal cord injury, or radical pelvic surgery that interrupts innervation to the detrusor muscle). Bladder outlet and urethral obstruction can also cause overdistention and overflow.

KEY POINTS

1. Spastic bladder implies an upper motor neuron problem due to lesions involving the frontal lobes, pons, or suprasacral spinal cord. Symptoms include incontinence with urgency. Urodynamics show decreased capacity and reduced compliance.
2. Atonic bladder implies a lower motor neuron lesion at the level of the conus medullaris, cauda equina, or sacral plexus; or it may reflect peripheral nerve dysfunction. It is characterized by overflow incontinence and increased capacity and compliance.
3. Sphincter dyssynergia produces an increased PVR with fluctuating voiding pressures and varying flow rate.
4. A small PVR is good; a large PVR with spastic or atonic bladder is not. It can cause increased intrabladder pressure with deleterious effect on the ureters and kidneys.

Incontinence in the Neurologic Patient

The evaluation of urinary incontinence in the neurologic patient requires a detailed physical and neurologic exam in an attempt to define the level of the lesion: supraspinal, spinal, peripheral, or mixed.

Supraspinal Diseases

Supraspinal diseases usually result in a hyperreflexic bladder, causing urge incontinence, reduced bladder capacity, and small PVR, with no deleterious effects on the upper urinary tract because voiding is unobstructed.

CEREBROVASCULAR DISEASE

Large strokes (particularly frontal or pontine) produce an upper motor neuron bladder (hyperreflexic and small with urgency and frequency). Urinary incontinence after stroke is common and is associated with overall poor functional outcome.

PARKINSON'S DISEASE

Voiding dysfunction occurs in 40 to 70% of patients with Parkinson's disease. DH is the most common finding. Pseudodyssynergia occurs as a consequence of sphincter bradykinesia. Urologic causes, such as benign prostatic hypertrophy, are frequently associated.

Spinal Cord Diseases

Spinal cord diseases are the most common cause of neurogenic bladder dysfunction. In a clinical study, 74% of patients with neurogenic bladder dysfunction had some form of spinal cord disease.

Following disconnection from the pons, the sphincter tends to contract when the detrusor is contracting (dyssynergia). New reflexes emerge to drive bladder emptying and cause DH. During spinal shock, the bladder is acontractile, but gradually, over weeks, reflex detrusor contractions develop in response to low filling volumes.

SPINAL CORD INJURY

Spinal cord injury produces DH, loss of compliance, and detrusor-sphincter dyssynergia.

MULTIPLE SCLEROSIS

About 75% of patients with multiple sclerosis (MS) have bladder dysfunction. About 65% complain of irritative symptoms, 25% of obstructive symptoms, and 10% of mixed symptoms. DH occurs in 50 to 90% of patients, among whom 50% also have detrusor-sphincter dyssynergia.

Peripheral Nerve Diseases

Because of the bladder's extensive autonomic innervation, its dysfunction is most often seen in those generalized polyneuropathies involving small (autonomic) nerve fibers. Urodynamic studies show impaired detrusor contractility, decreased bladder sensation, decreased flow rate, and increased PVR. A classic example is diabetic cystopathy, in which a progressive loss of bladder sensation and impairment of bladder emptying eventually results in chronic low-pressure urinary retention. The situation is similar in other types of neuropathies such as amyloidosis, immune-mediated polyneuropathies (25% of Guillain-Barré patients have bladder symptoms), and inherited neuropathies. Injury to pelvic nerves (e.g., by local radiation or surgery) can produce similar symptoms.

> ### KEY POINTS
> 1. Stroke and spinal cord disease usually produce an upper motor neuron bladder or spastic bladder with or without sphincter dyssynergia.
> 2. Small-fiber neuropathies can produce a neurogenic atonic bladder with high PVR.

Treatment

Therapy for a neurogenic bladder includes pharmacologic and nonpharmacologic approaches. Some of the behavioral techniques that may help with the treatment of this condition include toileting assistance, bladder retraining, and pelvic muscle rehabilitation.

Pharmacologic agents are available to treat bladder dysfunction. The choice of therapy is based on an understanding of the underlying mechanism of the dysfunction and therefore the site of the neural injury. Table 9-2 summarizes treatments for urinary incontinence.

> ### KEY POINTS
> 1. Therapy of urinary incontinence is individualized and often requires adjustments.
> 2. The main management goals are preservation of upper urinary tract function and improvement of the patient's urinary symptoms that impair quality of life.

▄ ERECTILE DYSFUNCTION

The sexual response cycle of excitement, plateau, orgasm, and resolution requires the integrated and coordinated activity of the somatic and autonomic nervous systems innervating the reproductive system. Erectile dysfunction (ED) is defined as the persistent inability to attain or maintain penile erection sufficient for sexual intercourse.

An estimated 10 to 20 million American men have some degree of ED. Biologic or organic causes are demonstrated in up to 80% of cases, though psychiatric or psychogenic factors are important.

Anatomy and Physiology

The pudendal nerves carry both motor and sensory fibers that innervate the penis and clitoris. The parasympathetic nerves are located in the sacral cord (S2 through S4) and participate in erection. The

■ **TABLE 9-2**

Treatment of Urinary Incontinence

Type	Therapy	Notes
Urge incontinence (spastic bladder)	1. Anticholinergic agents a. Tolterodine (Detrol), 2 mg tid b. Oxybutynin (Ditropan), 2.5–5.0 mg po tid/qid c. Propantheline, 7.5–30.0 mg tid/qid 2. Tricyclic antidepressants a. Imipramine, 25 mg po tid/qid 3. Desmopressin (DDAVP) spray or tablets 4. Intravesical capsaicin	Tolterodine is tolerated better than oxybutynin. Most frequent side effect: dry mouth. Others include headache, dyspepsia, dizziness, and urinary tract infections Desmopressin is used to treat diabetes insipidus; however, it produces a significant reduction in voiding frequency in the 6 hours following treatment. Use only *once* a day. Intravesical capsaicin is used for intractable detrusor hyperreflexia. It has a neurotoxic effect on the afferent C fibers that drive volume-determined reflex detrusor contractions. Lessening of urgency and frequency may last up to 6 months.
Stress incontinence	1. Alpha-adrenergic agonist drugs a. Phenylpropanolamine, 25–100 mg bid b. Pseudoephedrine, 15–30 mg tid 2. Estrogen therapy, oral or vaginal	Alpha-adrenergic agonist drugs stimulate smooth muscle alpha-adrenergic receptors. Estrogen therapy is adjunctive for postmenopausal women with stress or mixed incontinence.
Atonic bladder with overflow incontinence	1. Credé's maneuver or Valsalva maneuver to empty the bladder. 2. Intermittent self-catheterization is perhaps the mainstay of long-term treatment. 3. Pharmacotherapy is usually not an effective treatment modality. The cholinergic agent bethanechol (25–100 mg qid) is used.	Bethanechol stimulates cholinergic receptors, increasing detrusor muscle tone. Side effects include bronchospasm, diarrhea, abdominal pain, and flushing.
Detrusor dyssynergia	1. Intermittent catheterization 2. Suprapubic catheterization 3. Sacral nerve stimulation	

sympathetic nerves arise from cells in the T11 to T12 levels of the spinal cord through the hypogastric plexus and are important in ejaculation.

Local tissue mediators such as nitric oxide and cGMP are primarily released by parasympathetic activity, contributing to sustained erection.

Causes of Sexual Dysfunction

The etiology of sexual dysfunction can be multifactorial. Neurogenic causes include neuropathy, myelopathy, cauda equina lesions, and CNS dysfunction. Other causes include vascular disease, pelvic trauma, and endocrine disorders such as hypothyroidism, hypogonadism, and hyperprolactinemia. Chronic illness, psychogenic illness, and drugs (i.e., antihypertensives, anticholinergics, antidepressants, sedatives, and narcotics) are frequent causes. Metabolic and toxic disorders such as alcohol abuse, liver disease, and renal failure are also common causes.

Diagnostic Evaluation

The evaluation of a patient with ED includes a complete history and physical exam. Neurologic examination may provide evidence of cerebral, spinal cord, or peripheral nerve dysfunction. Laboratory evaluation includes an endocrine panel with levels of prolactin, testosterone, and gonadotropins. Sleep studies can be helpful [erection usually occurs with each episode of rapid-eye-movement (REM) sleep]. EMG and somatosensory evoked potentials can help in cases of myelopathy or peripheral nerve disease. Vascular studies evaluate the response of the penis to the injection of vasoactive agents such as papaverine.

Treatment

The management of ED requires recognition of the etiology and treatment of the underlying disease. Endocrine, metabolic, vascular, and psychogenic causes must be treated when present. If drugs are responsible, changes in medication may be beneficial. Discussion of most available medical and surgical treatments is beyond the scope of this chapter.

Pharmacologic therapy of ED includes selective inhibitors of cGMP-specific phosphodiesterases like sildenafil (Viagra) and vardenafil (Levitra), intraurethral suppositories, and intracavernosal injections of alprostadil (Caverject).

KEY POINTS

1. ED affects an estimated 10 to 20 million men in the United States.
2. ED is often multifactorial. Many neurogenic diseases can produce ED, including strokes, multiple sclerosis, and diabetes.
3. Medical and surgical therapies are available.

Headache is one of the most common symptoms encountered by physicians. Approximately 70 to 80% of the population have headaches at some time, and 50% have headaches at least once a month. The challenge of caring for patients with headache lies not only in finding the appropriate treatment but also in determining when headache represents a symptom of more serious disease. Therefore the approach to the patient with headache entails understanding the pathophysiology of head pain, performing a complete history and physical exam, generating a differential diagnosis, and pursuing treatment options.

Pathogenesis

Headache is caused by a disturbance or irritation of the pain-sensitive structures in the head. Within the cranium, pain-sensitive structures include blood vessels, meninges, and the cranial nerves. Outside the cranium, the pain-sensitive structures are the periosteum of the skull, muscles, nerves, arteries and veins, subcutaneous tissues, eyes, ears, sinuses, and mucous membranes. Of note, the brain parenchyma itself and bones are insensitive to pain. Tumors or hydrocephalus can cause pain by producing enough mass effect to result in stretching of pain-sensitive structures such as the meninges or blood vessels.

Irritation or damage to the pain-sensitive structures relays nociceptive information to the brain via CN V (trigeminal) or by the upper cervical roots. In addition to the dermatomal innervation of the trigeminal nerve (Figure 10-1), the anterior and middle cranial fossae are innervated by CN V, especially V_1, while the upper cervical roots innervate structures in the posterior fossa. Thus, painful stimulation of structures in the anterior or the middle fossa is often referred to the eye or front or side of the head, whereas painful stimulation of structures in the posterior fossa results in pain that is referred to the back of the head and upper part of the neck.

KEY POINTS

1. Pain-sensitive structures inside the skull include blood vessels, meninges, and the cranial nerves.
2. CN V relays nociceptive information from the pain-sensitive structures inside the skull to the brain.

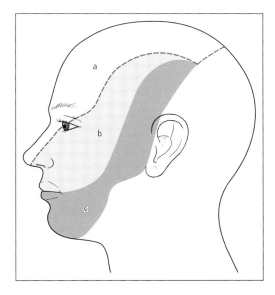

Figure 10-1 • Sensory division of the trigeminal nerve (cranial nerve V): (a) ophthalmic division, or V_1; (b) maxillary division, or V_2; (c) mandibular divison, or V_3.
(Reproduced with permission from Ginsberg L. Lecture Notes Neurology. 8th ed. Oxford: Blackwell Publishing, 2005:29.)

Clinical Manifestations

History and Physical Examination

Generally, headaches should be classified into three major categories:

1. Primary headaches that represent the common headache syndromes such as migraine, cluster, and tension headaches. These headaches are not generally associated with an underlying structural cause.
2. Headaches related to serious neurologic diseases such as brain tumor, meningitis, and aneurysm.
3. Headaches or pain from structures in the skull and face such as the eyes, sinuses, and mouth.

The history and physical exam should be aimed at differentiating the above possibilities. Onset and frequency aid in the diagnosis of chronic headache. A sudden severe headache that has never occurred before may be a symptom of subarachnoid hemorrhage from aneurysm rupture. A progressively worsening headache over the preceding month or so may indicate a slowly expanding tumor, whereas a frequent headache that has been present for 20 years without neurologic signs or symptoms usually implies a benign etiology.

Location of pain, such as tenderness over the sinuses (sinusitis) or the temporomandibular joint, can help differentiate these conditions from a primary headache disorder. Migraine and cluster headaches are often unilateral, whereas tension headaches are usually bilateral. Prodromal symptoms such as scintillating scotomas or gradually spreading paresthesias can be associated with classic migraine headaches. Precipitating factors are also an important guide to identifying the etiology of headache. Alcohol is often a trigger for cluster headache, whereas nitrite-containing foods (hot dogs, salami, and other preserved meats) and cheeses containing tyramine can trigger migraine headaches.

Description of pain is also useful in characterizing headache or facial pain. Lancinating or shooting pain in a V_2 or V_3 distribution of the trigeminal nerve is characteristic of trigeminal neuralgia (tic douloureux). Unilateral throbbing pain is common in migraine, whereas a dull, band-like, or tightening pain can be part of tension headache. A sharp, stabbing pain, especially behind one eye, is common in cluster headaches.

Associated symptoms and neurologic signs are extremely important aids in the diagnosis of headache and facial pain conditions. Nausea and vomiting can be associated either with migraine headaches or raised ICP from hydrocephalus or a tumor. Photophobia, phonophobia, or increased frequency of the headache at menstruation can be associated with migraine. Systemic symptoms such as fever can suggest meningitis or a local infection such as a dental abscess as the cause of pain. Unilateral lacrimation or rhinorrhea is associated with cluster headaches.

Warning signs during the history that should alert one to the possibility of a more serious cause of the headache are sudden onset of a new headache or a progressively worsening headache. Headaches associated with a change in level of consciousness can be due to tumor or subarachnoid hemorrhage. Fever, neurologic symptoms or signs, or new headache after the age of 50 should prompt consideration for a serious cause of the headache.

The physical exam should be complete, including registration of vital signs to exclude fever, but particular attention should be focused on the head and neck. Inspection of the entire head should be performed, noting the shape of the head (especially in children who may have hydrocephalus) and identifying signs of trauma. The conjunctiva or iris can appear irritated with primary ocular disorders or with cluster headaches. Auscultation of the carotid arteries may reveal bruits, and auscultation with the bell over the orbits may reveal bruits from an arteriovenous malformation. Palpation can demonstrate tight and tender cervical muscles, which are often found in patients with tension headaches. Tenderness of a temporal artery in an elderly person may indicate temporal arteritis, while palpation of the temporomandibular joints when the jaw is opened and closed may indicate temporomandibular joint dysfunction. Sinus tenderness during palpation may indicate sinusitis, and tenderness to palpation of the teeth may indicate a dental abscess. Signs of meningeal irritation (see Chapter 21) should be sought, especially in patients with fever. Detailed cranial nerve examination should be performed, including funduscopic examination to look for papilledema as a sign of increased intracranial pressure. Partial oculomotor nerve (CN III) palsy identified along with a unilateral dilated pupil can be associated with uncal herniation or an aneurysm of the posterior communicating artery. A unilateral Horner syndrome can be seen with cluster headache or carotid artery dissection. Trigger points causing pain in the trigeminal nerve distribution (especially V_2 and V_3) or in the pharynx can suggest trigeminal neuralgia or glossopharyngeal neuralgia, respectively.

PRIMARY HEADACHE DISORDERS

Headaches that do not have an underlying structural cause are called primary headaches. These headaches are diagnosed based on their clinical features, which reinforces the importance of a good history. The main types of primary headaches are migraine, tension-type, and cluster.

■ MIGRAINE

Migraine headaches are generally unilateral and pulsing or throbbing in quality. They affect women more commonly than men. Age of onset is typically in the teens or early twenties, and migraines are often associated with nausea and vomiting, photophobia, and phonophobia. The symptoms are typically worsened by physical activity and relieved by lying down in a dark room.

Common migraine headache (without aura) represents the majority of migraine. Migraine can, however, be associated with an aura, a transient focal neurologic symptom that usually precedes the headache and lasts between 15 minutes and 1 hour. Migraine with aura is also called classic migraine. The most common type of aura is visual and can consist of flashing lights or zigzag lines that march across the patient's visual field. Sensory or motor symptoms can also occur. Most auras develop in a marching fashion, in which the symptoms spread gradually. The headache usually follows the aura within 20 to 60 minutes and lasts between 4 and 72 hours. Some patients have aura only. The march of symptoms is the most useful distinction between the focal neurologic deficits caused by migraine aura and those caused by stroke (sudden onset) or seizure (spread over seconds).

Treatment of migraine is aimed at either preventing or aborting an attack. Prevention can be attempted by avoiding triggers such as aged cheese, red wine, and other foods that precipitate an attack. Prophylactic medications such as beta blockers (propranolol), calcium channel antagonists (verapamil), tricyclic antidepressants (amitriptyline), and some anticonvulsants (valproic acid, topiramate, and lamotrigine) can decrease the frequency and severity of attacks.

Abortive therapy is used to stop an acute attack. Simple analgesics such as acetaminophen, aspirin, or prescription-strength nonsteroidal anti-inflammatory drugs (NSAIDs) may be effective if taken early during headache symptoms. Ergot alkaloids and selective serotonin ($5-HT_1$) agonists (triptans) also abort migraine but have limited time windows in which they can be used and are contraindicated in patients with uncontrolled hypertension or coronary artery disease because of their vasoconstrictive properties. Antiemetics such as prochlorperazine or chlorpromazine are also useful abortive treatments. Status migranosus, a migraine that lasts longer than 24 hours, may benefit from corticosteroid treatment.

■ TENSION-TYPE HEADACHE

Tension-type headache is the most common type of primary headache disorder. It is described as a bilateral headache with a pressing or squeezing quality, often in a band-like distribution and involving the back of the neck. The underlying pathophysiologic mechanism of the headache is unknown. Muscle spasm may be involved, but controversy exists as to whether the muscle spasm is an epiphenomenon or causal.

Many of the same medications used in treating migraine are effective for tension-type headaches. In addition to pharmacologic treatment with these analgesics, muscle relaxants such as cyclobenzaprine, physical therapy, stress management, biofeedback, and psychotherapy may be beneficial.

■ CLUSTER HEADACHES

Unlike the other primary headache disorders, cluster headaches affect men approximately six times more frequently than women. As the name implies, the headaches usually occur in cyclic clusters. Headaches usually occur one to three times per day during a cluster, which can last up to several months. The remission period can be months to years. The pain typically occurs after work or within several hours of sleep onset and is always unilateral, behind one eye or over the lateral part of the nose. The pain can be extremely severe, and patients commonly have ipsilateral conjunctival injection, lacrimation, nasal congestion, and, less frequently, Horner syndrome. It is believed that cluster headache pathophysiology is focused in the superior pericarotid cavernous sinus plexus.

Treatment is aimed at avoiding possible precipitants such as alcohol or strenuous exercise during an attack. For prophylaxis, verapamil and lithium can be used. Symptomatic treatment of cluster headache is inhalation of pure oxygen, which is over 90%

effective. Triptans, dihydroergotamine, and cortico-steroids can also be used.

PAROXYSMAL HEMICRANIA

Paroxysmal hemicrania occurs mostly in young adults and affects women more than men. The disorder is characterized by daily attacks of severe unilateral pain in the periorbital or temporal regions that last approx-imately 20 minutes each. Like cluster headaches, paroxysmal hemicrania is accompanied by autonomic features such as lacrimation, ptosis, conjunctival injec-tion, and rhinorrhea ipsilateral to the pain. The response of paroxysmal hemicrania to indomethacin is a defining feature of the syndrome. The demographic profile of patients with paroxysmal hemicrania and their dramatic response to indomethacin help to dif-ferentiate it from cluster headache.

CHRONIC DAILY HEADACHE AND REBOUND HEADACHE

Chronic daily headache occurs in a subset of patients with both migraine and tension-type headaches. The headaches occur daily, and the symptoms may resemble those of migraine or tension headaches or a combina-tion. Chronic daily headache is often associated with analgesic overuse and caffeine dependence. These headaches are very difficult to treat and often respond better to nonmedical therapies—such as biofeedback, meditation, massage, ultrasound, and physical therapy—than they do to medical therapies. Rebound headache occurs in the setting of analgesic overuse for the acute relief of headache. Like chronic daily headache, rebound headache is more effectively treated with nonmedical therapies and rapid tapering of analgesics.

KEY POINTS

1. Primary headaches do not have underlying struc-tural causes.
2. Table 10-1 summarizes the features of primary headaches.

SECONDARY HEADACHES

As mentioned previously, headache can result from a myriad of underlying etiologies. The following examples

TABLE 10-1

Features of Headache Disorders

Headache Type	Male-Female Ratio	Age of Onset	Typical Clinical Features
Migraine	F > M	Teen years	Can be unilateral or bilateral, typically throbbing.
Tension	M = F	Any age	Usually bilateral and occipital or frontal. Pain is typically dull or band-like.
Cluster	M > F	Middle age	Stabbing pain behind one eye associated with ipsilateral conjunctival injection, lacrimation, nasal congestion, and occasional Horner syndrome.
Chronic paroxysmal hemicrania	F > M	Middle age	Similar to cluster headache.
Increased intracranial pressure	F = M	Any age	Pain worse in the morning, with cough, bending over, or Valsalva.
Low-pressure headache	F = M	Any age	Pain worse when sitting or standing up.
Trigeminal neuralgia	F = M	Middle age	Lancinating pain typically at border of V_1 and V_2 or V_2 and V_3.
Subarachnoid hemorrhage	F = M	Middle age	Sudden onset, terrible headache.
Chronic daily headache	F > M	Middle age	Associated with analgesic overuse. Symptoms are a combination of migraine and tension-type headaches.

are not all-inclusive but illustrate either common neurologic causes of headache or particularly dangerous causes that should be considered in the differential diagnosis.

SUBARACHNOID HEMORRHAGE

A nontraumatic subarachnoid hemorrhage (SAH) is caused by rupture of an aneurysm or bleeding from an arteriovenous malformation (see Chapter 14). These headaches are sudden, typically severe, and often represent the worst headache of the patient's life. Vomiting, neck stiffness, cessation of activity, and loss of consciousness are common features. About one-third of patients with aneurysmal SAH have premonitory, or "sentinel" headaches in the days or weeks prior to the event. CT or LP looking for evidence of hemorrhage or heme breakdown in the CSF makes the diagnosis. Treatment in the acute setting involves stabilization in an intensive care unit for management of blood pressure, to ensure adequate brain perfusion, and monitoring for vasospasm and acute obstructive hydrocephalus caused by the subarachnoid blood. Definitive treatment involves surgical resection or clipping of the aneurysm by a neurosurgeon or coiling by an interventional neuroradiologist.

TEMPORAL ARTERITIS

Temporal arteritis (giant cell arteritis) is a subacute granulomatous inflammatory condition involving medium- and large-sized arteries, especially the temporal arteries. This disorder occurs almost exclusively in the elderly and is rare in patients below 50 years of age. It is characterized by headache that can be unilateral or bilateral, particularly over the temporal arteries. Scalp tenderness and jaw pain during chewing (jaw claudication) are classic findings. Polymyalgia rheumatica—a disorder characterized by pain and stiffness in the shoulders and pelvis, fever, malaise, and weight loss—is frequently associated with temporal arteritis. Temporal arteritis is a neurologic emergency that can produce sequential blindness of both eyes by involvement of the ophthalmic arteries. Thus the diagnosis must be considered in an elderly patient with a new or worsening headache, especially one involving the temporal region.

Temporal arteritis is usually associated with an elevated erythrocyte sedimentation rate (ESR), often to 100 or more. Definitive diagnosis, however, is made by temporal artery biopsy demonstrating vasculitis.

Multiple biopsies may be required because the vessel can be affected in a patchy manner, and the first site of biopsy may miss the inflamed portion of vessel. Treatment is prednisone, initially at a dose of 1 mg/kg/day, followed by tapering over the next 1 to 2 years.

TRIGEMINAL NEURALGIA

Trigeminal neuralgia (tic douloureux) is a facial pain syndrome in which brief, severe, electrical shock–like pains occur in the distribution of one of the branches of the trigeminal nerve. The second and third divisions of the trigeminal nerve are involved most commonly. Trigeminal neuralgia is more common in middle-aged and elderly patients. Movement, a cold breeze, or tactile stimulation in a trigger zone on the face can precipitate an attack. The etiology is not completely known, but it is due to microvascular compression of the trigeminal nerve in some patients. MS (by way of lesions in the trigeminal entry zone in the pons) and tumors (by compression) can cause similar pain episodes and should be ruled out, particularly in younger patients. Carbamazepine is particularly effective in treating trigeminal neuralgia. If the neuralgia is refractory to medical therapy, microvascular decompression of the trigeminal root or radiofrequency ablation can be considered.

IDIOPATHIC INTRACRANIAL HYPERTENSION (PSEUDOTUMOR CEREBRI)

Idiopathic intracranial hypertension (IIH) can affect individuals of any age group but is more common in patients in the second to fourth decades of life. It is more common in women, and there is an association with obesity. In addition to headache, there are often associated visual symptoms that tend to be bilateral and can include fleeting loss of visual acuity, scotomas, or double vision. Neurologic exam is normal except for papilledema, which may be present on funduscopic exam. CT or MRI of the head is normal, and LP shows elevated pressure that is typically greater than 250 mm H_2O.

The pathophysiology of IIH is not known. Corticosteroids, tetracycline antibiotics, and excesses of vitamins A or D may predispose to IIH. Treatment usually includes acetazolamide, a carbonic anhydrase inhibitor. Alternatively, the diuretic furosemide or oral steroids can be used. Weight loss should be encouraged. Serial lumbar punctures to reduce the CSF pressure can also be performed. If visual symptoms or high pressure persists or worsens, a surgeon can perform fenestration of the optic nerve sheath or shunting of the CSF to improve visual function or prevent further progression. If treatment is not effective, patients may be left with permanent visual loss.

■ POST–LUMBAR PUNCTURE OR LOW-PRESSURE HEADACHE

Low-pressure headache usually develops in the upright position and is relieved by recumbency. LP is the most common cause of low-pressure headache. The headache usually starts within 48 hours of the LP. The headache is usually relieved when the patient lies down and, with bed rest and rehydration, typically resolves in several days. If the headache continues, medications such as intravenous caffeine or a blood patch can alleviate it. The blood patch is a procedure in which peripheral blood is injected into the epidural space at the site of the lumbar puncture. A clot is formed, which seals the small puncture site in the thecal sac where CSF leakage resulted in traction of pain-sensitive structures in the head.

■ OTHER NEUROLOGIC CAUSES

Other neurologic causes of headache are numerous and include brain tumors, increased intracranial pressure from a variety of causes including meningitis, and some types of seizures and strokes. These topics are discussed in more detail in other chapters of this book.

KEY POINTS

1. Sudden onset of severe headache is suspicious for subarachnoid hemorrhage due to aneurysmal rupture.
2. Temporal arteritis occurs in the elderly and requires urgent evaluation because it can cause blindness.
3. Temporal arteritis is often associated with pain over the temporal arteries and an elevated ESR.

Part Three

Neurologic Disorders

Aphasia and Other Disorders of Higher Cortical Function

Disorders of higher cortical function are among the most interesting in neurology to both physicians and laypersons. Stories of patients who have lost particular aspects of language or who mistake a wife for a hat, for example, continue to intrigue medical students and residents.

It is not hard to understand why this might be. Although primary vision, sensation, and motor control are clearly brain functions that are essential for day-to-day survival, it is the more developed cognitive functions that allow us to carry out the activities that seem **human**. The fact that these functions reside in some fairly discrete areas of the brain and can be quite selectively damaged by lesions in these areas contributes to our fascination with them.

■ APHASIA

Aphasia refers to any acquired abnormality of language, usually from a focal brain lesion. The problem must be a primary disorder of language; not everyone who cannot communicate properly is aphasic. For example, diffuse problems with consciousness, attention, or initiative may prevent a patient from communicating by oral or written means, but this would not necessarily qualify as aphasia. Likewise, problems with speech, such as dysarthria (slurring) or stuttering, or problems with motor control of the mouth may prevent oral communication, but pronunciation deficits should not be confused with aphasia.

Diagnostic Evaluation

There are several recognized forms of aphasia (Table 11-1) that are typically caused by lesions in particular brain locations (Figure 11-1) and can be distinguished from each other by testing certain aspects of language, such as fluency, comprehension, and repetition (Table 11-2).

A sensitive test for detecting an aphasia of any kind is to test naming, since **anomia** (impaired naming) is a feature of essentially all aphasias. Severely aphasic patients may not be able to name common or high-frequency objects (e.g., watch, necktie), while less severely afflicted patients may have trouble only with low-frequency objects or parts (e.g., dial of the watch, lapel). In addition, no aphasic patient writes normally. Screening for aphasia by asking patients to write a paragraph is quite effective.

KEY POINTS

1. **Aphasia** is an acquired abnormality of language, usually from a focal brain lesion.
2. Other causes of impaired communication—including problems with attention, initiative, or articulation—are not truly aphasias.
3. Problems with naming or writing are features of almost all types of aphasia.

Broca's Aphasia

Broca's aphasia is primarily a problem of language production. Speech is nonfluent, meaning that the patient cannot produce a reasonably long string of words. Attempted speech output is punctuated by hesitations and ill-fated attempts at beginnings of words ("tip-of-the-tongue" phenomenon). A Broca's aphasia patient's speech may be telegraphic, in that conjunctions, prepositions, and the like may be omitted and only key nouns and verbs strung together (e.g., "want go store"). Patients' speech may include paraphasias (word substitution errors), often of the

■ TABLE 11-1

Aphasias

Type	Fluency	Repetition	Comprehension	Commonly Associated Signs	Lesion Location
Broca's	Impaired	Impaired	Relatively preserved	Right hemiparesis (especially face)	Broca's area
Wernicke's	Preserved	Impaired	Impaired	Right upper visual field cut	Wernicke's area
Conduction	Preserved	Impaired	Preserved	—	Arcuate fasciculus
Transcortical motor	Impaired	Preserved	Preserved	Right hemiparesis	Near Broca's area
Transcortical sensory	Preserved	Preserved	Impaired	—	Near Wernicke's area
Global	Impaired	Impaired	Impaired	Severe right hemiparesis	Large left hemisphere lesion
Subcortical	Variable	Preserved	Variable	Hypophonia	Left basal ganglia, thalamus

phonemic type (substitution based on sound, like "spool" for "spoon"). An important feature of Broca's aphasia is that patients are quite aware of and almost invariably frustrated by their language problem. Oddly, overused phrases (e.g., "how do you do"), expletives, and lyrics sung to music may be relatively preserved. Broca's aphasia patients cannot repeat phrases said to them. Although the most prominent deficit is with language output, Broca's aphasia patients have subtle deficits of comprehension, particularly for complex grammatical constructions involving prepositions or the passive voice. For example, Broca's aphasia patients may not be able to follow a command such as "under the paper put the pen" or understand which animal is dead if "the lion was killed by the tiger."

Classically, Broca's aphasia arises from lesions that include the posterior part of the inferior frontal gyrus in the dominant (usually left) hemisphere, a region known as Broca's area. Most often these are relatively large strokes in the territory of the superior division of the middle cerebral artery (MCA), although tumors, hemorrhages, and other lesions in this area can cause an identical syndrome. Strokes here typically are associated with some weakness of the contralateral side, particularly involving the face and arm.

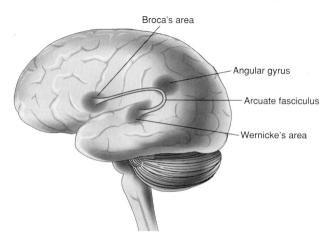

Figure 11-1 • Higher cortical centers in the left hemisphere.

Labels: Broca's area, Angular gyrus, Arcuate fasciculus, Wernicke's area

KEY POINTS

1. **Broca's aphasia** is a problem of language production.
2. Patients are frustrated and have nonfluent, hesitant, telegraphic speech output, with an inability to repeat but relatively preserved comprehension.
3. Broca aphasia is typically caused by lesions in the posteroinferior frontal lobe (the Broca area).

Wernicke's Aphasia

Although Wernicke's aphasia is often characterized as a problem with language comprehension, it features difficulty with both the output and input of language. Patients cannot understand what is said to them and thus may not be able to follow even the simplest

■ **TABLE 11-2**

Examination of Language Function

Function	Testing
Fluency	Listen to patient's spontaneous speech to see if words are strung together into phrases. Overused phrases (e.g., "how do you do") do not count.
Repetition	Least challenging: Ask patient to repeat single words.
	Most challenging: Ask patient to repeat complex sentence, such as "no ifs, ands, or buts about it."
Comprehension	Least challenging: Ask patient to follow simple midline commands, such as "close your eyes" or "open your mouth."
	Most challenging: Ask patient to follow multistep appendicular commands that cross the midline, such as "point to the ceiling, then touch your left ear with your right hand."
Naming	Least challenging: Ask patient to name high-frequency objects, like watch or tie.
	Most challenging: Ask patient to name low-frequency objects or parts of objects, like dial of watch or lapel.
Reading	Ask patient to read written material aloud, and to follow written instructions.
Writing	Ask patient to write a spontaneous sentence, or a sentence dictated by the examiner. Simply having the patient write his name does not count, as that is an overlearned task.

commands. Their spontaneous speech is fluent but nonsensical, so that they can string words together, but the sequence or content may not make sense ("word salad"). Wernicke's aphasia patients produce many paraphasias, particularly of the semantic type (substitution based on meaning, like "fork" for "spoon") as well as neologisms (nonexistent words). The cadence and fluency of speech are preserved, but the content is often incomprehensible. One might not be able to recognize that a speaker of a foreign language had a Wernicke's aphasia, because all but the content of language would be intact. Wernicke's aphasia patients cannot repeat. Unlike patients with Broca's aphasia, those with Wernicke's aphasia seem unaware of their deficit initially and can become quite angry or paranoid when it becomes obvious that others have difficulty understanding them.

Classically, Wernicke's aphasia arises from lesions in the posterior part of the superior temporal gyrus in the dominant hemisphere, known as Wernicke's area. Most commonly, these are strokes involving the inferior division of the MCA, and a high percentage of them are due to emboli from proximal locations such as the heart or the internal carotid artery. However, other nonvascular lesions in this area can cause an identical syndrome. Lesions causing Wernicke aphasia may not be accompanied by weakness or sensory loss, but there may be a contralateral homonymous superior quadrantanopia.

KEY POINTS

1. **Wernicke's aphasia** is a problem with language comprehension that results in difficulties with both output and input of language.
2. Patients have fluent but very abnormal speech output ("word salad"), frequent paraphasias and neologisms, and an inability to comprehend or repeat.
3. Wernicke aphasia is typically caused by lesions involving the posterior part of the superior temporal gyrus (Wernicke area).

Other Aphasias

A distinct form of aphasia called **conduction aphasia** is characterized by an inability to repeat what is said, with preserved fluency and comprehension. Classic teaching states that the lesion responsible lies in the arcuate fasciculus, the white matter connections between Broca's and Wernicke's areas. However, there is little anatomic evidence to support this idea, and in fact lesions involving the temporal or parietal lobes (but sparing Wernicke's area) can lead to this syndrome. Patients with conduction aphasia also make many paraphasic errors, which we all normally correct "on the fly" as we monitor our own speech—a function they cannot perform.

Lesions in the frontal lobe slightly superior to Broca's area can cause a nonfluent aphasia very similar to Broca's aphasia except that repetition is preserved, because the path between and including Broca's and Wernicke's areas is unaffected. Such a **transcortical motor aphasia** can also be caused by lesions in the supplementary motor area and in the anterior portions of the basal ganglia.

Similarly, a **transcortical sensory aphasia** is caused by lesions in the inferior portion of the left temporal lobe and is characterized by fluent speech with impaired comprehension but preserved repetition. Infarcts in the territory of the left posterior cerebral artery (PCA) as well as small temporal lobe hemorrhages and contusions are the most common causes.

A distinction, therefore, is made between perisylvian (around the sylvian fissure) aphasias (Broca's, Wernicke's, and conduction), in which repetition is impaired, and transcortical aphasias (motor and sensory), in which repetition is preserved.

KEY POINTS

1. **Conduction aphasia**, primarily characterized by an inability to repeat, is caused by lesions involving the temporal and parietal lobes but sparing the Wernicke area.
2. **Transcortical motor and sensory aphasias** resemble Broca's and Wernicke's aphasias, respectively, except that repetition is preserved.

Global aphasia, typically caused by large dominant hemispheric lesions affecting the frontal and temporal lobes including Broca's and Wernicke's areas, results in problems with language production, comprehension, and repetition.

Subcortical aphasias are acquired language deficits associated with lesions in deep dominant hemispheric structures, such as the basal ganglia and thalamus. These typically do not fall easily into the aphasia classification given above, although more anterior subcortical lesions have a tendency to produce aphasias that resemble Broca's aphasia and more posterior lesions lead to aphasias that resemble Wernicke's aphasia. Often, subcortical aphasias are accompanied by hypophonia of the voice.

Disorders of Written Communication

Reading and writing are commonly affected in all of the aphasias. Typically, reading parallels comprehension of spoken language, while writing parallels production of spoken language, although the respective difficulties with written language are typically much worse than those with spoken language. Thus Broca's aphasia patients may be able to understand simple commands by reading them, though they cannot read them aloud or write them.

A unique syndrome called **alexia without agraphia**, or **pure alexia**, is characterized by an inability to read despite a preserved ability to write. This leads to the surprising finding that a patient may not be able to read back the words she has just written well. The responsible lesion is situated in the dominant occipital lobe but also involves the splenium of the corpus callosum. In this way the fibers connecting visual cortex (on either side) to Wernicke's area in the dominant hemisphere are interrupted, thus preventing input of language through visual means. A contralateral homonymous hemianopia is typically an associated finding.

■ APRAXIA

Apraxia is defined as an inability to carry out a learned motor task despite preservation of the primary functions needed to carry out the task, such as comprehension, motor ability, sensation, and coordination.

A patient with an apraxia, for example, might not be able to demonstrate how to hammer a nail, despite sufficient language comprehension to understand the command and sufficient motor strength, sensation in the hands, and coordination to carry out the command. It is as if the patient could not imagine or execute the motor program for the task.

Terminology regarding different types of apraxias—including names such as **ideational, ideomotor,** and **limb-kinetic**—is confusing. It is more enlightening simply to describe what the patient can and cannot do. In one type of apraxia, patients can recognize when others are carrying out the task correctly rather than incorrectly, but they cannot perform the motor task themselves. Sometimes these patients can carry out the task with the actual objects given to them (e.g., using a real hammer and nail), but they cannot mimic the task without the actual objects. In another type of apraxia, patients cannot even recognize when others are carrying out the task correctly.

Diagnostic Evaluation

There are three basic ways to test for apraxia: asking patients to pretend they are performing an action, to mimic the examiner performing an action, or to use actual objects in performing an action. Examples of bedside tests include asking the patient to wave good-bye, salute, brush his teeth, or comb his hair. Two-handed tasks, such as hammering in a nail or slicing a loaf of bread, are more demanding. Some patients who have a specific form of apraxia involving oral movements may be unable to demonstrate whistling or blowing out a match. Many patients with apraxia will have a tendency to use their limbs as objects (e.g., running their fingers through their hair when asked to demonstrate how to use a comb).

Etiology

Apraxias are typically associated with either frontal or parietal lesions in the dominant hemisphere. Frontal lesions typically cause apraxias in which patients are able to recognize the task done correctly by others but cannot perform it themselves, whereas parietal lesions typically result in apraxias in which patients cannot recognize the task done correctly.

KEY POINTS

1. **Apraxia** is the inability to perform a learned motor task despite preservation of the necessary basic motor, sensory, and cognitive capacities.
2. Examples of bedside tests for apraxia include asking a patient to mimic the motions necessary to brush her teeth, comb her hair, hammer in a nail, or slice a loaf of bread.
3. Apraxia is typically caused by lesions in the frontal or parietal lobes of the dominant hemisphere.

■ AGNOSIA

Agnosia refers to an inability to recognize objects through one or more sensory modalities despite the preserved functioning of those primary sensory modalities.

Diagnostic Evaluation

A patient with visual agnosia, for example, might not be able to recognize objects placed in his vision, though all other aspects of his vision, such as acuity and fields, are intact. The same patient would be able to recognize those objects when allowed to touch them. With his vision, he might be able to describe specific features of the object, but he would not be able to recognize the object as a whole.

Etiology

Agnosias are typically caused by lesions in the sensory association areas of the brain, processing areas that lie next to the primary sensory areas and are responsible for integrating primary sensory information into higher-order complex forms. For example, the visual association area lies in the occipitotemporal region anterior and inferior to the primary visual cortex and is responsible for the recognition of objects using primary visual information. Lesions here can cause a visual agnosia. A specific form called **prosopagnosia**, an inability to recognize faces, can occur with right hemispheric or bilateral lesions in the visual association area.

KEY POINTS

1. **Agnosia** is the inability to recognize objects despite preservation of the basic sensory modalities being used.
2. Agnosia is typically caused by lesions in the sensory association areas.

■ GERSTMANN'S SYNDROME

Lesions in the inferior parietal lobule of the dominant hemisphere, and specifically in the angular gyrus (see Figure 11-1), can cause **Gerstmann's syndrome**, a constellation of problems in higher cortical function. These are agraphia, the inability to write; acalculia, the inability to calculate; right-left confusion; and finger agnosia, the inability to recognize one's own or the examiner's individual fingers. One explanation is that this area of the parietal lobe is responsible for the symbolic representation of body parts as well as orthographic and numerical symbols.

KEY POINTS

1. **Gerstmann's syndrome** is characterized by four elements: agraphia, acalculia, right-left confusion, and finger agnosia.
2. Gerstmann's syndrome is typically caused by lesions in the angular gyrus of the dominant hemisphere.

Neglect

There are times when it seems that all interesting higher cortical functions reside in the dominant hemisphere. Neglect, however, one of the most fascinating cortical disorders, is usually the result of damage to the nondominant (usually right) hemisphere.

Neglect is directed inattention, or a relative lack of attention, paid to one hemispace. Patients with neglect will tend to be less aware (or completely unaware) of objects or actions in one side of the world (usually the left). It is not that a patient has a hemianopia and cannot see that side or a primary motor or sensory deficit for that side; rather, there is decreased attention toward the left side.

Diagnostic Evaluation

Those with the most severe forms of neglect ignore the left side completely and deny that such a side even exists. They may leave their left side ungroomed, unshaven, and undressed; they may leave food on the left side of their plates untouched. They may deny having a left hand, and when confronted with it, may claim that it is actually the examiner's. When asked to describe their surroundings or draw a picture, they may omit items on the left side (Figure 11-2).

Patients with milder neglect may not have such gross abnormalities but may perform actions involving their left side only with encouragement or after repeated prodding. When asked to bisect a line, they may err toward the right. When asked to cross out letters scattered across a page, they may leave some on the left side unmarked.

The most sensitive sign of neglect, which may be the only finding seen in patients with the mildest form,

is extinction to double simultaneous stimulation. This phenomenon occurs when sensory stimuli applied singly to either side are felt properly; but when both sides are stimulated simultaneously, only the stimulus on the nonneglected side is felt. Extinction may exist with tactile, visual, or auditory stimulation.

Etiology

Neglect is typically caused by lesions in the right hemisphere, particularly the right frontal or parietal lobes. It is most commonly seen as an acute finding after a stroke, though other lesions in these areas can cause a similar clinical syndrome. Lesions in the right frontal lobe may cause more of a motor neglect, in which the patient has a tendency to not use the left side for motor actions, whereas lesions in the right parietal lobe may cause more of a sensory neglect, in which stimuli from the left side tend to be ignored.

KEY POINTS

1. **Neglect** is directed inattention or a relative lack of attention paid to one hemispace, usually the left.
2. Patients with severe neglect may fail to describe objects on the left, may fail to dress or shave the left side, or may even deny that their left arms are theirs.
3. Those with milder forms may not bisect lines or cancel out letters properly, or they may exhibit extinction to double simultaneous stimulation.
4. Neglect is usually caused by lesions in the right frontal or parietal lobe.

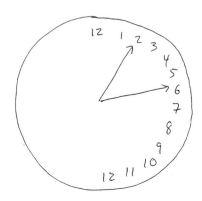

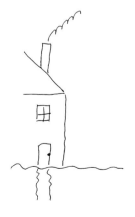

Figure 11-2 • Drawing demonstrating neglect of the left side.

OTHER NONDOMINANT HEMISPHERIC SYNDROMES

The semantic elements of language (those associated purely with meaning) reside in the language-dominant (usually left) hemisphere, as described in the discussion on aphasias above. However, some of the other elements of successful oral communication, such as changing the inflection of one's voice when asking a question or when making an angry statement, reside in the nondominant (usually right) hemisphere. These elements are collectively referred to as *prosody*, and patients with right hemispheric lesions may have difficulty with this part of communication. Some may have difficulty applying the proper inflection to their own speech output, for example, and sound fairly monotone. Others may have difficulty understanding the speech inflections of those speaking to them and cannot distinguish between a statement said to them in anger or in jest.

Some patients with right hemispheric lesions have a tendency to be unaware of their deficits, a condition termed **anosognosia**. A patient with a complete left hemiplegia, for example, may insist on immediate discharge from the hospital because he feels that nothing is wrong. A patient with a dense left hemianopia may wonder why she keeps bumping into others when she notices nothing wrong with her vision. As expected, these patients tend to have more difficult and unsuccessful rehabilitations.

Dementia

Dementia is a common cause of morbidity and mortality in the elderly and has many different etiologies. It implies an intellectual and cognitive deterioration of sufficient severity to interfere with normal functioning. Memory, orientation, visuospatial perception, language, and higher executive functions (planning, organizing, and sequencing) may be impaired in dementia.

The terms **delirium** and **acute confusional state** imply a global disturbance of mental functions, in general reversible, accompanied by altered level of consciousness. These conditions are often acute and reversible; they are discussed further in Chapter 3.

Epidemiology

Dementia is most common in the elderly but can occur at a younger age (particularly in those with a hereditary component). Approximately 5% of people between ages 65 and 70 have dementia; this increases to more than 45% above age 85. Alzheimer's disease accounts for 50 to 70% of cases of dementia. Cerebrovascular disease accounts for about 15 to 20%, and the other causes presented in Box 12-1 account for most of the rest. Dementia has a considerable social cost (over $50 billion in the United States every year).

Clinical Manifestations

There is a known cognitive decline with old age, and sometimes the differentiation between a dementing illness and age-related cognitive decline is difficult. In general, most patients with dementia start having problems with short-term memory, followed by an indolent deterioration of cognitive functions that may involve language, praxis, and so forth. Many dementing illnesses manifest characteristic symptoms and clinical findings that are helpful in establishing an etiologic diagnosis.

Diagnostic Evaluation

The initial recognition of dementia is difficult. Normal aging can mimic some of its features. Rarely, the patient is aware of cognitive deterioration; in most cases, the family brings the patient to the doctor months or years after problems have started. The most important information in the diagnosis of dementia is the clinical history (including reports by relatives) and the physical exam (with a very detailed mental status examination). Then, the diagnosis of the cause of dementia consists of matching the major clinical features of the individual patient with characteristics of known dementing illnesses.

It is important to rule out an underlying depression, because depression can mimic dementia ("pseudodementia"), and the associated cognitive abnormalities of depression can constitute a true dementia. Not rarely, when a patient complains of features suggesting dementia, depression is the problem. Correspondingly, it is often a family member who brings a patient with dementia to the physician.

The use of laboratory tests depends on the clinical history and exam, the tentative diagnosis, and the possibility of finding reversible causes. Box 12-2 summarizes some tests to consider. Most are used to rule out reversible causes of dementia.

KEY POINTS

1. Symptoms and signs of dementia include memory loss, abnormalities of speech, difficulties with problem solving and abstract thinking, impaired judgment, personality changes, and emotional lability.
2. The diagnosis of the cause of dementia requires a detailed history and neurologic and physical examination.

BOX 12-1   CAUSES OF DEMENTIA

Degenerative
  Alzheimer's disease
  Huntington's disease
  Parkinson's disease
  Lewy body dementia
  Pick's disease
  Progressive supranuclear palsy
  Spinocerebellar degeneration
  Amyotrophic lateral sclerosis with dementia
  Olivopontocerebellar atrophy
  Frontotemporal dementia associated with
    chromosome 17 (FTD-17)
Metabolic
  Wilson's disease
  Hypothyroidism
  Vitamin B_{12} deficiency
  Hypercalcemia
  Addison's disease
Lipid storage diseases and leukodystrophies
Toxic
  Drug intoxication
  Alcohol
  Arsenic, mercury, and lead intoxication
Infectious
  Creutzfeldt-Jakob disease
  AIDS
  Syphilis
  Subacute sclerosis panencephalitis (post-measles)
Neoplastic and paraneoplastic
Vascular
  Vascular dementia
  Vasculitis
Hydrocephalus
Traumatic
  Severe head injury
  Boxer's encephalopathy (punch drunk)
  Chronic subdural hematoma
Undetermined
Mixed (Alzheimer's plus vascular)

BOX 12-2   TESTS TO CONSIDER IN A PATIENT WITH DEMENTIA

Hematologic screening, including ESR
Vitamin B_{12} and folate
Blood calcium
Liver function tests, including ammonia
Electrolytes
Serum urea nitrogen and creatinine levels
Infection workup, including syphilis, HIV, TB, etc.
Thyroid function tests

EEG: Should not be ordered routinely in a dementia assessment. Its use is justified when the patient has evidence of fluctuations in cognitive status that could represent seizures. The EEG may be useful at the initial presentation in patients with suspected Creutzfeldt-Jakob disease (CJD).

CT or MRI of the brain (rule out structural abnormalities such as tumor, subdural hematoma, and hydrocephalus and evaluate cortical atrophy).

Neuropsychological assessment: Useful in early stages to establish the diagnosis of dementia and to use as a comparison tool in the progression of the disease.

Brain biopsy: Only indicated in specific cases such as CJD, HIV, CNS vasculitis, and so on, to confirm the diagnosis and find or exclude possible treatable causes.

CAUSES OF DEMENTIA

■ ALZHEIMER'S DISEASE

In 1907, Alois Alzheimer, a German clinician and neuropathologist, published the landmark case of a 51-year-old woman with deterioration of her mental state. Her autopsy disclosed the classic pathology of Alzheimer's disease (AD): neurofibrillary tangles and senile plaques in the cerebral neocortex and hippocampus.

Epidemiology

Nearly 4% of people older than 65 years have severe Alzheimer's disease (AD) and are incapacitated. Recent estimates suggest that more than 2 million people have AD in the United States alone. Because of increased life expectancy, the population at risk for AD is the fastest-growing segment of society. Annually, approximately 100,000 people die of Alzheimer's disease and more than $25 billion is spent on the institutional care of patients with AD.

Etiology and Risk Factors

Many factors are associated with an increased frequency of AD, including age, female sex, history of severe head trauma, and Down syndrome.

There are also many putative genetic risk factors. The gene for ApoE4 (on chromosome 19) has been shown to be associated with both early- and late-onset AD of both sporadic and familial varieties. Early-onset AD has been associated with mutations in the amyloid precursor protein (APP) on chromosome 21, and presenilin 1 (PS1) and presenilin 2 (PS2) on chromosomes 14 and 1, respectively. More than 65 mutations in these genes are described. Another mutation in a gene on chromosome 12 that encodes α_2-macroglobulin has been associated with AD. The ApoE alleles and the α_2-macroglobulin mutation predispose individuals to early onset of sporadic AD and even more to late-onset AD. The other mutations in APP, PS1, and PS2 are associated with early onset of the disease in the third through sixth decades.

Amyloid–beta precursor protein (AβPP) mutations may cause increased amyloid-beta (Aβ) production with subsequent aggregation in the neurons. This mutation changes the normal structure of the protein, altering its recognition by metabolizing enzymes like alpha-secretase and utilizing alternative pathways for degradation, leading to a progressive accumulation of the peptide. Other pathophysiologic mechanisms have been described, including inflammatory, oxidative, metabolic, nutritional, and immune mechanisms.

Clinical Manifestations

"Doctor, my mother is 75 years old and over the last 3 years I have noted that she is having more difficulty with her memory. She remembers her marriage 50 years ago but she does not remember that we were here yesterday. She asks the same questions constantly and forgets my answers. She is unable to balance her checkbook, and yesterday she could not find the way home from the drugstore." This history illustrates characteristic features of AD. At the beginning of the illness, the exam shows no difficulty with language, reasoning, or performance of normal social and personal behaviors. Only those close to the patient notice small slip-ups suggesting that something is wrong (becoming lost while driving, misplacement of objects, the kitchen left unattended, missed appointments, loss of social and interpersonal interactions). Later, the patient has more difficulty with activities of daily life.

As the disease progresses, other aspects of cognitive function are lost, including the ability to speak, understand, think, and make decisions. Characteristically, in contrast to patients with vascular dementia, elementary neurologic functions (motor, visual, somatosensory, and gait) remain normal until very late in the disease. Psychiatric manifestations are common at this time: personality changes (apathetic or impulsive), aggressive behavior (physical or verbal), paranoid thoughts and delusions (persecution, things being stolen), sleep disturbances (the word "sundowning" is used to describe worsening psychiatric manifestations during the evening and night), hallucinations (uncommon and in general a side effect of medications), and depression. The course is relentlessly progressive; the patient usually succumbs over 5 to 10 years due to a combination of neurologic and medical problems.

Diagnostic Evaluation

Except for brain biopsy, there are no tests that definitively establish the diagnosis of AD in living patients. The diagnosis is suggested by the clinical features and by the insidiously progressive course. Investigations are designed to exclude other causes of dementia (see Box 12-2). Elevated tau protein and low Aβ-42 levels in the CSF have been suggested as early diagnostic markers for AD. MRI-based volumetric measurements may show reduction of up to 40% in the size of the hippocampus, amygdala, and thalamus. Functional neuroimaging such as PET and SPECT (single-photon emission computed tomography), used to quantify cerebral metabolism and blood flow, may help to differentiate AD from other dementias. In Alzheimer disease, PET and SPECT scans show bilateral temporoparietal hypometabolism, but this is not specific enough to be diagnostic.

Pathology

The major pathologic features of AD are brain atrophy, senile plaques, and neurofibrillary tangles (NFTs), associated with substantial loss of neurons in the cerebral cortex and gliosis. NFTs represent intracellular accumulation of phosphorylated tau protein. Senile plaques are extracellular deposits of amyloid surrounded by dystrophic axons.

Treatment

At present there is no satisfactory treatment for patients with Alzheimer's disease.

Therapy consists of the following:

- **Preventing associated symptoms:** Treatment of depression, agitation, sleep disorders, hallucinations, and delusions.
- **Preventing or delaying progression:** This includes therapy with acetylcholinesterase inhibitors such as donepezil or rivastigmine, as well as the newer agent memantine, an *N*-methyl-D-aspartate (NMDA) receptor antagonist.
- **Prophylaxis:** No data from randomized clinical trials are available. Use of vitamin E, NSAIDs, and estrogens has been proposed.

Table 12-1 provides information regarding therapy of AD and other dementias.

KEY POINTS

1. AD is the most common neurodegenerative disease of the brain and accounts for 50 to 70% of all instances of dementia.
2. Risk factors for developing AD include older age, female sex, head trauma, and family history.
3. Potentially treatable causes of dementia should be excluded through laboratory testing and brain imaging.
4. The average length of time from onset of symptoms until diagnosis is 2 to 3 years. The average duration from diagnosis to nursing home placement is 3 to 6 years. AD patients typically spend 3 years in nursing homes before death. Thus, the total duration of AD is roughly 9 to 12 years.

■ TABLE 12-1

Dementia Therapy

	Dose	Comments
Alzheimer's disease		
Donepezil (Aricept)	5–10 mg po qid	Equal efficacy and fewer side effects than tacrine. Rare: hepatic toxicity. Common: diarrhea and abdominal cramps
Rivastigmine (Exelon)	6–12 mg/day, given po bid; start 1.5 mg po bid	GI disturbances during dose adjustment. Rare: hepatic toxicity. Recently approved by FDA.
Tacrine	10 mg po qid	Hepatic toxicity. Check ALT every 2 weeks during dosage titration.
Ibuprofen	400 mg po tid	Targeting the anti-inflammatory theory of AD. Not proven different from placebo in recent studies
Vitamin E	800–2000 IU po daily	Mild anticoagulant effect, particularly with patients on coumadin.
Conjugated estrogens	0.625 mg po daily	Women only. Not proven in recent clinical trials to alter the course of the disease.
Vascular dementia		
Antihypertensive medications	Any	Maintain systolic BP below 160 and diastolic between 85 and 95. Treatments that lower diastolic BP may worsen cognitive function
Warfarin (Coumadin)	Variable	Check INR and maintain value between 2 and 3. Indicated in patient with atrial fibrillation and strokes.
Aspirin	81–325 po mg qD	Consider warfarin if atrial fibrillation is present.
Clopidogrel (Plavix)	75 mg po qD	Can produce TTP. Can be used in combination with aspirin.
Dipyridamole and aspirin (Aggrenox)	1 capsule (200–225 mg) po bid	Same indications as aspirin.
Vitamin E	800–2000 IU daily	Mild anticoagulant effect, particularly with patients on coumadin.

ALT, alanine aminotransferase; BP, blood pressure; INR, international normalized ratio; TTP, thrombotic thrombocytopenic purpura.

◼ VASCULAR DEMENTIA

This dementia (previously referred to as multi-infarct dementia) may develop in patients with cerebrovascular disease. There are two recognized types: macrovascular, related to large infarcts, and microvascular, in which the pathophysiologic mechanism of brain injury is subcortical ischemia associated with cerebral small vessel disease (lacunes or deep white matter changes on MRI). Vascular dementia has the risk factors of cerebrovascular disease, including hypertension, diabetes, age, embolic sources, and extensive large artery atherosclerosis. It is not infrequent for vascular dementia and other diseases (AD, Lewy body disease) to coexist in the same patient. For this reason, it is unclear exactly how commonly dementia can arise from a purely vascular etiology.

Clinical Manifestations and Diagnostic Evaluation

The criteria for diagnosis of vascular dementia include presence of dementia and two or more of the following: focal neurologic signs on physical examination; onset that was abrupt, stepwise, or stroke-related; or brain imaging study showing multiple strokes, lacunes, or extensive deep white matter changes. Most patients with vascular dementia are hypertensive or diabetic. The diagnosis requires investigation of the cause of stroke. Cardiac and hypercoagulable workups should be considered in selected cases.

Treatment

The prevention and treatment of vascular dementia are essentially the same as prevention and treatment of stroke (see Table 12-1 and Chapter 14).

KEY POINTS

1. Vascular dementia may be a common cause of dementia, but it often coexists with other causes.
2. Vascular dementia is associated with Binswanger's disease (microvascular disease), a lacunar state, and large strokes.

DEMENTIAS ASSOCIATED WITH EXTRAPYRAMIDAL FEATURES

This group of dementias includes dementia with Lewy bodies, progressive supranuclear palsy, corticobasal degeneration, striatonigral degeneration, Huntington's disease, and Wilson's disease.

◼ DEMENTIA WITH LEWY BODIES

This is now thought by many to be the second most common cause of dementia after Alzheimer's disease. The clinical picture is that of a parkinsonian dementia syndrome with visual hallucinations. Sometimes it is very difficult to differentiate this from the disease of a Parkinson's disease patient who develops dementia.

Clinical Manifestations

The major features are cognitive impairment (severe problems of visuospatial perception and visual memory), marked fluctuations of alertness, prominent visual hallucinations (up to 80% of cases) and delusions, extrapyramidal symptoms, and an extraordinary sensitivity to neuroleptics (i.e., marked worsening with drugs like haloperidol).

Diagnostic Evaluation

The pathologic hallmark is the Lewy body (found in Parkinson's disease in the substantia nigra), an eosinophilic intracellular inclusion of alpha synuclein. In dementia with Lewy bodies (unlike in Parkinson's disease), the Lewy body is found in cortical neurons. Other pathologic abnormalities can also be present, including varying degrees of AD-type abnormalities such as NFTs and senile plaques.

Treatment

Management of dementia with Lewy bodies can be complex, since treatment of the parkinsonian syndrome may worsen neuropsychiatric dysfunction, and treatment of the neuropsychiatric disorder may exacerbate the parkinsonian syndrome. Low doses of atypical neuroleptics such as risperidone and clozapine have been used to treat behavioral symptoms.

KEY POINTS

1. Dementia with Lewy bodies may be the second most common type of dementia.
2. Fluctuations of alertness, visual hallucinations, and an extraordinary sensitivity to neuroleptics are the three key distinguishing features of dementia with Lewy bodies.
3. Death ensues after 10 to 15 years.

PROGRESSIVE SUPRANUCLEAR PALSY

Also known as the Steele-Richardson-Olszewski syndrome, progressive supranuclear palsy (PSP) may account for 2 to 3% of dementias. No clear predisposing or genetic factors have been identified.

Clinical Manifestations

The main features are supranuclear ocular palsy (mainly failure of vertical gaze), dysarthria, dysphagia, extrapyramidal rigidity, gait ataxia, and dementia. In the early stages of PSP, falls and gait abnormalities are prominent. Dementia may occur early or develop later. Frontal lobe abnormalities predominate. Patients become apathetic and talk and act less frequently. In early stages, PSP may be mistaken for AD.

Diagnostic Evaluation

The pathology shows atrophy of the dorsal midbrain, globus pallidus, and subthalamic nucleus. NFTs, neuronal loss, and gliosis in many subcortical structures are characteristic. The course is progressive, with a median survival of 6 to 10 years.

KEY POINTS

1. PSP is a form of subcortical dementia with prominent extrapyramidal features.
2. The characteristic clinical findings are palsy of vertical gaze, abnormal gait, and frequent falls.
3. Median survival is 6 to 10 years.

HUNTINGTON'S DISEASE

Huntington's disease (HD) is an autosomal dominant neurodegenerative disorder with predominant abnormalities of the basal ganglia.

Clinical Manifestations

Symptoms usually appear between the ages of 35 and 45 and include the triad of chorea, behavioral changes or personality disorder (frequently obsessive-compulsive disorder), and dementia. The three may occur together at onset, or one may precede the others by years.

Diagnostic Evaluation

Diagnosis is by family history, clinical signs, atrophy of the caudate on brain imaging, and the demonstration of more than 40 CAG repeats in chromosome 4.

Pathology

Pathologic examination shows severe destruction of the caudate and putamen (striatal and nigral GABA-ergic neurons) and loss of neurons in the cerebral cortex (layer 3). HD is linked to chromosome 4p16.3 on the HD gene, encoding for a protein named **huntingtin.** The mutation produces an unstable CAG repeat. This induces aberrant processing of cell proteins with formation of deposits in the nucleus and activation of intracellular mechanisms of cell death.

Treatment

Pharmacologic management of dementia and chorea often involves dopaminergic antagonists, including neuroleptic drugs, but it is far from adequate. Genetic counseling is fundamental.

KEY POINTS

1. Huntington disease is characterized by chorea, dementia, and personality and behavioral changes.
2. Death occurs 10 to 20 years after onset.
3. Suicide is not rare in at-risk and early-onset HD patients.

Parkinson's Disease

Parkinson's disease (PD) may produce subcortical dementia. Cognitive impairment develops in about 30% of patients with idiopathic PD. The distinction from other types of dementia is based on the natural history and the presence of associated symptoms. The clinical manifestations include those of subcortical dementia, with marked psychomotor involvement.

Frontotemporal Dementia

Frontotemporal dementia (FTD) encompasses a group of degenerative disorders characterized by significant alterations in personality, social behavior, and language.

Clinical Manifestations

Unlike Alzheimer's disease, FTD often presents initially with cognitive and behavioral deficits other than memory loss, because the frontal and/or temporal cortices are affected early. For example, patients may neglect social and personal responsibilities, present failure in judgment, and show defective sequencing and organization. FTD includes Pick's disease, primary progressive aphasia, and semantic dementia. In addition, there are forms of FTD associated with parkinsonism and with motor neuron disease.

Pick disease is a rare form of progressive dementia characterized by personality change, speech disturbance, inattentiveness, and sometimes extrapyramidal signs. The diagnosis is made by clinical history and the presence of circumscribed frontotemporal lobar atrophy. Argyrophilic round intraneuronal inclusions (Pick bodies) represent the characteristic pathologic change. Abnormal tau protein with tau-positive inclusions is found in neurons and glial cells. Senile plaques are generally not present. Primary progressive aphasia is a form of FTD in which language deficits appear early.

KEY POINTS

1. Frontotemporal dementia is uncommon.
2. Anterior lobar atrophy is characteristic.
3. Personality changes early in the disease are characteristic, in contrast to Alzheimer disease.

DEMENTIAS CAUSED BY INFECTIOUS AGENTS

■ PRION-RELATED DISEASES

Prion-related diseases include CJD (familial and sporadic); Gerstmann-Straüssler-Scheinker syndrome; and fatal familial insomnia.

These so-called spongiform encephalopathies are a group of disorders characterized by spongy degeneration, neuronal loss, gliosis, and astrocytic proliferation resulting from the accumulation in the brain of a mutated protease-resistant prion protein.

CJD is the most common of these disorders. It is characterized by a rapidly progressive dementia with pyramidal signs, myoclonus, cerebellar or extrapyramidal signs, and periodic sharp waves in the EEG. MRI with DWI (diffusion-weighted images) may show evolving cortical and basal ganglial abnormalities during the course of the disease. CSF is typically normal, but the presence of protein 14-3-3 is relatively sensitive and specific for CJD. There is no therapy. This syndrome evolves over weeks to months, and death usually occurs within a year.

KEY POINTS

1. CJD is rare.
2. CJD presents as a rapidly progressive dementia with focal neurologic signs and myoclonus.
3. EEG and MRI are not diagnostic, but they become more specific in the setting of the appropriate clinical history.

■ HIV-ASSOCIATED DEMENTIA COMPLEX

Most patients with human immunodeficiency virus (HIV) disease have CNS involvement. The virus can produce an encephalitis and also makes the individual susceptible to CNS infections such as toxoplasmosis, tuberculosis, and syphilis, which can cause dementia as well. HIV-associated dementia complex is a clinical entity recognized in HIV patients (usually with low CD4 cell counts) and is characterized by progressive deterioration of cognitive function.

Clinical Manifestations

Patients report memory problems, difficulty with concentration, and poor attention. The pathophysiologic bases for this cognitive impairment have not been clarified.

Diagnostic Evaluation

MRI usually shows cortical and subcortical atrophy.

Treatment

Zidovudine (AZT) treatment is controversial. Currently, selegiline and memantine (an NMDA antagonist) are being evaluated. High-dose antiretroviral therapy may be helpful in retarding cognitive loss.

KEY POINTS

1. HIV-associated dementia is common in HIV patients with low CD4 cell counts.
2. Therapy includes AZT, selegiline, and memantine.

METABOLIC CAUSES OF DEMENTIA

Vitamin B_{12} deficiency may present as a progressive dementing illness. However, there are usually many other neurologic features, including dysfunction in the spinal cord (subacute combined degeneration) and peripheral nervous system, such that the diagnosis becomes clearer. The most common neurologic symptoms are those of neuropathy (paresthesias in hands and feet, sensory ataxia, visual loss, orthostatic hypotension) and memory loss. Systemic symptoms include anemia and sore tongue. Appropriate replacement of vitamin B_{12} should suffice in the treatment. Other metabolic causes of dementia are mentioned in Box 12-1.

PHYSIOLOGY

Normal sleep is divided into two states: REM and non-REM. Usually, REM sleep alternates with non-REM sleep in 90-minute cycles (Figure 13-1), with vivid dreaming occurring during REM sleep. These sleep cycles are under cerebral influence. Thus, sleep medicine is an interdisciplinary specialty usually comprising internists, pulmonary specialists, and neurologists. Polysomnography is the main tool that sleep specialists use in order to distinguish sleep states. Recordings are derived from EEGs, EMGs to demonstrate muscle tone, and electro-oculograms to determine eye movements. In addition, other physiologic measures—such as nasal and oral airflow, respiratory effort, and cardiac rhythm—are monitored.

In using polysomnography, non-REM sleep is divided into four stages (I, II, III, and IV). During the awake state, the EEG usually shows an 8- to 13-Hz ("alpha") rhythm, predominantly in the posterior portions of the brain. Stage I sleep is characterized by diminished alpha rhythms, which are replaced by 4- to 7-Hz (theta) rhythm activity, with some 12- to 14-Hz activity. Stage II sleep is characterized by sleep spindles (bursts of 12- to 14-Hz activity) and K complexes (high-voltage waves of both positive and negative polarity, best seen in EEG leads at the vertex of the head). Stages III and IV sleep are characterized by slow-wave activity of 4-Hz or slower (delta) waves. Stage III is defined as 20 to 50% of a set period consisting of delta waves; stage IV sleep occurs when greater than 50% of that period is occupied by delta waves.

Normal people progress in an orderly fashion through the four stages of non-REM sleep, with stage IV (delta sleep) occurring 30 to 45 minutes after sleep onset. REM sleep occurs 60 to 90 minutes after sleep onset, and the EMG shows loss of tone in all muscles except for respiratory and ocular muscles. The EEG shows mixed frequencies, and respirations and heart rate are irregular. Dreaming occurs primarily in REM sleep. At the end of REM sleep, the first

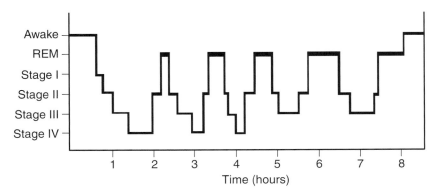

Figure 13-1 • Stages of sleep. Rapid-eye-movement (REM) sleep and the four stages of non-REM sleep alternate throughout the night in cycles that last approximately 90 minutes. There are typically four to six cycles each night in a healthy young adult.

cycle of sleep is completed. Thereafter, in a normal, healthy young adult, non-REM sleep continues to alternate with REM sleep for a total of four to six cycles through the night (see Figure 13-1).

KEY POINTS

1. Sleep is divided into REM and non-REM sleep.
2. Non-REM sleep is divided into four stages (I, II, III, and IV).
3. REM sleep is characterized by loss of muscle tone except in the respiratory and eye muscles. It is also characterized by dreaming.

SLEEP DISORDERS

The International Classification of Sleep Disorders defines four major categories of sleep disorders: dyssomnias, parasomnias, sleep disorders associated with medical and psychiatric conditions, and proposed sleep disorders. The more common sleep disorders from the first three categories are covered below.

◼ DYSSOMNIAS

Dyssomnias are primary sleep disorders that produce either difficulty initiating and maintaining sleep (insomnia) or excessive daytime sleepiness. A detailed history including medications, caffeine use, alcohol consumption, and drug use can often reveal the cause of insomnia.

Narcolepsy

Narcolepsy is a disorder characterized by excessive daytime sleepiness, often associated with cataplexy and other REM sleep phenomena such as hypnagogic hallucinations or sleep paralysis. The onset of narcolepsy is typically between 15 and 25 years of age, with a family history in two-thirds of cases. The cardinal feature of narcolepsy is excessive daytime sleepiness that can occur at inappropriate times or places. The patient may take frequent naps; these usually last from a few minutes to 15 to 30 minutes and are remarkably refreshing. Patients can go on to develop cataplexy, which is a brief loss of muscle tone during which the patient will fall to the ground or her head may slump forward for a few seconds. These attacks are often triggered by emotion such as laugh-

ter or anger. Consciousness is preserved, but prolonged episodes may be followed immediately by REM sleep.

Hypnagogic hallucinations are hallucinations that occur at the beginning of sleep and can involve the visual, auditory, or vestibular system. These hallucinations are a manifestation of the sudden onset of inappropriate REM sleep. Another feature of narcolepsy, sleep paralysis, is an inability to move voluntary muscles during sleep-wake transitions. This can occur normally on awakening from REM sleep, but patients with narcolepsy usually experience the sensation at sleep onset as well.

The diagnosis of narcolepsy can be made clinically with a history of excessive daytime sleepiness, especially if associated with cataplexy. In those with an unclear history, a type of polysomnographic study called a multiple sleep latency test (MSLT) is appropriate. This test measures the tendency to sleep during the day as well as the type of sleep the patient obtains during brief naps. The patient is scheduled to take a number of brief naps during the day, and the latency to sleep onset is measured. The mean latency to sleep onset in patients with narcolepsy is typically less than 5 minutes. In addition, a diagnosis of narcolepsy requires that two out of five of the naps demonstrate REM sleep of rapid onset. Treatment is typically with amphetamine-like drugs, including methylphenidate, methamphetamine, or dextroamphetamine. Pemoline can also be used, but because of possible hepatic failure, it should be reserved until other medications have failed. Modafinil is a newer drug that treats sleepiness effectively with a relative paucity of side effects. Unlike the amphetamines, modafinil does not treat cataplexy. Therefore an additional medication—such as clomipramine, a tricyclic antidepressant, or venlafaxine, a norepinephrine-serotonin reuptake inhibitor (SSNRI)—may be needed to treat cataplexy, especially if it is severe or frequent.

Obstructive Sleep Apnea

Another disorder in the family of dyssomnias is obstructive sleep apnea, which is characterized by repetitive episodes of upper airway obstruction during sleep. Other cardinal features include oxygen desaturation during the apneic spell, sleep disruption, and excessive daytime sleepiness. In severe cases, patients can fall asleep at inappropriate times, as when driving or while at work. Diagnosis requires polysomnography throughout the night in order to measure the degree of sleep disruption, oxygen desaturation, and number of apneas. Treatment is with nasal continuous positive airway pressure (CPAP), which helps maintain upper airway patency during sleep. Also, alcohol and sedating drugs that can decrease upper airway tone should be avoided or discontinued. Weight loss may be beneficial in reducing symptoms, because obesity is a strong risk factor for obstructive sleep apnea. Surgical treatment may be indicated if there is excessive tissue, such as enlarged tonsils, in the posterior pharynx.

Restless Legs Syndrome

Restless legs syndrome, another dyssomnia, is characterized by disagreeable leg sensations, usually prior to sleep onset, that cause an almost irresistible urge to move the legs. All patients with restless legs syndrome also suffer from periodic limb movement disorder, but some can have the latter condition without the former. Patients with periodic limb movement disorder have recurrent periodic leg jerks involving the flexor muscles of the legs. These twitches can occur every 20 to 40 seconds throughout the night and are usually noticed by the bed partner. Both these limb disorders can be caused by metabolic abnormalities such as iron deficiency, chronic alcohol use, or uremia. Treatment is with iron replacement if there is a deficiency or with dopamine agonists or benzodiazepines such as clonazepam.

KEY POINTS

1. Dyssomnias are primary sleep disorders that produce either difficulty initiating and maintaining sleep (insomnia) or excessive daytime sleepiness.
2. Narcolepsy is characterized by excessive daytime sleepiness. It is often associated with cataplexy.
3. The MSLT, a type of polysomnographic test, shows early sleep onset as well as early REM sleep in patients with narcolepsy.
4. Narcolepsy is treated with modafinil, methylphenidate, or pemoline.
5. Obstructive sleep apnea is characterized by repetitive episodes of upper airway obstruction.
6. Obstructive sleep apnea is treated with nasal CPAP or surgery.
7. Restless legs syndrome is characterized by disagreeable leg sensations causing an almost irresistible urge to move the legs and by recurrent periodic leg jerks during the night.

PARASOMNIAS

Parasomnias are undesirable events that occur during sleep or are exacerbated by sleep. The more common parasomnias are sleepwalking, sleep terrors, and sleep bruxism. Sleepwalking consists of complex behaviors initiated during slow-wave sleep and results in walking during sleep. Patients are in a confused state and can perform complex, automatic acts. Sleep terrors are characterized by sudden arousal from slow-wave sleep with a scream or cry accompanied by automatic and behavioral manifestations of intense fear. Sleep bruxism is a stereotyped movement disorder characterized by grinding or clenching of the teeth during sleep. This is a common disorder that can result in disrupted sleep, damaged teeth, morning headaches, and temporomandibular joint dysfunction. A nocturnal tooth guard can alleviate symptoms.

There are also several parasomnias that are associated specifically with REM sleep. Examples include nightmares, sleep paralysis, and REM sleep behavior disorder. Nightmares are frightening dreams that occur during REM sleep and usually awaken the sleeper. Sleep paralysis consists of a period of inability to perform voluntary movements at either sleep onset (hypnagogic) or upon awakening during the night or in the morning (hypnopompic). This represents a partial arousal and entry into REM sleep, such that the brain is awake and conscious but the atonia associated with REM sleep is present. REM sleep behavior disorder is characterized by the loss of the atonia associated with REM sleep and the appearance of elaborate motor activity associated with dreaming. This allows patients to enact dreaming by running, kicking, or punching. Bed partners can be injured. Vocalization may be associated as well. Medications such as antidepressants and alcohol withdrawal can be precipitating causes.

KEY POINTS

1. Parasomnias are undesirable events that occur during sleep or are exacerbated by sleep.
2. Common parasomnias are sleepwalking, sleep terrors, and sleep bruxism.
3. Parasomnias associated with REM sleep include nightmares, sleep paralysis, and REM behavior disorder.

◼ SLEEP DISORDERS ASSOCIATED WITH MEDICAL, NEUROLOGIC, OR PSYCHIATRIC CONDITIONS

Sleep disorders occur during many psychiatric illnesses. For example, in patients with depression, there is often difficulty initiating and maintaining sleep, with early morning awakening. Patients with mania may have prolonged periods of inability to sleep. Neurologic illnesses such as epilepsy are often exacerbated by sleep disturbances, and neurologic degenerative processes such as Parkinson's disease may have associated disrupted sleep patterns. In addition, 25 to 60% of patients with Parkinson's disease or other degenerative neurologic diseases such as multiple system atrophy, or Lewy body dementia can have associated REM sleep behavior disorder. It is thought that the disease process involves degeneration of some of the midbrain structures (such as striatal connections to the midbrain, neurons in the dorsal raphe nucleus, and neurons in the locus ceruleus) involved not only in movement and movement disorders but also in sleep-wake cycles. Interestingly, REM sleep behavior disorder can precede the development of Parkinson's disease by years. Other medical conditions—such as pain from arthritis or peptic ulcer disease and paroxysmal nocturnal dyspnea from congestive heart failure—can result in nocturnal arousal and disrupted sleep patterns. Therefore a complete medical history is important in all patients who present with complaints of sleep disruption.

14 Vascular Disease

Stroke is the third leading cause of death in the United States, surpassed only by heart disease and cancer. Each year, approximately 750,000 people in the United States will have strokes, and one-third to one-fourth of these patients will die from complications of those strokes. Furthermore, stroke is associated with significant morbidity from emotional disability and loss of independence.

Stroke causes acute damage to the nervous system due to an abnormality of the blood supply. Ischemia is the cause of approximately 80% of strokes, and hemorrhage is responsible for the remaining 20%. The term **transient ischemic attack** (TIA) was used in the past to define a stroke-like episode with symptoms lasting less than 24 hours. Because the pathophysiology and risk for future stroke are similar in both TIA and "completed" stroke, TIA is being redefined to describe an event that generally lasts less than 1 hour.

Risk factors for stroke include older age, male sex, family history, hypertension, diabetes, smoking, hypercholesterolemia, heavy alcohol use, and cardiac or peripheral vascular disease. Race is correlated with an increased risk of particular types of stroke. For example, Caucasian men have an increased risk of extracranial occlusive disease causing stroke compared to African Americans and Asians, who have a higher risk of intracranial stenosis and intracerebral hemorrhage.

■ VASCULAR ANATOMY

To understand the varied clinical presentations of stroke, one must have a detailed knowledge of the anatomy and blood supply of the brain. It will then be possible to localize the lesion on the basis of clinical features and examination findings. General neuroanatomic features and the vascular supply of the brain will be reviewed in order to elucidate the more commonly encountered stroke syndromes.

The arterial circulation to the brain is divided into the anterior and posterior circulations. **Anterior circulation** refers to the territory ultimately supplied by the carotid arteries, and **posterior circulation** refers to the territory ultimately supplied by the vertebral and basilar arteries (Figure 14-1).

Anterior Circulation

The anterior circulation begins at the bifurcation of the common carotid artery to form the origin of the internal carotid artery. As the internal carotid artery enters the skull, it follows an S-shaped curve called the **siphon**, which gives rise to its first branch, the ophthalmic artery. An embolus from the bifurcation of the carotid artery or the siphon can travel to the ophthalmic artery, resulting in transient monocular blindness, also called **amaurosis fugax.** The internal carotid artery then penetrates the dura and gives rise to the anterior choroidal and posterior communicating arteries before it bifurcates to form the anterior cerebral artery, which courses anteriorly, and the MCA, which courses laterally.

The anterior cerebral arteries supply the parasagittal cerebral cortex (Figure 14-2) and are connected to each other via the anterior communicating artery (Figure 14-3). The MCA travels laterally and gives off the lenticulostriate artery branches, which supply blood to the basal ganglia and internal capsule. As the MCA continues through the sylvian fissure, it gives off several branches that supply most of the cerebral hemisphere (see Figure 14-1).

Posterior Circulation

The posterior circulation is formed by a vertebral artery from each side. The two vertebral arteries unite in the midline at the junction of the medulla and

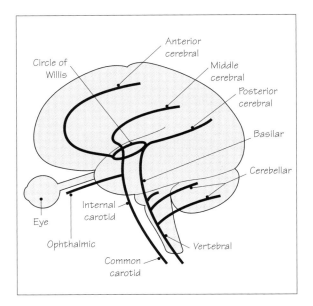

Figure 14-1 • Schematic diagram of the vessels of the brain, including the anterior and posterior circulation.
(Reproduced with permission from Wilkinson I, Lennox G. Essential Neurology. 4ᵗʰ ed. Oxford: Blackwell Publishing, 2005:27.)

pons to form the basilar artery. The vertebral arteries are the first branch from each subclavian artery and travel through the transverse foramina of the cervical vertebrae. The vertebral arteries give off posterior and

anterior spinal artery branches and the posterior inferior cerebellar artery (PICA). The vertebral arteries then join, forming the basilar artery, which gives off bilateral anterior inferior cerebellar arteries (AICA) and superior cerebellar arteries (SCA). The basilar artery also gives off small branches that penetrate the brainstem and supply it with blood. The basilar artery then divides at the junction of the pons and midbrain to form the posterior cerebral artery (PCA), which give off branches to the midbrain and thalamus before supplying the occipital lobes and inferior portions of the temporal lobes (see Figure 14-3). The intracranial blood supply communicates via the circle of Willis (see Figure 14-3).

KEY POINTS

1. The arterial circulation to the brain is divided into the anterior and posterior circulation. The anterior circulation is the territory ultimately supplied by the carotid arteries, and the posterior circulation is the territory ultimately supplied by the vertebral and basilar arteries.
2. Amaurosis fugax usually results from an embolus to the ophthalmic artery.

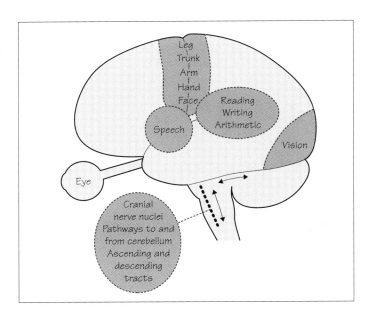

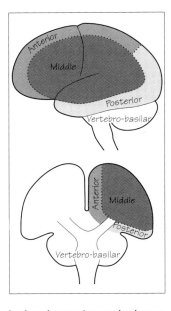

Figure 14-2 • Arterial territories supplied by the anterior cerebral, middle cerebral, and posterior cerebral arteries, with corresponding localization of function.
(Reproduced with permission from Wilkinson I, Lennox G. Essential Neurology. 4ᵗʰ ed. Oxford: Blackwell Publishing, 2005: 28–29.)

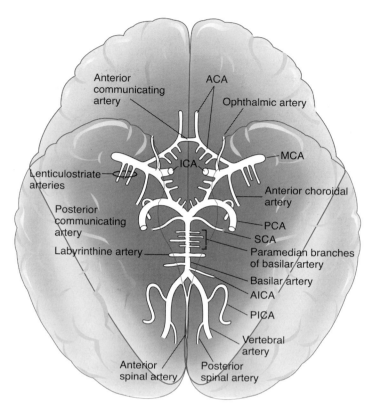

Figure 14-3 • Arteries of the circle of Willis.

◼ BRAIN ISCHEMIA

Ischemic stroke is caused by a lack of blood flow to the brain. It can be subdivided further into three different mechanisms: thrombosis, embolism, and decreased perfusion.

Thrombosis

Thrombosis refers to an obstruction of blood flow due to a localized occlusion within a blood vessel. By far the most common cause of thrombus formation is atherosclerotic disease. Other sources of thrombus include primary hematologic diseases such as a systemic hypercoagulable state or thrombocytosis. In African-American children, sickle cell disease is an important cause of thrombotic stroke. Other causes of thrombosis include fibromuscular dysplasia (caused by hyperplasia of the media of the blood vessel wall), arteritis, and arterial dissection. Clinically, neurologic symptoms from thrombi tend to evolve over minutes or hours and often have a stuttering or fluctuating course.

Embolism

An **embolus** is material that is formed elsewhere within the vascular system and travels to distant sites where it becomes lodged, resulting in ischemia. Common sources of emboli are the heart (the most common); major arteries such as the aorta, carotid, or vertebral arteries; and systemic veins.

Emboli from the heart can originate from the heart valves and are especially likely in the setting of atrial fibrillation. Emboli from arteries can be composed of red blood cells, clumps of platelets, or fragments of ruptured atherosclerotic plaques. Systemic veins like those in the legs can be the source of clots in the setting of a patent foramen ovale or atrial septal defect. In this situation, **paradoxical emboli** bypass the lungs and enter the left side of the heart and the cerebrovascular circulation. Clinically, embolic strokes tend to produce neurologic deficits that are maximal at onset.

Decreased Perfusion

Decreased systemic perfusion results from either systemic hypotension (hypovolemia or blood loss) or cardiac failure (caused by myocardial infarction or arrhythmia). The decreased perfusion usually leads to a more generalized neurologic dysfunction in both cerebral hemispheres than that caused by an embolus or thrombus. Typically, the areas of the brain that are most vulnerable to hypoperfusion are the watershed or border-zone regions, which are areas of brain at the periphery of two different vascular territories (e.g., between the ACA and MCA).

KEY POINTS

1. Stroke can be either ischemic or hemorrhagic.
2. Ischemic stroke can be caused by embolism, thrombosis, or hypoperfusion.
3. A cardiac source is the most common cause of embolism.
4. Hypoperfusion results from hypovolemia or cardiac failure.

■ COMMON ISCHEMIC STROKE SYNDROMES

Armed with this knowledge of neuroanatomy and the function of the nervous system (as discussed elsewhere, particularly Chapters 4 to 8 and 11), one can usually correlate the findings of the neurologic exam with one of seven common localization patterns.

Left Hemispheric Lesion

This lesion can be caused by occlusion of the left internal carotid artery or the MCA. Clinical symptoms can include right-sided weakness and sensory loss, right visual field defect, inability to gaze to the right, and aphasia. The patient may also have impairment of reading, writing, and calculation. If the lesion is isolated to the ACA, the main finding will be right leg weakness.

Right Hemispheric Lesion

Similarly, the right hemispheric lesion results from occlusion of the right internal carotid artery or the MCA. Clinical symptoms can include left-sided weakness and sensory loss, gaze deviation to the right, neglect of the left visual space, corticosensory defects (such as extinction of visual or tactile stimuli on the left side when presented simultaneously to both sides), difficulty drawing or copying, and aprosodic speech.

Lesion of the Left PCA

Occlusion of the left PCA usually results in a right-sided visual field defect, sensory loss on the right side (if the thalamus is involved), difficulty naming colors presented visually, and alexia without agraphia (inability to read with preserved ability to write) if the splenium of the corpus callosum is also involved.

Lesion of the Right PCA

Occlusion of the right PCA results in a left-sided visual field defect and left-sided sensory loss if the thalamus is involved. There may also be associated neglect of the left side.

Vertebrobasilar Artery Infarction

Occlusion of a vertebral or basilar artery will present with either isolated or combined cerebellar and brainstem signs. These can include vertigo, diplopia, nystagmus, weakness or numbness of the extremities, ataxia, vomiting, occipital headache, or crossed motor or sensory findings.

A classic example of a vertebrobasilar stroke is Wallenberg's syndrome. This is a dorsolateral medullary infarction usually caused by vertebral artery occlusion: the signs and symptoms typically include ipsilateral ataxia, ipsilateral Horner's syndrome, and ipsilateral facial sensory loss with contralateral impairment of pain and temperature in the arm and leg (i.e., crossed sensory loss). Also, the patient typically has nystagmus and vertigo and may have hiccups or difficulty swallowing. There is no associated motor weakness because the corticospinal tracts travel anteriorly in the medulla and are spared.

Pure Motor Stroke

A pure motor stroke involving the face, arm, and leg on one side of the body that is fairly equal in severity in the affected body parts is usually caused by a lesion in the contralateral posterior limb of the internal capsule, corona radiata, or base of the pons. There should not be associated impairment of higher cortical functions or sensory or visual loss.

Pure Sensory Stroke

A pure sensory stroke typically involves numbness of the face, arm, and leg on one side of the body and is usually caused by a lesion in the contralateral thalamus. There should not be associated weakness or impairment of higher cortical functions or visual loss.

Diagnostic Evaluation

Once the clinical diagnosis of stroke is made, one considers tests to confirm the diagnosis and exclude other possible causes for the neurologic deficits, such as tumor or brain abscess, and to clarify the underlying cardiovascular or hematologic cause. Therapeutic options are highly dependent on the etiology of the stroke. Therefore the evaluation of patients with brain ischemia includes brain and vascular imaging studies and routine blood work (i.e., CBC; serum electrolytes including glucose, coagulation profiles, serum cholesterol, and lipids; and other tests as warranted by the history) to confirm the diagnosis.

CT scans of the head are good for identifying hemorrhagic strokes because blood appears hyperdense on CT (Figure 14-4); they are also useful for identifying ischemic strokes, which appear hypodense (Figure 14-5). CT scans, however, are somewhat limited in identifying acute ischemic strokes, because these lesions

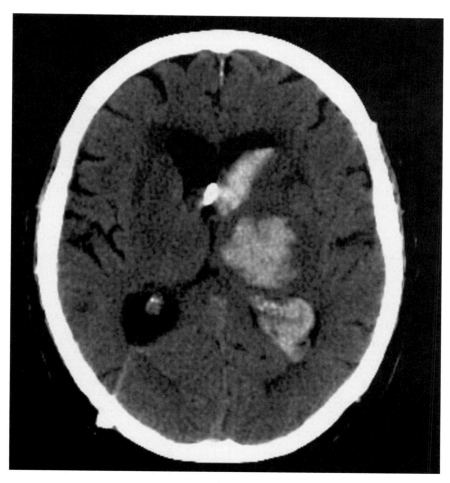

Figure 14-4 • CT scan of the head shows hyperdensity originating in the left thalamus and basal ganglia and filling the lateral ventricles.

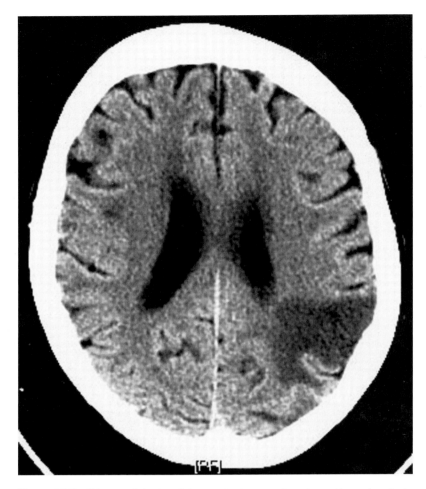

Figure 14-5 • CT scan of the head demonstrates a wedge-shaped hypodensity in the distribution of a branch of the left middle cerebral artery.

are often not visualized until 12 to 24 hours after the onset of symptoms. Also, CT scans are not as sensitive at identifying strokes in the brainstem or cerebellum because of artifact from surrounding bone.

MRI of the head, especially with diffusion-weighted imaging (DWI), is especially sensitive for identifying acute ischemic strokes, with a bright DWI signal (restricted diffusion) in the area of infarction (Figure 14-6). The MRI scan is also sensitive for detecting infarcts in the brainstem or cerebellum. Additionally, with susceptibility sequences, the MRI can reliably identify cerebral hemorrhages, which appear black.

If an ischemic stroke is identified, one must consider whether the cause is an embolus or thrombus. In the case of hypoperfusion, a history of myocardial infarction with significantly reduced cardiac output

or hypotension is usually apparent. The location of thrombus or source of embolus can be investigated noninvasively with MRA or CT angiography of the head and neck, which can visualize stenotic lesions in the ICA or in the vessels of the circle of Willis. Doppler ultrasonography is another noninvasive method of investigating for carotid stenosis, and transcranial Doppler (TCD) ultrasound can be used to look for the presence of intracranial stenosis and monitor for emboli passing under the probe.

Other tests include echocardiography to assess for the possibility of a thrombus in the heart or an atrial septal defect allowing for a paradoxical embolus. The ECG can assess the possibility of a myocardial infarction causing the stroke and rule out atrial fibrillation, which is associated with an increased risk of embolism.

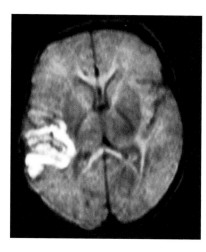

Figure 14-6 • Bright signal is seen on a diffusion-weighted MR image (DWI), indicating a recent infarction. (Reprinted with permission from Patel PR. Lecture Notes on Radiology. Oxford: Blackwell Science, 1998:244.)

The tests discussed above are aimed at confirming the diagnosis and establishing a mechanism of injury. The etiology of the stroke may also be suggested by the neurologic findings. For example, pure sensory and motor strokes are typically caused by small lacunar strokes in the thalamus and internal capsule, respectively. Lacunar strokes are often thought to be caused by lipohyalinosis, occlusion of small penetrating arteries, in turn caused by chronic hypertension. Microatheromas can also obstruct penetrating arteries, causing branch infarcts and lacunes.

> ### KEY POINTS
>
> 1. DWI is the most sensitive imaging study for identifying acute strokes.
> 2. Vascular imaging is essential to define the cause of stroke.
> 3. Cardiac and hematologic tests are often important.

Treatment

Thrombolysis with intravenous recombinant tissue-type plasminogen activator (rt-PA) can reverse damage caused by ischemic stroke and improve long-term outcome. This agent works best in patients who have embolic occlusions of intracranial arteries and do not already have large areas of infarction soon after symptom onset, when rt-PA is given (usually within 3 hours). Hemorrhage is the major risk of rt-PA administration. Contraindications include recent surgical intervention and elevated prothrombin time.

Most patients with ischemic strokes are not eligible for rt-PA, as they will have modest deficits, usually present more than 3 hours into the course of their strokes, or meet one of the exclusionary criteria. Treatment, then, is targeted at the underlying pathophysiologic process. For example, patients with greater than 70% stenosis of the carotid artery on the side responsible for TIAs or a stroke should be considered for carotid endarterectomy. This has been shown to decrease the risk of future ipsilateral strokes. If there is no evidence of carotid artery stenosis, antiplatelet agents such as aspirin, clopidogrel, or dipyridamole are used commonly. Aspirin and clopidogrel provide essentially equivalent benefit in stroke prophylaxis. The combination of aspirin and dipyridamole (Aggrenox) is more effective than aspirin alone in preventing stroke recurrence. Anticoagulation with heparin (acute treatment) or warfarin (long term) is considered if there is evidence of atrial fibrillation or another cardiac source of embolism. However, the benefit of anticoagulation must be weighed against the risk of hemorrhagic complications. Cholesterol-lowering agents like atorvastatin should be used if the patient has an abnormal lipid profile. Evaluations for hypercoagulability should be performed in young patients with strokes. Rehabilitation for stroke patients at a dedicated facility is often necessary.

> ### KEY POINTS
>
> 1. Treatment should be tailored to the individual patient based on the diagnostic evaluation for the underlying etiology.
> 2. rt-PA can be used if the patient presents soon after symptom onset.
> 3. Treatment options include antiplatelet agents.
> 4. Anticoagulation with heparin or warfarin should be considered for patients with a cardiac source of embolism.

■ CEREBRAL HEMORRHAGE

Cerebral hemorrhages can be subdivided into four types: subarachnoid, intracerebral, epidural, and subdural. Epidural and subdural hematomas are often traumatic and are discussed elsewhere (see Chapter 17).

Hemorrhage leads to brain dysfunction through a variety of mechanisms, including destruction of tissue, mass effect, and compression of blood vessels leading to ischemia.

Subarachnoid Hemorrhage

SAH is a neurologic emergency often caused by rupture of an intracranial aneurysm, but it can also be caused by trauma, bleeding from arteriovenous malformations (AVMs), or drug use. In the case of aneurysmal rupture, blood is released rapidly into the subarachnoid space, resulting in increased ICP. Aneurysms are commonly found at the junction between the anterior communicating artery and the anterior cerebral artery, at the bifurcation of the MCA, in the PCA, at the apex of the basilar artery, and at the origin of the PICA (Figure 14-7). A sudden, severe headache (commonly described as the worst headache of the patient's life) is the typical clinical presentation, rather than focal neurologic deficits. As ICP rises, the patient may become lethargic, have other signs of altered mental state, and may vomit.

The focus of SAH evaluation is to determine whether an aneurysm is present. CT is usually the first diagnostic step in the evaluation of patients with suspected SAH (Figure 14-8). It can demonstrate blood in the subarachnoid space and next to the likely site of aneurysmal rupture. LP should be performed to look for red cells or xanthochromia (a yellowish tinge caused by heme breakdown) in the CSF if the CT is negative and the suspicion for SAH is high. Angiography is the "gold standard" for defining the presence and location of an aneurysm. Definitive treatment is coiling or clipping

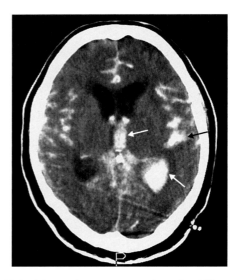

Figure 14-8 • CT scan demonstrates subarachnoid hemorrhage. (Reproduced with permission from Patel PR. Lecture Notes Radiology. 2nd ed. Oxford: Blackwell Publishing, 2005:278.)

of the aneurysm. These patients require close monitoring in an intensive care setting.

Intraparenchymal Hemorrhage

Intraparenchymal hemorrhage is bleeding directly into the brain parenchyma itself. Hypertension is the most common cause. Acute rises in blood pressure can lead to rupture of penetrating arteries. Also, long-standing hypertension damages small intracerebral arterioles and can result in the leakage of blood. Other causes of intracerebral hemorrhage include anticoagulants such as heparin or warfarin, use of drugs such as cocaine or amphetamines, vascular malformations, and diseases affecting the blood vessel walls, such as amyloid angiopathy. Other causes include hemorrhage into an underlying brain tumor.

The location of the hemorrhage and clinical history (i.e., history of anticoagulation or drug use) can be helpful in determining the etiology of the hemorrhage. For example, hemorrhages caused by hypertension are most often found in the basal ganglia, thalamus, pons, and cerebellum (in order of decreasing frequency).

Lobar hemorrhages occur in the subcortical white matter in any cerebral lobe (frontal, temporal, parietal, and occipital). They can be caused by a bleeding diathesis, trauma, or an underlying lesion. Amyloid angiopathy is a predisposition to bleeding in the cerebral hemispheres, especially the parietal and occipital lobes, caused by the deposition of amyloid in small

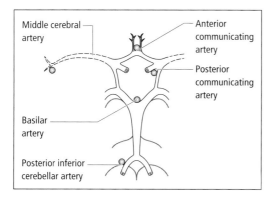

Figure 14-7 • Common sites of aneurysm in the circle of Willis. (Reproduced with permission from Ginsberg L. Lecture Notes Neurology. 8th ed. Oxford: Blackwell Publishing, 2005:87.)

arteries and arterioles. It is much more common in older patients.

The clinical presentation of patients with intraparenchymal hemorrhage includes focal symptoms that may progress, headache, and loss of consciousness (with large hematomas). Herniation may also result from large intracerebral hemorrhages (see Chapter 17). Seizures are not common but occur more frequently in patients with intracerebral hemorrhage than in other types of strokes. Additionally, hemorrhages may originate in the ventricles of the brain, in which case patients may present with headache, vomiting, decreased level of arousal, and neck stiffness.

As in the case of SAH, CT is the first diagnostic step in the workup of intraparenchymal hemorrhage (see Figure 14-4). Patients with sizable hemorrhages require admission to an intensive care unit. Reversal of anticoagulation (if applicable) should be performed aggressively by discontinuing anticoagulants, administering vitamin K, and transfusing fresh frozen plasma. Cautious control of blood pressure is advised: too high a blood pressure may increase the ICP or size of the hemorrhage, while too low a pressure may result in ischemia. Mechanical ventilation and an osmotic diuretic like mannitol may help reduce ICP. Surgical drainage, if the hematoma is expanding and accessible, can be lifesaving, as can placement of an intraventricular drain. Chronic management includes modification of risk factors such as hypertension.

KEY POINTS

1. SAHs are often caused by aneurysmal rupture.
2. If a head CT scan is negative and the index of suspicion for SAH is high, an LP must be performed.
3. Hemorrhages related to hypertension are most commonly found in the basal ganglia, thalamus, pons, and cerebellum.

◼ ARTERIOVENOUS MALFORMATIONS AND OTHER VASCULAR ANOMALIES

Arteriovenous malformations (AVMs) are congenital lesions composed of tangled arteries and veins with intervening sclerotic tissue. They present in a variety of ways including seizure, hemorrhage, headache, and mass lesions causing progressive neurologic deficits. Approximately 2 to 3% of AVMs bleed per year, with a mortality rate of 10% per bleed. Treatment involves surgery for small AVMs in noneloquent cortex with superficial draining patterns or catheter-directed embolization for larger lesions. **Cavernous angiomas** are composed of entangled capillaries. They bleed much less frequently than AVMs. Surgical removal of symptomatic cavernous angiomas in accessible locations is curative. **Developmental venous anomalies** are the most common vascular malformation. They are composed of an enlarged collection of veins and have a minimal propensity to bleed. Surgical resection can lead to venous infarction and is not recommended. **Capillary telangiectasias** are clinically silent collections of capillaries interspersed amid normal brain. No treatment is indicated for these lesions.

KEY POINTS

1. The four types of vascular anomalies are AVMs, cavernous angiomas, developmental venous anomalies, and capillary telangiectasias.
2. Surgery is indicated for selected patients with AVMs or cavernous angiomas.

15 Seizures

Seizures are among the most common problems in neurology. Up to 10% of the population will have a seizure at some point in their lives. In addition, seizures can be among the most dramatic forms of nervous system dysfunction. Although seizures have many different causes and manifestations, by definition a seizure is an abnormal hypersynchronous electrical discharge of neurons. Epilepsy is defined as a condition in which there is a tendency toward recurrent unprovoked seizures. Practically, the diagnosis of epilepsy is often applied after a patient has had two unprovoked seizures.

Classification

Seizures can arise from one portion of the brain (**partial**) or from the entire brain at once (**generalized**). Those that arise from one portion of the brain can evolve and spread to involve the whole brain (**secondarily generalized**). Among partial seizures, those in which awareness is impaired are termed **complex**, whereas those in which awareness is preserved are termed **simple**.

Simple Partial Seizures

By definition, simple partial seizures begin in a focal area of the brain and do not impair awareness. In general, such seizures lead to positive rather than negative neurologic symptoms (e.g., tingling rather than numbness, hallucinations rather than blindness). The manifestations of simple partial seizures depend on their site of origin in the brain. Focal motor seizures, in which one part of the body may stiffen or jerk rhythmically, stem from the motor cortex in the frontal lobe. The classic jacksonian march occurs when the electrical discharge spreads along the motor strip, leading to rhythmic twitching that spreads along body parts following the organization of the motor homunculus. Simple partial seizures from other regions of the brain can cause sensory phenomena (parietal), visual phenomena (occipital), or gustatory, olfactory, and psychic phenomena (temporal). The latter may include déjà vu, jamais vu, or sensations of depersonalization ("out of body") or derealization.

Complex Partial Seizures

Complex partial seizures have a focal onset and involve an impairment of awareness. They commonly arise from the temporal lobe, although some may originate in the frontal lobe as well. Complex partial seizures may include automatisms (stereotyped motor actions without clear purpose) such as lip-smacking, chewing movements, or picking at clothing. The patient may have speech arrest or may speak in a nonsensical manner. By definition the patient does not respond normally to the environment or to questions or commands. Occasionally the patient may continue the activity she was participating in at the onset of the seizure, sometimes to remarkable lengths: patients may continue folding the laundry during a seizure or even finish driving home. Complex partial seizures of frontal lobe origin may involve bizarre bilateral movements, such as bicycling or kicking, or behavior such as running in circles.

Generalized Tonic-Clonic Seizures

Generalized tonic-clonic (GTC) seizures were formerly called **grand mal** seizures and are the seizure type with which the lay public is most familiar. They typically begin with a tonic phase, lasting several seconds, in which the entire body becomes stiff (including the pharyngeal muscles, sometimes leading to a vocalization known as the epileptic cry).

This is followed by the clonic phase, in which the extremities jerk rhythmically, more or less symmetrically, typically for less than 1 to 2 minutes. Toward the end of the clonic phase, the frequency of the jerking may peter out until the body finally becomes flaccid. The patient may bite his tongue and become incontinent of urine during a GTC seizure. There is typically a postictal state after the seizure, lasting minutes to hours, during which the patient may be tired or confused, before returning slowly back to normal.

Absence Seizure

An absence seizure is a generalized seizure that most commonly occurs in children and is characterized primarily by an unresponsive period of staring that lasts for several seconds, with immediate recovery afterward. Absence seizures can occur tens or even hundreds of times a day and may first be diagnosed by schoolteachers as daydreaming or difficulty concentrating. A classic 3-Hz spike-and-wave EEG pattern accompanies absence seizures (Figure 15-1). Hyperventilation is a common trigger.

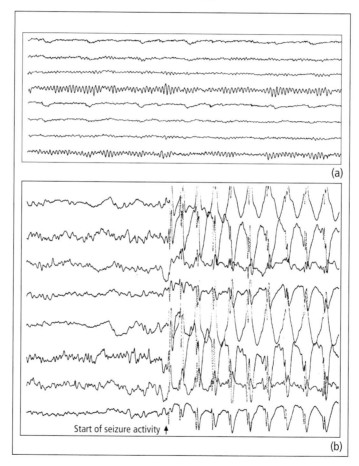

Figure 15-1•Characteristic EEG findings in the absence seizures. (a) This tracing demonstrates a normal EEG recording in an awake adult. The top four channels are derived from electrodes over the left side of the head, from front to back, while the bottom four are derived from the right side of the head. A normal sinusoidal alpha rhythm is seen most prominently over the posterior head regions bilaterally (fourth and eighth channels). (b) Midway through the tracing, rhythmic 3-Hz generalized spike-and-slow-wave discharges appear. This is the typical EEG pattern of an absence seizure; during these discharges, the patient may stare and be unresponsive. (Reproduced with permission from Ginsberg L. Lecture Notes Neurology. 8th ed. Oxford: Blackwell Publishing, 2005:75.)

Other Seizure Types

Rarer seizure types include atonic, tonic, and myoclonic seizures, all of which are generalized in onset.

KEY POINTS

1. A seizure is an abnormal hypersynchronous electrical discharge involving neurons in the brain.
2. Epilepsy is a tendency to have recurrent unprovoked seizures.
3. Seizures may manifest with motor, sensory, or psychic phenomena and are usually characterized by positive rather than negative neurologic symptoms.
4. Partial seizures originate in a focal area of the brain but may become secondarily generalized; awareness is preserved during simple partial seizures and impaired during complex partial seizures.
5. Generalized seizures originate in the entire brain at once; tonic-clonic and absence seizures are examples of such seizures.

Epidemiology and Etiologies

Seizures often have their onset in the very young and the very old (Figure 15-2). Etiologies vary depending on age of onset. In infants, a variety of neonatal infections, hypoxic-ischemic insults, and genetic syndromes are common causes of seizures.

Febrile seizures are a special case. They are the most common cause of seizures in children, affecting up to 3 to 9% of this age group. They occur between 6 months and 5 years of age in the setting of a febrile illness without evidence of intracranial infection and are usually generalized in onset. The risk of future epilepsy is very small unless the seizures are prolonged or partial in onset or if other neurologic abnormalities or a family history of epilepsy is present.

Older children may also develop seizures related to head injury or meningitis; genetic syndromes continue to be a significant etiology in this age group. Among young adults, head injury and alcohol are common causes of new-onset seizures, but brain tumors become one of the most common etiologies by middle age. Finally, in the elderly, strokes become the most common etiology, and metabolic disturbances from systemic problems such as hepatic or renal failure are a frequent cause as well.

Frequently, seizures occur in children (and sometimes adults) as part of a syndrome that may include specific seizure types, EEG patterns, and associated neurologic abnormalities. The diagnosis of a specific syndrome may have implications both for genetic testing and for the proper choice of pharmacologic treatments. Examples of epilepsy syndromes are outlined in Table 15-1.

KEY POINTS

1. The incidence of new-onset seizures is highest among the very young and the very old.
2. Common etiologies of new-onset seizures differ depending on age of onset.
3. Febrile seizures in children are common and generally carry a benign prognosis.
4. Seizures may occur as part of specific epilepsy syndromes characterized by distinctive seizure types, EEG patterns, or associated neurologic abnormalities.

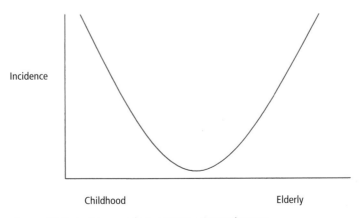

Figure 15-2 • Incidence of new-onset seizures by age.

■ TABLE 15-1

Selected Epilepsy Syndromes

	Age of Onset	Seizure Types	Associated Findings	EEG Findings	Treatment
Lennox-Gastaut syndrome	Childhood	Tonic, atonic, myoclonic, generalized tonic-clonic, absence	Mental retardation	Slow (1–2 Hz) spike-and-wave	Valproic acid, lamotrigine, felbamate
Benign rolandic epilepsy	Childhood	Simple partial involving mouth and face, generalized tonic-clonic	Nocturnal preponderance of seizures	Centrotemporal spikes	Carbamazepine; sometimes no treatment
Absence epilepsy	Childhood and adolescence	Absence, generalized tonic-clonic	Hyperventilation as trigger	3-Hz spike-and-wave	Ethosuximide, valproic acid
Juvenile myoclonic epilepsy	Adolescence and young adulthood	Myoclonic, absence, generalized tonic-clonic	Early morning preponderance of seizures	4- to 6-Hz polyspike-and-wave	Valproic acid, lamotrigine

Clinical Manifestations

History

The diagnosis of seizures is a clinical one. Most commonly the patient will be seen after an event has occurred and the diagnosis will have to be made on the history alone. In these cases the patient (and more importantly, witnesses, if the seizure was not simple partial) must be pressed for an exact description of the event itself, any premonitory symptoms, and the character of the recovery period in order for the clinician to decide whether the event was a seizure, and if so, what type of seizure it was. It is these clinical details that should allow for the differentiation of seizures from other paroxysmal neurologic events (Table 15-2).

■ TABLE 15-2

Characteristics of Partial Seizures and Other Paroxysmal Neurologic Events

	Partial Seizures	Transient Ischemic Attacks (TIAs)	Migraines
Onset	Progression of symptoms over seconds	Sudden onset of symptoms	Progression of symptoms over 15–20 minutes
Neurologic symptoms	Positive motor or sensory symptoms, "psychic" symptoms such as déjà vu	Negative motor, sensory, or visual symptoms	Positive sensory or especially visual symptoms, such as scintillating scotomata
Duration	Usually less than a few minutes	Usually less than 30 minutes, always less than 24 hours	Symptoms for 15–20 minutes, followed by headache for up to hours
Consciousness	Impaired (if complex)	Preserved	Preserved
Headache	Occasionally postictal	None	Throbbing pain following progression of symptoms
Recovery	Postictal confusion, sleepiness	Immediate	Fatigue common
Risk factors	Structural brain lesion, family history of seizures	Hypertension, hyperlipidemia, smoking, diabetes	Family history of migraines

Physical Examination

Examination will be of diagnostic benefit in the rare instances in which the patient is seen during the event or shortly thereafter. In the latter case, a postictal hemiparesis, or Todd's paralysis, may be detected after a secondarily generalized seizure. Such a finding indicates that the seizure was of partial onset, even if that was not apparent to onlookers at the time. Other abnormalities on neurologic exam may also suggest the presence of a focal brain lesion. Of course, the general physical exam may yield findings suggestive of infection or other systemic disease that might explain a new-onset seizure. In particular, signs of meningitis should be sought in any patient who has had a seizure.

Diagnostic Evaluation

Laboratory Studies

Laboratory testing may reveal an underlying metabolic abnormality that might explain a new-onset seizure, such as hyponatremia or hypocalcemia. There is commonly a lactic acidosis, resulting in decreased serum bicarbonate, after a GTC seizure. In cases where infection is suspected, an LP should always be performed.

Radiographic Imaging

An uncomplicated seizure in a patient with known epilepsy does not generally warrant head imaging. However, with rare exceptions, neuroimaging should usually be performed in patients with new-onset seizures. For seizures of probable partial onset, an MRI is typically a necessary part of the diagnostic workup, so as to look for a structural abnormality that may serve as a focus for a partial seizure. A head CT may suffice in the urgent setting, however.

Electroencephalography

An EEG may be useful for several reasons: It may identify a potential focus of seizure onset, it may reveal characteristic findings that are diagnostic of a specific epilepsy syndrome, and it may establish whether a patient who has had a seizure and is still not waking up is merely postictal or is having continuous nonconvulsive seizures. However, the diagnosis of whether a particular paroxysmal event was a seizure or not must rest primarily on clinical grounds, because up to 50% of EEGs performed on known epilepsy patients may be normal.

KEY POINTS

1. The diagnosis of seizure is a clinical one and usually rests primarily on the history.
2. Certain elements of the history may help to differentiate seizures from other paroxysmal events.
3. Physical exam, laboratory studies, and neuroimaging may help to identify the cause of a new-onset seizure.
4. EEG may help to refine the diagnosis of seizures in particular settings.

Treatment

Drugs

The mainstay of epilepsy treatment is medical therapy. The number of available antiepileptic drugs (AEDs) has more than doubled in recent years, and there is now a large selection of agents from which to choose, each with its own set of indications and adverse effects (Table 15-3).

An AED is typically not started after a single seizure. This applies especially to symptomatic seizures, namely those that are due to a treatable or reversible condition, such as meningitis, alcohol withdrawal, or hyponatremia. Most neurologists would also not start an AED after a single seizure for which no underlying cause is found.

AED treatment is usually begun after two seizures that are not symptomatic or provoked. The primary goal of AED usage is monotherapy—that is, control of seizures using a single drug. Most neurologists increase the dosage of a single drug until either seizure control is achieved or adverse effects become intolerable. If the latter occurs, the dose is lowered and a second drug added if necessary. If seizure control is achieved, an attempt is then made to taper the first drug, leaving the second as monotherapy. For about 70% of epilepsy patients, seizures will be well controlled on monotherapy. For the remainder, two or more AEDs may be required, or the seizures may remain refractory to all medical therapy.

KEY POINTS

1. Most neurologists begin drug therapy after two unprovoked seizures.
2. Each drug has its own set of indications and adverse effects.
3. Monotherapy is the primary goal of antiepileptic therapy; most patients' seizures are well controlled on one medication.

■ TABLE 15-3

Selected Antiepileptic Drugs

	Site of Action	Seizure Types Treated*	Characteristic Side Effects
Phenytoin (Dilantin)	Na$^+$ channel	Partial	Gingival hyperplasia, coarsening of facial features, ataxia
Carbamazepine (Tegretol)	Na$^+$ channel	Partial	Hyponatremia, agranulocytosis, diplopia
Valproic acid (Depakote)	Na$^+$ channel, GABA receptor	Partial, generalized, absence	GI symptoms, tremor, weight gain, hair loss, hepatotoxicity, thrombocytopenia
Phenobarbital	GABA receptor	Partial, generalized	Sedation
Ethosuximide (Zarontin)	T-type Ca^{2+} channel	Absence	GI symptoms
Gabapentin (Neurontin)	Unknown	Partial	Sedation, ataxia
Lamotrigine (Lamictal)	Na$^+$ channel, glutamate receptor	Partial, generalized	Rash, Stevens-Johnson syndrome
Topiramate (Topamax)	Na$^+$ channel, GABA activity	Partial, generalized	Word-finding difficulty, renal stones, weight loss
Tiagabine (Gabitril)	GABA reuptake	Partial	Sedation
Levetiracetam (Keppra)	Unknown	Partial, generalized	Insomnia, anxiety, irritability
Oxcarbazepine (Trileptal)	Na$^+$ channel	Partial	Sedation, hyponatremia
Zonisamide (Zonegran)	Unknown	Partial, generalized	Sedation, renal stones, weight loss

* Drugs effective against partial seizures can also be used against seizures that are secondarily generalized.

Vagus Nerve Stimulation

The vagus nerve stimulator is a novel treatment device that has recently become available; it has been shown to be effective in the treatment of partial seizures. The device is implanted subcutaneously in the chest and stimulates the left vagus nerve through programmed electrical impulses delivered through leads placed in the neck.

Surgery

Patients refractory to medical management may be treated with epilepsy surgery. (Exactly what constitutes being medically refractory will depend on an individual patient's circumstances; contributing factors typically include seizure type and frequency, tolerance of AED therapy, number of AEDs tried, and effect on patient's quality of life.) The most common surgical procedure is resection of the epileptogenic area, typically following a presurgical evaluation in which continuous video-EEG monitoring combined with neuroimaging and other tests is used to identify the focus of seizure onset. For seizures of medial temporal lobe origin, the rate of seizure freedom following resective surgery may be as high as 90%. Other less commonly used surgical procedures include corpus callosotomy, hemispherectomy, or multiple subpial transection.

■ STATUS EPILEPTICUS

Status epilepticus (SE) is an abnormal state in which either seizure activity is continuous for a prolonged period or seizures are so frequent that there is no recovery of consciousness between them. There are several types of SE, including the generalized convulsive form (ongoing clonic movements of the extremities) and more subtle forms in which the patient may appear merely comatose or have subtle motor signs such as eyelid twitching or nystagmus. Potential etiologies of SE include acute metabolic disturbances, toxic or infectious insults, hypoxic-ischemic damage to the brain, and underlying epilepsy. Morbidity from SE can be high; outcome depends largely on etiology and duration. SE is a medical emergency, the management of which centers on stopping the seizure activity and preventing the occurrence of systemic complications (Figure 15-3). It is important to note that a cluster of frequent seizures may warrant similarly aggressive management, particularly because this condition may evolve to SE quickly.

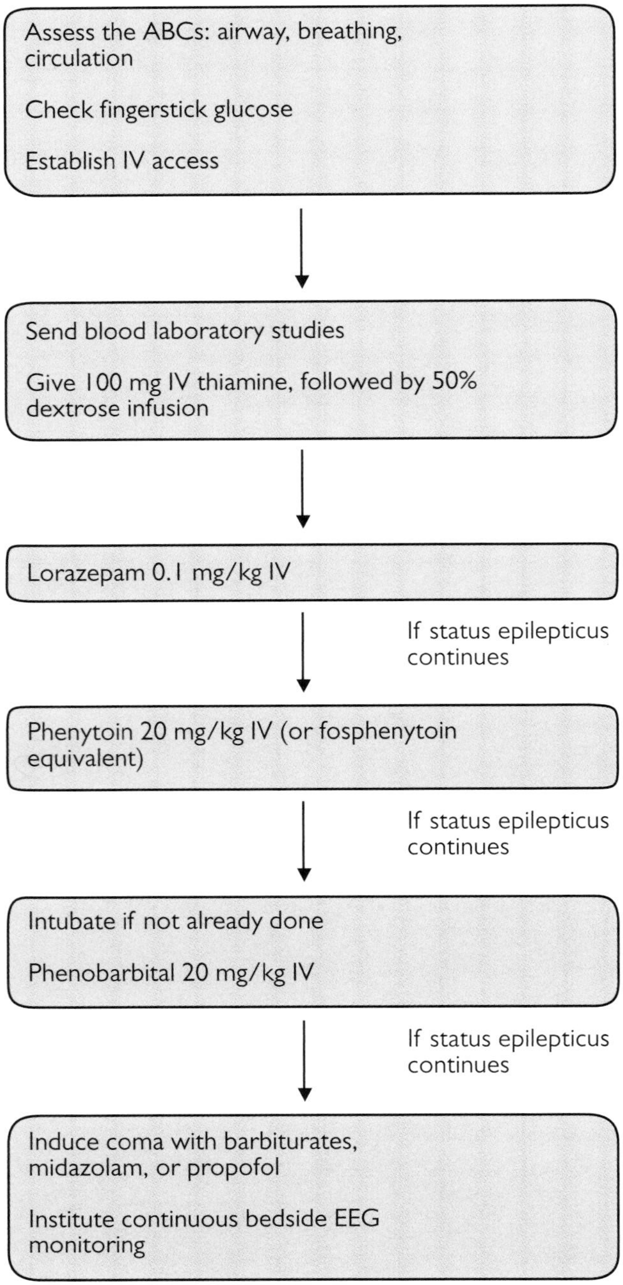

Assess the ABCs: airway, breathing, circulation

Check fingerstick glucose

Establish IV access

↓

Send blood laboratory studies

Give 100 mg IV thiamine, followed by 50% dextrose infusion

↓

Lorazepam 0.1 mg/kg IV

If status epilepticus continues ↓

Phenytoin 20 mg/kg IV (or fosphenytoin equivalent)

If status epilepticus continues ↓

Intubate if not already done

Phenobarbital 20 mg/kg IV

If status epilepticus continues ↓

Induce coma with barbiturates, midazolam, or propofol

Institute continuous bedside EEG monitoring

Figure 15-3 • Neurologic emergency: status epilepticus.

■ SPECIAL TOPICS

First Aid for Seizures

All physicians should be familiar with first aid measures for those having a seizure. In general, the goal is to prevent the patient from becoming injured and to prevent well-meaning bystanders from intervening unwisely. The patient with complex partial seizures may wander or make semipurposeful movements; if necessary, she should be gently guided out of harm's way. More aggressive attempts at restraint may provoke a violent reaction. The patient with GTC seizures should be laid on his side, if possible, so that vomiting does not lead to aspiration. Tight clothing should be loosened. **Nothing should be placed in the mouth.** Most GTC seizures stop within 1 to 2 minutes; immediate medical attention should be sought if a seizure becomes more prolonged.

Seizures and Driving

Each state has its own licensing requirements for those with epilepsy; physicians who care for seizure patients should be aware of these. Most states require a specific seizure-free interval before a patient may drive; exceptions can sometimes be made for purely nocturnal seizures or those with a prolonged simple partial onset that provides the patient with a warning without impaired awareness. A few states require physicians to report patients with seizures to the department of motor vehicles.

Antiepileptic Drugs and Pregnancy

Women taking AEDs have a somewhat higher risk of fetal malformations than the general population, though the absolute risk is still low. Valproic acid specifically has been associated with a higher rate of neural tube defects. All women with epilepsy who are considering becoming pregnant should take folic acid (1 mg or more per day). It is reasonable to consider modifying a woman's AED regimen prior to conception depending on the severity of her epilepsy, but the risk of anticonvulsant teratogenicity must be balanced with the risk of seizure occurrence during pregnancy.

Psychogenic Nonepileptic Seizures

A reported 10 to 30% of patients evaluated at tertiary referral centers for medically refractory epilepsy actually have events resembling seizures that have no EEG correlate and are felt to be psychogenic in nature. Some of these patients may also have true epileptic seizures at other times. Many patients with psychogenic events have comorbid psychiatric illnesses or a history of abuse. Continuous video-EEG monitoring to record the typical events may be the most reliable method of differentiating psychogenic events from epileptic seizures.

■ IDIOPATHIC PARKINSON'S DISEASE

Idiopathic Parkinson's disease (PD) is a chronic degenerative disorder with characteristic clinical findings, response to L-dopa replacement therapy, and pathologic changes in the brain. **Parkinsonism** is a term used to describe a heterogeneous group of conditions that share some of the clinical features of idiopathic PD but differ partially in their clinical expression, response to L-dopa therapy, and underlying pathologic substrates.

Epidemiology

PD is a common neurodegenerative condition. Most instances are sporadic, although there are reports of familial PD in which mutations in the α-synuclein, parkin, UCH-L1 (ubiquitin carboxy-terminal hydrolase 1) and DJ-1 genes have been described.

Pathology

PD is characterized by the progressive death of selected neuronal populations, notably the ventral tier of the neuromelanin-containing dopaminergic neurons of the substantia nigra pars compacta. The pathologic hallmark of PD is the Lewy body.

Clinical Manifestations

The four cardinal clinical features of idiopathic PD are tremor, rigidity, bradykinesia, and postural instability. Features that may be useful in distinguishing idiopathic PD from other parkinsonian syndromes are summarized in Table 16-1.

■ TABLE 16-1

Parkinsonian Syndromes

Parkinsonian Syndrome	Distinguishing Clinical Features
Progressive supranuclear palsy	Supranuclear ophthalmoplegia, with limitation of vertical more than horizontal gaze; axial rigidity and neck extension; early falls as a consequence of impaired postural reflexes, neck extension, and inability to look down
Corticobasal ganglionic degeneration	Apraxia, cortical sensory impairment and alien-limb phenomenon; severe unilateral rigidity; stimulus-sensitive myoclonus
Diffuse Lewy body disease	Early dementia; prominent visual hallucinations; extreme sensitivity to extrapyramidal side effects of antidopaminergic neuroleptic drugs
Vascular parkinsonism	"Lower-half" parkinsonism with rigidity in the legs and marked gait impairment; other evidence of diffuse vascular disease (corticospinal tract dysfunction, pseudobulbar palsy)
Multiple system atrophy	Early and prominent features of autonomic dysfunction; evidence of corticospinal tract dysfunction; cerebellar signs; stimulus-sensitive myoclonus; vocal cord paresis

The tremor is slow (3 to 5 Hz) and most prominent when the limb is at rest. It affects the distal arm more often than the leg and is described as "pill rolling." It may also affect the lips, chin, and tongue. Rigidity typically affects the distal limbs more than the axial musculature and is described as "lead pipe" or "cogwheel." Slowness of movement (bradykinesia) and thought (bradyphrenia) are common features in idiopathic PD. Postural instability is the result of impaired postural reflexes and is largely responsible for falls. Dementia is increasingly recognized as an important feature of PD and occurs in 25 to 30% of patients as the disease advances.

Treatment

Replacement of the deficient dopamine with its precursor L-dopa is the mainstay of treatment. L-Dopa is administered because dopamine does not cross the blood-brain barrier. It is given together with a peripheral decarboxylase inhibitor (e.g., carbidopa) in a combined formulation (e.g., Sinemet). Carbidopa prevents the peripheral conversion of L-dopa to dopamine and thus reduces the incidence of peripheral dopaminergic side effects such as nausea, vomiting, and hypertension.

Dopaminergic agonists have been proposed as alternative initial agents for symptomatic treatment, but the evidence that early therapy with dopaminergic agonists (e.g., ropinirole) may reduce the subsequent risk of dopa-induced dyskinesias is controversial.

Several other agents have been used in early PD. The anticholinergics may be particularly useful in the treatment of tremor-predominant disease. Amantadine may be helpful for the early treatment of bradykinesia, rigidity, and gait disturbance. The selective monoamine oxidase B inhibitor selegiline may also provide early symptomatic benefit. The catechol-O-methyl transferase inhibitors are the most recent addition to the antiparkinsonian armamentarium. They decrease removal of L-dopa and thereby augment its effects. The pharmacologic agents used in the treatment of PD are summarized in Table 16-2, and an approach to commonly encountered clinical scenarios is outlined in Table 16-3.

There has been a recent resurgence in lesioning and deep brain stimulation for the treatment of PD. These procedures target the motor thalamus, the internal segment of the globus pallidus, or the subthalamic nucleus.

KEY POINTS

1. Idiopathic PD results from loss of dopaminergic neurons in the substantia nigra.
2. The pathologic hallmark is the Lewy body.
3. Tremor, rigidity, bradykinesia, and postural instability are the four cardinal symptoms.

■ DRUG-INDUCED MOVEMENT DISORDERS

Drugs with dopamine receptor–blocking activity have a particular propensity for inducing a variety of movement disorders, including akathisia, acute dystonic reactions, parkinsonism, tardive dyskinesia, and the neuroleptic malignant syndrome.

Neuroleptic malignant syndrome (NMS) is an uncommon disorder characterized by muscular rigidity, fever, autonomic lability, altered level of consciousness, elevated creatine kinase level, and leukocytosis. Treatment involves discontinuation of the offending agent, antipyretics, rehydration, and occasionally the use of bromocriptine or dantrolene.

Akathisia is a dysphoric state characterized by the subjective desire to be in constant motion and is often associated with an inability to sit or stand still. Anticholinergics and beta blockers have been used with the most success in the treatment of this disorder.

Tardive dyskinesia is an orolinguomasticatory dyskinesia that occurs as the most common (late and persistent) movement disorder complicating neuroleptic use. Commonly observed are chewing movements, lip smacking, and rolling of the tongue inside the mouth and up against the inside of the cheek. The limbs and trunk may also be affected. A history of the use of dopamine receptor–blocking drugs is essential to the diagnosis. The offending drug should be discontinued when possible; further therapeutic benefit may be obtained from dopamine-depleting agents such as reserpine and tetrabenazine. Some tardive dyskinesias remain unresponsive to any treatment.

KEY POINTS

1. Antipsychotics (haloperidol as well as the newer atypical agents) are the most common cause of drug-induced movement disorders.
2. The propensity of a drug to cause these movement disorders is related to its D_2-receptor–blocking activity.

■ TABLE 16-2

Pharmacologic Treatment of Parkinson Disease

Drug	Mechanism of Action	Dosing	Side Effects
Levodopa/carbidopa	Dopamine precursor/dopa decarboxylase inhibitor	Start with a half of a 25/100 tablet twice daily Increase dose as needed Typically dosed 3 to 5 times a day	Anorexia, nausea, psychosis, hallucinations, orthostatic hypotension, dyskinesia
Trihexyphenidyl	Anticholinergic	Start with 1 mg at mealtime Increase to 2 mg thrice daily as needed	Dry mouth, constipation, urinary retention, confusion, hallucinations, narrow-angle glaucoma
Benztropine	Anticholinergic	Start with 0.5–1 mg at bedtime Increase to 2 mg qid as needed	As above
Amantadine	NMDA antagonist	100 mg twice daily	Hallucinations, leg edema, livedo reticularis
Bromocriptine	Dopamine agonist	Start with a half 2.5-mg tablet twice daily Titrate gradually to 5–7.5 mg/day	Nausea, orthostatic hypotension, psychosis, hallucinations, dyskinesia
Pergolide	Dopamine agonist	Start with 0.05 mg/day Titrate gradually to 0.75–3 mg/day divided into three doses	As above
Pramipexole	Dopamine agonist	Start with 0.125 mg thrice daily Titrate gradually to 1.5 mg thrice daily	As above
Ropinirole	Dopamine agonist	Start with 0.25 mg thrice daily Titrate gradually to 1 mg thrice daily	As above
Tolcapone	COMT inhibitor	100–200 mg thrice daily	Nausea, vomiting, insomnia, orthostatic hypotension, confusion, dyskinesia
Entacapone	COMT inhibitor	200 mg with each L-dopa dose	As above

■ STIFF-PERSON SYNDROME

Stiff-person (or stiff-man) syndrome is a rare disorder characterized by fluctuating and progressive muscle rigidity with spasms. It may occur as an autoimmune or paraneoplastic process. Symptoms usually begin with stiffness of the axial and trunk muscles, with spread to the proximal limb muscles over time. Patients develop a lumbar hyperlordosis with restricted movements of the hip and spine that leads to the description of the gait as like that of a tin man. Superimposed on this background rigidity, they develop paroxysmal painful muscle spasms, often provoked by sudden movement or startle.

Diagnosis rests on the characteristic clinical profile and the demonstration of continuous motor unit activity without evidence of neuromyotonia, pyramidal or extrapyramidal dysfunction, or structural spinal cord disease. CSF is usually normal, and antibodies directed against glutamic acid decarboxylase (GAD) may be present.

Benzodiazepines and baclofen are the most useful antispasticity agents. The presence of anti-GAD antibodies and the occurrence of the stiff-man

■ TABLE 16-3

Therapeutic Strategies in Parkinson's Disease

Scenario/Problem	Therapeutic Approach
Initial treatment	Levodopa/decarboxylase inhibitor or dopamine agonist
Poor or no response to initial treatment	Increase dose and consider alternative diagnoses
Tremor-predominant disease	Anticholinergic or amantadine
Early-morning stiffness	Consider overnight controlled-release preparation of L-dopa
L-dopa–induced hallucinations	Discontinue concurrent therapy with anticholinergics, amantadine, selegiline, or dopamine agonists Decrease dose of levodopa Low-dose atypical antipsychotic
"Wearing off"	Combine levodopa and dopamine agonist Switch dopamine agonist Smaller doses, more frequent dosing Add anticholinergic Add COMT inhibitor
Dyskinesia	Reduce dose of levodopa Add or increase dose of dopamine agonist Change dopamine agonist Discontinue selegiline Add amantadine Consider surgery

syndrome as a paraneoplastic syndrome have led some to use immunosuppressive therapy (steroids, plasmapheresis, or intravenous immunoglobulins), with varying success.

KEY POINTS

1. Stiff-person syndrome is characterized by chronic axial muscle rigidity and stiffness with superimposed painful muscle spasms.
2. Stiff-person syndrome may be associated with anti-GAD antibodies.

■ TREMOR

Tremor is an involuntary rhythmic oscillation of a body part (arm, leg, head, jaw, lips, or palate). Tremor is described as **resting** (present while the body part is not moving), **postural** (emerges during sustained maintenance of a posture), or **action** (appears during a voluntary movement). Action tremor may increase as the target is approached (**intention** tremor). Common causes of the various types of tremors are summarized in Box 16-1.

Essential tremor (ET) is a condition in which postural tremor is the only symptom. It may begin at any age, develops insidiously, and progresses gradually. A family history is common but not invariable. ET almost always affects the hands but may also affect the head, face, voice, trunk, or legs. It is almost always bilateral. Improvement of the tremor with small quantities of alcohol is a characteristic feature.

BOX 16-1 TREMOR

Resting
  Idiopathic Parkinson's disease
  Other parkinsonian syndromes
Postural
  Essential tremor
  Physiological tremor
  Drugs (e.g., theophylline, β-agonists)
  Alcohol
Action
  Cerebellum and cerebellar outflow tract
    dysfunction (e.g., infarction, multiple sclerosis,
    tumor, Wilson's disease, drugs)

Primidone and propranolol are of proven benefit in the treatment of ET. Topiramate and gabapentin have also been used with some success.

KEY POINTS

1. Tremor is an involuntary rhythmic oscillation of a body part.
2. PD causes a resting tremor.
3. Essential tremor is the most common cause of postural tremor.
4. Action or intention tremor suggests disease of the cerebellum or its connections.

■ CHOREA

Chorea is defined as involuntary, abrupt, and irregular movements that flow as if randomly from one body part to another. Patients are often unaware of even severe chorea. One of the earliest symptoms may be clumsiness or incoordination. Involvement of bulbar muscles may cause dysarthria and dysphagia. Chorea is usually accompanied by an inability to maintain a sustained muscle contraction (motor impersistence). Classic examples include an inability to keep the tongue protruded (serpentine tongue) and the inability to maintain a tight handgrip (milkmaid grip).

There are many causes of chorea, and it is impossible to determine the etiology based simply on the phenomenology of the abnormal movements. It is necessary to consider the age and relative acuity of onset, the presence or absence of a family history, the presence of associated symptoms, and the distribution of the movements. The different causes are summarized in Box 16-2.

For treatment, haloperidol has been used with greatest success.

KEY POINTS

1. Chorea comprises involuntary, abrupt, and irregular movements that flow randomly from one body part to another.
2. Huntington's disease, poststreptococcal infection, systemic lupus erythematosus, thyrotoxicosis, and pregnancy are among the more common causes of chorea.

BOX 16-2	CHOREA

Hereditary
  Huntington's disease
  Neuro-acanthocytosis
  Wilson's disease
Drugs
  Neuroleptics
  Antiparkinsonian medications
Toxins
  Alcohol
  Anoxia
  Carbon monoxide
Metabolic
  Hyperthyroidism
  Hyperglycemia and hypoglycemia
  Hepatocerebral degeneration
Pregnancy
Immunologic
  Systemic lupus erythematosus
  Poststreptococcal (Sydenham's chorea)
Vascular
  Caudate infarction or hemorrhage

■ BALLISM

Ballism is defined as large-amplitude and poorly patterned flinging or flailing movements of a limb that are frequently unilateral (**hemiballismus**). It usually results from a contralateral lesion in the caudate, putamen, or subthalamic nucleus. Stroke is the most common cause.

Dopamine-depleting and blocking agents are the most useful treatment. When ballism is severe, contralateral thalamotomy or pallidotomy may be beneficial.

■ DYSTONIA

Dystonia is sustained muscle contraction leading to repetitive twisting movements or abnormal postures. The dystonias are classified as idiopathic or symptomatic. Recognition of secondary or symptomatic causes of dystonia is important because this may influence treatment.

A characteristic feature of dystonic movements is that they may be diminished by sensory tricks such as gently touching the affected body part (**geste antagoniste**). Dystonic movements tend to be exacerbated by fatigue, stress, and emotional states and may be suppressed by relaxation and sleep. Dystonia typically worsens during voluntary movement. At the time of onset, dystonia may be present only during a specific movement (action dystonia). With progression, however, the dystonia may emerge with other movements and eventually may be present at rest. Thus, dystonia at rest usually represents a more severe form than a pure action dystonia. Early onset of dystonia at rest should raise suspicion of an underlying cause ("secondary"). Other clinical features suggesting that the dystonia is symptomatic include the presence of associated neurologic abnormalities or involvement of one side of the body only (hemidystonia).

Idiopathic torsion dystonia is a primary dystonia and may occur as a familial condition. The spectrum of the disorder is broad and includes focal (blepharospasm, torticollis, spasmodic dysphonia, writer's cramp), segmental, and generalized forms. The gene for the autosomal dominant familial form has been located on chromosome 9q, and mutations have been identified in the ATP-binding protein designated *torsin A*. Botulinum toxin is the treatment of choice.

Secondary causes of dystonia include metabolic disorders (e.g., Wilson's disease), degenerative diseases (PD, progressive supranuclear palsy, corticobasal ganglionic degeneration, Huntington's disease, multiple-system atrophy), and nondegenerative CNS disorders (anoxia, head or peripheral trauma, prior stroke, multiple sclerosis, or drug-induced).

KEY POINTS

1. Dystonia is a sustained muscle contraction leading to repetitive twisting movements or abnormal postures.
2. Idiopathic torsion dystonia is a familial condition that may manifest as torticollis, writer's cramp, blepharospasm, or spasmodic dysphonia.

MYOCLONUS

Myoclonus is a sudden lightning-like movement produced by abrupt and brief muscle contraction (positive myoclonus) or inhibition (negative myoclonus or asterixis).

The four etiologic categories are essential, physiologic, epileptic, and symptomatic. **Essential** myoclonus is a nonphysiologic variety that occurs in isolation without evidence of other neurologic symptoms or signs. It may occur in familial and sporadic forms.

BOX 16-3 MYOCLONUS

Physiologic
  Hypnic jerks
  Anxiety and exercise induced
  Hiccups
Essential
Epileptic
  Primary generalized epilepsies (e.g., juvenile myoclonic epilepsy)
  Myoclonic epilepsies (often associated with encephalopathy or ataxia)
Symptomatic
  Metabolic encephalopathy (uremia, liver failure, hypercapnia)
  Wilson's disease
  Creutzfeldt-Jakob disease
  Hypoxic brain injury

Some patients may note a striking improvement with small quantities of alcohol. The causes of the other varieties of myoclonus are summarized in Box 16-3.

Clonazepam and valproate are used with greatest success in the management of myoclonus.

KEY POINTS

1. Myoclonus is a sudden, lightning-like movement produced by abrupt and brief muscle contraction.
2. Clonazepam is the most effective treatment for many patients.

TICS

Tics are abrupt, stereotyped, coordinated movements or vocalizations. They may vary in intensity and be repeated at irregular intervals. The individual will frequently describe an inner urge to move, may be able to suppress the movement temporarily at the expense of mounting inner tension, and then obtain relief from the performance of the movement or vocalization. Tics may be exacerbated by stress and relieved by distraction.

Tics may be motor or vocal and are classified as being either simple or complex. Examples of simple motor tics include eye blinking, shoulder shrugging, and toe curling. Spitting and finger cracking are examples of complex motor tics. Simple vocal tics may take the form of sniffing, throat clearing, snorting, or coughing. The best-recognized example of a complex vocal tic is coprolalia (involuntary obscene utterances). Tics may also be classified as idiopathic (the majority) or secondary. Secondary causes include head trauma, encephalitis, stroke, and various drugs.

Gille de la Tourette's syndrome is a genetic disorder characterized by motor and vocal tics with onset in childhood. Boys are affected more than girls, although there is some suggestion that obsessive-compulsive disorder (OCD) may represent the phenotypic expression of the same genetic defect in girls. The motor and vocal tics may change over time. There is a trend toward periodic remission and exacerbation. In general, the disease is most active in adolescence and tends to diminish in severity during adulthood. There is an association with learning disability and OCD.

Pediatric autoimmune neurologic disorders associated with streptococcal infection (PANDAS) is a relatively recently described syndrome in which children develop exacerbation of tics, OCD, or both following a group A β-hemolytic streptococcal infection. The proposed, although unproved, etiology is that the streptococcal infection triggers an autoantibody response that cross-reacts with components of the basal ganglia in susceptible individuals.

For treatment of tics, dopamine antagonists (haloperidol or the atypical antipsychotics) are most effective. Because of the adverse effect profile of these agents, however, less potent drugs such as clonazepam and clonidine should be tried first.

KEY POINTS

1. Tics are abrupt, stereotyped, coordinated movements or vocalizations.
2. Tourette's syndrome is a common genetic disorder with onset of motor and vocal tics in childhood.
3. Dopamine antagonists are often the most effective therapy for tics.

■ WILSON'S DISEASE

WD is an autosomal recessive disorder of copper metabolism. The clinical presentation is usually with liver dysfunction and neuropsychiatric symptoms.

WD results from mutation of a copper-binding protein, dysfunction of which results in impaired conjugation of copper to ceruloplasmin and entry of copper into the biliary excretory pathway. This results in accumulation of copper within the liver and spillover into the systemic circulation, with deposition in the kidney, cornea, and CNS.

Neurologic manifestations of WD include tremor, ataxia, dysarthria, dyskinesia, parkinsonism, and cognitive dysfunction as well as disturbances of mood and personality. The Kayser-Fleischer ring is a golden brown or greenish discoloration in the limbic region of the cornea that results from copper deposition in Descemet's membrane. Kayser-Fleischer rings are almost invariably present in untreated patients with neurologic involvement.

In diagnosing WD, increased serum copper and decreased serum ceruloplasmin levels are expected but not always present. Increased 24-hour urinary copper excretion is the most sensitive screening test. Diagnosis may be confirmed by demonstrating increased copper staining on liver biopsy. Examination by an ophthalmologist for Kayser-Fleischer rings can be very helpful.

Copper chelation with D-penicillamine has been the traditional therapy for WD. More recently, there has been a trend toward using a less toxic chelator, trientine, in conjunction with zinc. Therapy is lifelong. Given the inherited nature of this disorder, family members of an affected individual should be screened.

KEY POINTS

1. Wilson's disease is a disorder of copper metabolism.
2. Hyperkinetic and hypokinetic movement disorders as well as cognitive, personality, and mood disturbances are the most common neurologic manifestations of WD.
3. Kayser-Fleischer rings represent copper deposition in the cornea.
4. Elevated serum copper levels, low ceruloplasmin levels, and elevated 24-hour urinary copper are useful screening tests.

■ PAROXYSMAL DYSKINESIAS

The paroxysmal dyskinesias are a rare group of movement disorders characterized by recurrent attacks of hyperkinesis with preserved consciousness. In paroxysmal kinesogenic choreoathetosis (PKC), episodes of chorea, athetosis, or dystonia are triggered by sudden movements and last for seconds to minutes. Attacks of paroxysmal (nonkinesogenic) dystonic choreoathetosis (PDC) are longer, lasting minutes to hours, and are triggered by alcohol, fatigue, and stress. In paroxysmal exercise-induced dystonia, episodes of dystonia are induced by sustained exercise and may persist for a number of hours. PKC is most effectively treated with agents such as carbamazepine.

17 Head Trauma

Trauma is the leading cause of mortality and morbidity for people aged 1 to 44 years in the United States. Head injury can result in seizures, permanent physical disability, or cognitive impairment. In more than half of trauma-related deaths, head injury is a significant contributor to mortality. There are approximately 500,000 new cases of traumatic brain injury per year in the United States; these figures do not include the cases that do not come to medical attention. Of the 500,000 patients with traumatic brain injury, approximately 50,000 die before reaching the hospital. Of the remaining patients, 80% have mild injury and 10% each have either moderate or severe injury.

Despite the serious nature of injury, mortality associated with severe head injury has decreased from 50% in the 1970s to 30% in the 1990s. The improvement is thought to be due in part to widespread use of CT scanners, establishment of trauma centers, better-trained medical personnel, and aggressive neurocritical care. In order to manage the patient with traumatic brain injury, it is important to be able to recognize the type of brain injury and to classify the severity of injury.

■ CLASSIFICATION

The most commonly used scale to classify the degree of severity of brain injury is the Glasgow Coma Scale (GCS) (Table 17-1). The GCS score is the sum of three scores (eye opening, best verbal response, and best motor response). The maximum score is 15; the minimum is 3. Head injury is classified as mild if the GCS score is 14 to 15, moderate if 9 to 13, and severe if 3 to 8. This classification combined with the type of cerebral injury helps to determine the prognosis.

■ INITIAL MANAGEMENT

As for all patients in the emergency ward, the initial assessment and management of a patient with traumatic brain injury focuses on airway protection, breathing, and circulation. Most patients with severe brain injury have damage to at least one other system. Thus, while the patient is being stabilized with respect to the respiratory and cardiovascular systems, a general medical examination should be conducted. Particular attention should be paid to signs of basal skull fracture, such as raccoon's eyes (periorbital ecchymoses), Battle's sign (postauricular ecchymoses), hemotympanum, or signs of CSF leakage from the nose or ear. Initially, the neurologic examination should focus on the level of consciousness as measured by the GCS, pupillary light reflexes, and extraocular movements. After the patient's cardiovascular status is stabilized, a more detailed neurologic examination should be performed.

KEY POINTS

1. The GCS is used to classify the severity of traumatic brain injury.
2. Initial management is aimed at stabilizing the patient's respiratory and cardiovascular status.

■ TYPES OF BRAIN INJURIES

After the history is obtained and an examination performed, all patients with focal neurologic abnormalities on exam or who have a GCS score of less than 15 should have a head CT scan. A noncontrast CT scan of the head is particularly sensitive in detecting

TABLE 17-1

Glasgow Coma Scale

Points	Best Eye Opening	Best Verbal	Best Motor
6	—	—	Obeys commands
5	—	Oriented	Localizes pain
4	Spontaneous	Confused	Withdraws to pain
3	To speech	Inappropriate	Decorticate posturing
2	To pain	Incomprehensible	Decerebrate posturing
1	None	None	None

hemorrhage. Patients who are older than 14 years with a perfect GCS score of 15, no loss of consciousness, and a normal neurologic examination can be discharged home without further testing provided that there is someone at home who can observe the patient for signs of deterioration.

For patients with a focal neurologic exam or a GCS score less than 15, the CT scan along with the neurologic exam will help determine the type and severity of injury to the brain. The major types of cerebral injuries are described below. Obvious lesions such as penetrating wounds from gunshot and stabbing are not covered here.

Acute Subdural Hematoma

Acute subdural hematoma (Figure 17-1) is the most common focal intracerebral lesion in patients with severe brain injury, with an incidence of approximately 30%. Tearing of the bridging veins between the cerebral cortex and the venous sinuses causes subdural hematomas and can occur spontaneously or with mild trauma, particularly in older people. Traumatic subdural hematomas are often associated with cerebral contusions, intracerebral hematomas, and brain lacerations. Acute subdural hematomas can be associated with high morbidity and mortality due to parenchymal damage underlying the hematoma and raised intracranial pressure caused by the additional volume occupied by the hematoma. Presentation can be varied and can include focal neurologic deficits, headache, or altered mental status.

Epidural Hematoma

In the majority of cases, epidural hematoma results from a skull fracture that lacerates the middle meningeal artery and causes accumulation of blood between the dura and the skull. The classic presentation of a patient with an epidural hematoma is brief loss of consciousness followed by a lucid interval for several hours and then deterioration in the level of consciousness, with hemiparesis on the side opposite the hematoma as well as ipsilateral pupillary dilation. On CT, scan, epidural hematomas are hyperdense with a biconvex (lenticular) shape (Figure 17-2). Usually, patients require emergency surgery. Mortality and

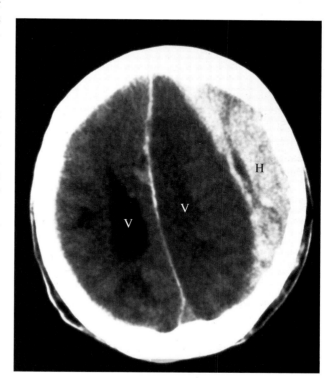

Figure 17-1 • Typical CT scan appearance of a large subdural hematoma (H) on the left cerebral hemisphere with compression of the lateral ventricle (V) and shift of the midline. (Reproduced with permission from Armstrong P, Wastie M, Rockall A. Diagnostic Imaging. 5th ed. Oxford: Blackwell Publishing, 2004:416.)

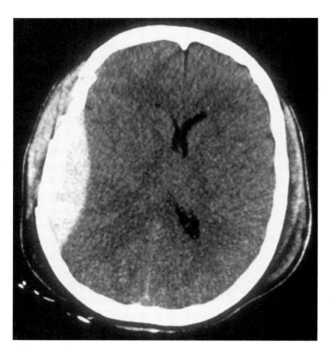

Figure 17-2 • CT scan of the head demonstrating the typical hyperdense lens-shaped appearance of an epidural hematoma. (Courtesy of David M. Dawson, MD, Brigham and Women's Hospital, Boston, MA.)

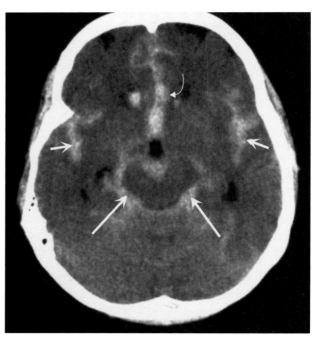

Figure 17-3 • Subarachnoid hemorrhage demonstrated on CT scan of the brain characterized by hyperdensity in the subarachnoid space. The blood outlines the brainstem in the basal cisterns (long arrows), sylvian fissures (short arrows), and falx (curved arrow). (Reproduced with permission from Armstrong P, Wastie M, Rockall A. Diagnostic Imaging. 5th ed. Oxford: Blackwell Publishing, 2004:410.)

morbidity are relatively low (5 to 10%) provided the hematoma is diagnosed and treated with surgical drainage within a few hours.

Contusions

Contusions and intracerebral hematomas are a continuum and are high-density areas on head CT, representing bruises of the brain parenchyma. As such, they typically occur in areas where sudden deceleration of the head causes the brain to impact on bony prominences. Therefore the majority of contusions occurs in the inferior frontal or temporal lobes. Contusions are sometimes described as **coup** (abnormalities seen directly below the site of impact) and **contrecoup** (abnormalities located on the opposite side of the brain as it is thrust against the skull). These patients are typically followed clinically and with follow-up head CT scans. Surgery is reserved for patients with significant mass effect and clinical deterioration.

Subarachnoid Hemorrhage

SAH is caused by bleeding into the subarachnoid space (Figure 17-3). Head trauma is the most common cause

of SAH. In patients with traumatic brain injury, SAH is usually found in association with either contusions or hematomas. Management of patients with SAH involves monitoring for cerebral vasospasm, increased intracranial pressure (ICP), and acute hydrocephalus (for further discussion, see Chapter 14).

Diffuse Axonal Injury

Diffuse axonal injury or diffuse axonal shearing is a lesion caused by rotational acceleration and deceleration of the head. This is most commonly seen with patients who have been injured in motor vehicle accidents. It is also the most common presumed cause of coma in patients with closed head injury in the absence of cerebral hemorrhage or other space-occupying lesion on head CT scan. Diffuse axonal injury is characterized by gross and microscopic axonal changes in the cerebral white matter and small hemorrhagic lesions of the corpus callosum and brainstem (Duret hemorrhages).

KEY POINTS

1. Subdural hematoma is the most common intra-cerebral lesion in patients with severe traumatic brain injury.
2. Epidural hematoma results from bleeding from the middle meningeal artery; this is usually a surgical emergency.
3. Contusions can be described as coup and contre-coup.
4. Contusions typically occur at the inferior frontal lobes or temporal lobes.
5. Subarachnoid hemorrhage can result in cerebral vasospasm, hydrocephalus, and increased ICP.

■ HERNIATION SYNDROMES

The cranial cavity is essentially a closed space with a set volume that must contain the brain parenchyma, blood supply to the brain, and CSF. If a mass lesion is present, either from tumor or blood, ICP will rise because the total volume is constant. The rise in ICP occurs after initial compensatory mechanisms, such as squeezing out of venous blood and CSF, have failed. Once ICP starts to rise, it does so in an exponential fashion. As ICP continues to rise, it results in distortion and displacement of the brain, which can in turn result in compression of critical brain structures, giving rise to the following herniation syndromes.

Uncal (Tentorial) Herniation

Uncal herniation occurs with mass lesions of the middle cranial fossa. The uncus, the inferomedial portion of the temporal lobe, herniates downward into the posterior fossa between the rostral brainstem and the tentorium cerebelli. Typically, the third cranial nerve is entrapped, resulting in a unilateral dilated pupil. As the herniation progresses, hemiparesis and alteration of consciousness can occur, with eventual brainstem signs and changes in respiratory patterns. In the latter stages of herniation, death is imminent.

Cingulate Herniation

Cingulate herniation occurs when there is a mass lesion, usually in the frontal lobes, causing displacement of the cingulate gyrus across the falx cerebri in the frontal midline. There are no specific signs or symptoms of this type of herniation, but it can frequently be seen on CT scan.

Central (Transtentorial) Herniation

Central herniation occurs when a large supratentorial mass causes downward displacement of the diencephalon and midbrain through the tentorial opening. Clinical findings include altered consciousness, bilateral small reactive pupils, and decorticate posturing followed by decerebrate posturing. Cheyne-Stokes respirations (crescendo-decrescendo pattern followed by a respiratory pause) can be seen. Cheyne-Stokes respirations are nonspecific and imply bilateral cerebral dysfunction from a variety of causes ranging from increased ICP to an underlying metabolic abnormality. In the terminal stage, tone is flaccid and respirations become slow and irregular.

Tonsillar Herniation

Tonsillar herniation occurs when a posterior fossa mass causes herniation of the cerebellar tonsils through the foramen magnum. The cerebellar tonsils compress the medulla, resulting in eventual respiratory arrest. Usually, tonsillar herniation is rapidly fatal.

KEY POINTS

1. The four major herniation syndromes are cingulate, uncal (tentorial), central (transtentorial), and tonsillar.
2. Uncal herniation is commonly recognized by a unilateral dilated pupil.
3. Herniation is a medical emergency requiring prompt recognition and management.

■ MANAGEMENT OF HEAD INJURY AND RAISED ICP

Once a patient is discovered to have a hemorrhage or herniation syndrome, consultations with neurology and neurosurgery should be obtained for further management of the patient. In addition to the initial management decisions of the patient with head injury described earlier in this chapter, the patient should have an urgent CT scan of the head if herniation or increased ICP is suspected. If suspicion for a herniation syndrome or increased ICP is high, the head of the patient's bed should be elevated to greater than 30 degrees in order to displace CSF. In addition, the patient should be hyperventilated to achieve a P_{CO_2} between 25 and 30 mm Hg, which causes cerebral vasoconstriction and a reduction of intracranial volume, which in turn decreases ICP. Both of these interventions are effective short-term measures that reduce ICP within minutes. Additionally, mannitol (0.25–2.0 g/kg) can be administered. This is an osmotic diuretic that decreases intracranial volume and pressure temporarily. Additionally, a loop diuretic, such as furosemide (20–40 mg), can cause additional diuresis. Both of these medications are effective short-term treatments for raised ICP; the effects are seen within a half hour to 1 hour. It must be remembered that these measures treat the symptoms of increased ICP causing herniation but that the underlying cause may need to be treated in additional ways. For example, a large parenchymal hemorrhage or epidural hematoma will likely require surgical drainage or placement of a shunt. Additionally, if raised ICP is caused by a tumor with surrounding edema, corticosteroids such as dexamethasone can be administered at a dose of 16 mg/day divided into a two- or four-times-per-day dosing schedule. Corticosteroids are effective in reducing ICP caused by vasogenic edema surrounding a tumor, but this may take days. There are also potential complications of steroid use, such as gastrointestinal ulcers and bleeding, myopathy, hyperglycemia, behavioral changes, avascular necrosis of the hip, and increased susceptibility to infections.

Systemic and Metabolic Disorders

The CNS and peripheral nervous system may be affected by a range of systemic and metabolic diseases. A few of these disorders have been selected for more detailed description in this chapter. Table 18-1 summarizes the more common neurologic manifestations of some systemic disorders that are not discussed below.

■ HEPATIC ENCEPHALOPATHY

"Hepatic encephalopathy" is a general term used to describe the altered mental state that accompanies liver failure. It encompasses two entities: the encephalopathy of fulminant hepatic failure and the portosystemic encephalopathy that is associated with cirrhosis and portal hypertension or that may develop following portacaval shunting.

Clinical Manifestations

The encephalopathy of fulminant hepatic failure progresses rapidly, within days, from mild inattention to stupor and coma. The essential feature of portosystemic encephalopathy is the presence of waxing and waning cerebral dysfunction in the setting of liver failure. Traditionally, hepatic encephalopathy is graded in severity on a scale from 0 (normal) to 4 (coma). The intermediate stages are characterized by impaired attention and concentration, altered sleep patterns, abnormal visuospatial perception, and subtle personality changes. Asterixis (negative myoclonus) is usually present. Other neurologic findings may include increased muscle tone, hyperreflexia, and extensor plantar responses.

■ TABLE 18-1

Neurologic Manifestations of Systemic Disease

Disease	Manifestations
Polyarteritis nodosa	Mononeuropathy multiplex, seizures, stroke
Churg-Strauss	Mononeuropathy multiplex, encephalopathy, stroke, chorea
Giant cell arteritis	Headache, blindness, polyneuropathy, stroke
Wegener's granulomatosis	Mononeuropathy multiplex, cranial neuropathy, basal meningitis
Rheumatoid arthritis	Myelopathy
Sjögren's syndrome	Sensory polyneuropathy
Behçet's disease	Aseptic meningoencephalitis
Cryoglobulinemia	Transient ischemic attack, stroke, peripheral neuropathy
Disseminated intravascular coagulation	Encephalopathy
Thrombotic thrombocytopenic purpura	Encephalopathy, seizures, stroke
Whipple's disease	Dementia, seizures, myoclonus, ataxia, supranuclear ophthalmoplegia, oculomasticatory myorhythmia

Pathogenesis

The pathophysiology of hepatic encephalopathy is incompletely understood but is thought to result from the accumulation of neurotoxic substances (e.g., ammonia), leading to increased brain glutamine concentrations, depressed glutamatergic neurotransmission, and increased expression of the peripheral-type benzodiazepine receptors. Manganese deposition in the basal ganglia may also play a pathogenic role.

Pathology

The Alzheimer type II astrocyte is the pathologic hallmark of this disorder. These astrocytes appear to be metabolically hyperactive, which has led to the suggestion that hepatic encephalopathy is a primary astrocytopathy.

Diagnostic Evaluation

The diagnosis is usually suspected clinically on the basis of the encephalopathy in the context of liver failure. Hepatic synthetic function is impaired, with low serum albumin and prolonged prothrombin time (PT) and partial thromboplastin time (PTT). The EEG usually shows background slowing and may demonstrate triphasic waves, and MRI may reveal increased T1 signal in the basal ganglia, but these findings are not specific. In a patient with known liver disease who develops encephalopathy, it is important to identify underlying precipitating factors such as gastrointestinal hemorrhage, infection, increased dietary protein intake, drugs, constipation, or hypokalemia.

Treatment

Treatment should be directed toward the underlying cause of the liver disease when possible and to the alleviation of precipitating factors. Lactulose, titrated to produce two to three stools per day, is the mainstay of symptomatic therapy.

KEY POINTS

1. The essential feature of portosystemic encephalopathy is the presence of waxing and waning cerebral dysfunction in the setting of liver failure.
2. Asterixis is frequently present.
3. Hepatic encephalopathy is thought to be a primary astrocytopathy.
4. Lactulose and the treatment of precipitating factors are the mainstays of therapy.

■ NEUROSARCOIDOSIS

Sarcoidosis is a multisystem granulomatous disorder of unknown etiology. Pulmonary disease is most common, and involvement of the nervous system occurs in around 5% of cases. It is very uncommon for sarcoidosis to involve the nervous system in the absence of other systemic disease.

Clinical Manifestations

Sarcoidosis may involve almost any part of the CNS or the peripheral nervous system. Cranial neuropathy due to chronic basal meningitis is the most common presentation of neurosarcoidosis, with the facial and optic nerves most frequently affected. Facial neuropathy may also occur due to parotid inflammation. Visual changes are common and may be due to direct involvement of the optic nerve or its meningeal covering or to uveitis. Raised intracranial pressure with papilledema may result from a space-occupying lesion, diffuse meningeal involvement, or hydrocephalus. Meningoencephalitis may manifest itself with cognitive and affective symptoms, and hypothalamic involvement may cause hypopituitarism, diabetes insipidus, sleep disturbance, obesity, and thermoregulatory disturbance. Space-occupying lesions may become apparent because of seizures or focal deficits. Myelopathy may result from an infiltrating or focal granulomatous process. Peripheral nerve involvement may become manifest as a symmetric distal polyneuropathy or mononeuropathy multiplex.

Pathology

The typical pathology is that of noncaseating granulomata.

Diagnostic Evaluation

Definitive diagnosis of neurosarcoidosis requires positive histology from affected tissue. Since there is often reluctance to obtain brain parenchymal or meningeal biopsy, the diagnosis is often presumptive, based on a consistent clinical presentation and histology from an alternative site. CSF is frequently abnormal, with elevated protein and lymphocytic pleocytosis, but it may be normal in the context of focal parenchymal disease. Serum angiotensin converting enzyme (ACE) concentration may be elevated. CSF ACE levels are often difficult to interpret in the context of elevated CSF protein. MRI may demonstrate white matter lesions, hydrocephalus, parenchymal mass lesion, nodular meningeal enhancement, or involvement of the optic nerve or spinal cord.

Treatment

Steroids are the mainstay of therapy. Although used often, there are limited data regarding the use of steroid-sparing agents such as methotrexate and azathioprine.

KEY POINTS

1. Sarcoidosis is a multisystem granulomatous disorder.
2. The nervous system is mostly affected in conjunction with systemic disease, but it may be affected in isolation.
3. Cranial neuropathy and basal meningitis are common.

■ DIABETES MELLITUS

Diabetes mellitus is common in patients with neurologic disease, primarily because the nervous system is susceptible to the damaging effects of impaired glycemic control. However, there are also a number of disorders that are characterized by both diabetes and neurologic symptoms. These include mitochondrial diseases, myotonic dystrophy, Friedreich's ataxia, and the stiff-man syndrome.

Peripheral neuropathy is the most common complication of diabetes mellitus and takes many forms (Box 18-1). Distal symmetric sensory polyneuropathy is the most common. Onset of this neuropathy is insidious, and it may often be asymptomatic. There is a predilection for involvement of small myelinated and unmyelinated fibers, with the result that loss of temperature and pinprick sensation are the most commonly reported symptoms. There may be associated distal motor neuropathy, but it is invariably minor. Once established, this neuropathy is largely irreversible. The incidence of this complication is reduced in type 1 diabetic patients by strict glycemic control. There is frequently an associated autonomic neuropathy, the common symptoms of which include gustatory sweating, orthostatic hypotension, diarrhea, and impotence. Neurogenic bladder and gastroparesis occur less frequently.

BOX 18-1 DIABETIC NEUROPATHIES

Hyperglycemic neuropathy
Generalized neuropathies
    Distal symmetric predominantly sensory
      polyneuropathy
    Autonomic neuropathy
    Chronic inflammatory demyelinating
      polyradiculopathy (CIDP)
Focal neuropathies
    Cranial neuropathies (especially III, IV, and VI)
    Thoracolumbar radiculopathy
    Focal compression and entrapment neuropathies
    Proximal diabetic neuropathy (diabetic amyotrophy)
    Mononeuropathy multiplex

Focal peripheral neuropathies also occur more commonly in diabetic patients. These include cranial neuropathies (most commonly affecting cranial nerves III, IV, and VI) and focal compression neuropathies, such as distal median neuropathies (carpal tunnel) and meralgia paresthetica (compression of the lateral cutaneous nerve of the thigh). Radiculopathy, especially thoracic, occurs with greater frequency in diabetic patients. Typically, these radiculopathies manifest with nonradicular pain, truncal sensory loss, and focal weakness of the muscles of the anterior abdominal wall. Spontaneous recovery usually occurs within a few months.

The entity of proximal diabetic neuropathy is well recognized but poorly understood. Another term that has been used to describe at least some of the patients with this disorder is **diabetic amyotrophy.** At least some of these proximal neuropathies are immune-mediated, perhaps involving a vasculitis, and respond to treatment with steroids and other immunosuppressive therapies. Finally, chronic inflammatory demyelinating polyradiculopathy (CIDP) occurs more commonly in patients with diabetes.

Hyperglycemia may affect both the peripheral nervous system and the CNS. There is a syndrome of an acute distal sensory neuropathy that presents with dysesthesias and pain in the feet. This typically resolves with establishment of the euglycemic state. Nonketotic hyperglycemia (common in type 2 diabetes mellitus) may produce lethargy and drowsiness as well as focal or generalized seizures. An uncommon manifestation of nonketotic hyperglycemia is a syndrome of dystonia and chorea associated with reversible T1 signal hyperintensity in the basal ganglia. Finally, cerebral edema may complicate diabetic ketoacidosis. Children are particularly susceptible to this potentially fatal complication.

Many of the symptoms of hypoglycemia are referable to the nervous system, including headache, blurred vision, dysarthria, confusion, seizures, and coma. Repeated episodes of hypoglycemia may produce injury to the anterior horn cells of the spinal cord and result in a syndrome similar to amyotrophic lateral sclerosis. Recurrent and prolonged hypoglycemia may also lead to the development of permanent cognitive deficits.

Cerebrovascular disease (TIAs and stroke) is more common in diabetic patients, with hypertension being the main risk factor for stroke among patients with diabetes. Most ischemic strokes in diabetic patients are due to intracranial small vessel disease (lacunar stroke).

KEY POINTS

1. Distal, primarily sensory polyneuropathy is the most common neurologic complication of diabetes.
2. Hyperglycemia may cause seizures, focal neurologic deficit, transient painful peripheral neuropathy, and occasionally chorea.
3. Stroke occurs more commonly in diabetic patients.

■ ALCOHOL AND NUTRITIONAL DISORDERS

Alcohol may affect the nervous system adversely in many ways (Table 18-2), and the manifestations of vitamin deficiency (Table 18-3) are frequently associated with alcoholism. Two of the better-known syndromes that result from alcohol abuse and vitamin deficiency are presented in more detail below.

Wernicke's Encephalopathy and Korsakoff's Syndrome

Wernicke's encephalopathy and Korsakoff's syndrome are related conditions that represent different stages of the same pathologic process. Wernicke's encephalopathy is characterized by the clinical triad of ophthalmoplegia, (truncal) ataxia, and confusion developing over a period of days to weeks. Associated signs and symptoms include impaired pupillary light response, hypothermia, postural hypotension, and other evidence of nutritional deficiency. The syndrome results from a deficiency of thiamine and may be precipitated by the administration of intravenous glucose. It is a clinical diagnosis and warrants immediate therapy with intravenous thiamine. Untreated, the condition is progressive and the mortality is high. Following the administration of thiamine, the ocular signs can resolve within hours and the confusion over days to weeks. The gait ataxia may persist. Once the global confusion has receded, isolated memory deficits may persist (Korsakoff's syndrome).

Subacute Combined Degeneration of the Spinal Cord

Subacute combined degeneration of the spinal cord results from vitamin B_{12} deficiency and derives its name from the degeneration of the posterior and lateral white matter tracts of the spinal cord. The

■ TABLE 18-2

Effects of Alcohol on the Nervous System

Condition	Manifestations
Peripheral neuropathy	Distal sensorimotor axonal neuropathy; recovery with abstinence is slow and incomplete
Cerebellar degeneration	Gait ataxia greater than limb ataxia, dysarthria, no nystagmus
Tobacco-alcohol amblyopia	Insidious and painless loss of vision; centrocecal scotoma
Marchiafava-Bignami syndrome	Frontal-type dementia, seizures, and pyramidal signs; focal demyelination and necrosis of corpus callosum
Acute intoxication	Impaired cognition, ataxia, dysarthria, nystagmus, diplopia
Acute withdrawal	Agitation, insomnia, tremulousness, hallucinations, seizures
Wernicke's encephalopathy	Confusion, ataxia, ophthalmoplegia
Korsakoff's syndrome	Isolated memory disturbance with confabulation

TABLE 18-3

Vitamin Deficiency Syndromes

Symptom	Deficient Vitamin
Confusion and encephalopathy	Thiamine, niacin
Dementia	Vitamin B_{12}, folate, niacin
Seizures	Pyridoxine, niacin
Ataxia	Vitamin E, niacin
Myelopathy	Vitamins B_{12} and E, niacin
Peripheral neuropathy	Thiamine, pyridoxine, vitamins B_{12} and E, niacin

clinical manifestations reflect disease within the dorsal columns and the lateral corticospinal tracts. The presentation is usually with insidious onset of paresthesias in the hands and feet. With time, weakness and spasticity may develop in the legs. Frequently, there is an associated large-fiber peripheral neuropathy (also due to the B_{12} deficiency). Hematologic abnormalities (macrocytic anemia) are variably present. Normal serum B_{12} levels do not preclude the diagnosis, and it may be necessary to measure levels of serum homocysteine and methylmalonic acid, the precursors of B_{12} (which are elevated when B_{12} is deficient). With B_{12} replacement therapy, partial improvement may be expected. Since folate is a necessary component to the B_{12} synthetic pathway, its deficiency (theoretically) may cause the same deficits as B_{12} deficiency. Typically, however, the hematologic abnormalities occur in isolation.

KEY POINTS

1. Wernicke's encephalopathy is characterized by the triad of confusion, ataxia, and ophthalmoplegia.
2. Subacute combined degeneration of the spinal cord refers to the damaging effects of vitamin B_{12} deficiency on the posterior and lateral columns of the spinal cord.

■ SYSTEMIC LUPUS ERYTHEMATOSUS

Systemic lupus erythematosus (SLE) is an inflammatory connective tissue disorder of unknown etiology. It occurs predominantly in young women, and neurologic involvement is common.

Clinical Manifestations

The neurologic manifestations of SLE are diverse, with both the peripheral nervous system and CNS affected. Neuropsychiatric manifestations, including psychosis and affective disorders, are most common, although their pathophysiology remains uncertain. Stroke, both venous and arterial, may result from the hypercoagulable state associated with antiphospholipid antibodies. Chorea and transverse myelitis may occur similarly in association with antiphospholipid antibodies. Headaches and seizures are other important symptoms of CNS dysfunction in SLE. The most common manifestation of peripheral nervous system involvement is a distal symmetric sensory polyneuropathy, although a mononeuropathy multiplex due to vasculitis may also occur.

Diagnostic Evaluation

The recognition that neurologic dysfunction is due to SLE is greatly facilitated by the presence of concurrent systemic manifestations (including but not limited to symmetric small joint arthritis, characteristic malar rash, proteinuria, etc.). Antinuclear antibody (ANA) titers are elevated in most patients with SLE. Isolated CNS lupus, manifesting with psychosis or depression, can be extremely difficult to recognize, as there is no diagnostic test.

Treatment

Treatment may be symptomatic (e.g., anticonvulsants for seizures) or directed at the underlying immune/inflammatory process. The decision to use immunosuppressant therapy depends on the severity of the disease but is usually warranted for neurologic manifestations. Corticosteroids, often in conjunction with cyclophosphamide, are the mainstay of therapy.

KEY POINTS

1. Neuropsychiatric manifestations of SLE, including psychosis and depression, are most common.
2. Other manifestations of CNS involvement include seizures, stroke, headache, chorea, and transverse myelitis.
3. Distal sensory polyneuropathy is the most common manifestation of peripheral nervous system involvement.

ANTIPHOSPHOLIPID SYNDROME

The antiphospholipid syndrome (APS) is a disorder in which venous or arterial thrombosis, recurrent fetal loss, and thrombocytopenia are associated with elevated titers of antibodies directed against phospholipids. The presence of these antibodies may be demonstrated by solid-phase immunoassay (e.g., anticardiolipin antibody) or by the in vitro prolongation of the partial thromboplastin time (lupus anticoagulant). The APS may occur in isolation (primary APS) or in association with an underlying autoimmune disorder, most commonly systemic lupus erythematosus (secondary APS). Involvement of the nervous system is not uncommon in the antiphospholipid syndrome.

Clinical Manifestations

Most thrombotic episodes in patients with antiphospholipid antibodies are venous; however, when thrombosis does occur in the arterial circulation, the brain is most commonly affected. Both small- and large-vessel stroke have been reported, and cardiac embolism may result in embolic stroke. In Sneddon's syndrome, cerebral ischemia and livedo reticularis are associated.

Diagnostic Evaluation

Antiphospholipid antibodies should be sought in young patients with stroke or in those with otherwise unexplained stroke, especially if any of the other features of the antiphospholipid syndrome are present. Diagnosis requires the demonstration of high-titer IgG antiphospholipid antibodies on two occasions at least 6 weeks apart.

Treatment

Long-term anticoagulation with warfarin to achieve an international normalized ratio (INR) of 3 to 4 is the recommended therapy.

KEY POINTS

1. Venous and arterial thrombosis, recurrent fetal loss, and thrombocytopenia are the major features of the antiphospholipid syndrome.
2. "Antiphospholipid antibody" is a general term that encompasses the lupus anticoagulant, anticardiolipin antibodies, and antibodies directed against a mixture of various phospholipids.
3. Anticoagulation is the treatment of choice for antiphospholipid-associated stroke.

THYROID DISEASE AND THE NERVOUS SYSTEM

The nervous system is more commonly affected by hypothyroidism than by hyperthyroidism. Neurologic signs and symptoms are very rarely the only manifestations of thyroid disease. The periodic paralyses and proximal myopathy associated with the hyperthyroid state are discussed in Chapter 24. Seizures, chorea, and dysthyroid eye disease may also result from hyperthyroidism, and there is an association with myasthenia gravis. The range of neurologic manifestations of hypothyroidism is summarized in Box 18-2.

CENTRAL PONTINE MYELINOLYSIS

Central pontine myelinolysis is a rare demyelinating disorder that occurs most often in alcoholic patients and may be precipitated by too rapid correction of hyponatremia. As the name indicates, the pons is most commonly affected, but the basal ganglia, thalamus, and subcortical white matter may also be involved. The clinical presentation includes an acute confusional state, spastic quadriparesis, locked-in syndrome, dysarthria, and dysphagia.

BOX 18-2 NEUROLOGIC MANIFESTATIONS OF HYPOTHYROIDISM

Mental state: Poor concentration and memory, dementia, psychosis, coma

Seizures

Headaches: Pseudotumor cerebri

Cranial nerves: Papilledema, ptosis, tonic pupil, trigeminal neuralgia, facial palsy, tinnitus, hearing loss

Cerebellar ataxia: Truncal and gait ataxia more than limb ataxia; dysarthria; nystagmus

Muscles: Cramps, pain and stiffness; proximal more than distal; creatine kinase level may be markedly increased

Neuromuscular junction: Worsening of myasthenia gravis

Nerves: Entrapment neuropathy (e.g., carpal tunnel), axonal polyneuropathy (improves with thyroxine replacement); delayed relaxation of deep tendon reflexes

Sleep apnea: Obstructive and central

■ METASTATIC TUMORS

Metastatic brain tumors are more common than primary brain tumors. It is estimated that there are now more than 100,000 new cases of metastatic brain tumors annually in the United States, compared with 16,800 new primary brain tumors in 1999. The most common metastatic intracranial tumor is from the lung, which accounts for almost half of the cases of metastases (Figure 19-1). Other common cancer types that metastasize to the brain are breast, melanoma, and renal cell carcinoma. Leptomeningeal metastases are most commonly caused by the acute leukemias, although lymphoma, breast cancer, melanoma, and lung cancer can also be responsible. Dura-based metastases are caused by breast cancer, prostate, and lymphoma. However, the focus of this chapter is on the primary brain tumors.

Etiology

The only clear risk factor for primary brain tumors is ionizing radiation. The latency between exposure and presentation can be 10 to 20 years. Radiation of the cranium can increase the incidence of tumors by up to a factor of 10, depending on the tumor type. There is no clear evidence that power lines, cell phones, and head trauma increase the risk of brain tumors. In most cases, the cause of a primary brain tumor is unknown.

Clinical Manifestations

Patients with brain tumors can present with either generalized or focal signs. Generalized signs are usually due to increased intracranial pressure (ICP) and consist of headache, papilledema, nausea, or vomiting. Headache is the presenting feature in 35% of

patients and develops in up to 70% during the course of the disease. The headaches can be on the same side as the tumor but can also be generalized; they are typically worsened with Valsalva maneuvers that can increase ICP. Seizures are the presenting symptom in 15 to 95% of patients, depending on the tumor type. For example, seizures are more commonly associated with low-grade gliomas and meningiomas than with

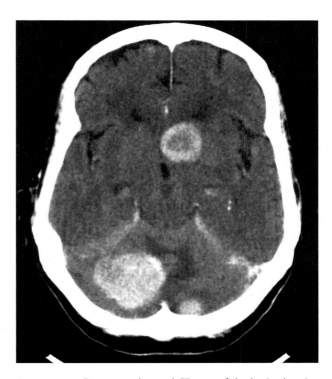

Figure 19-1 • Contrast-enhanced CT scan of the brain showing several metastatic lesions characterized by rounded areas of hyperdensity.
(Reproduced with permission from Armstrong P, Wastie M, Rockall A. Diagnostic Imaging. 5th ed. Oxford: Blackwell Publishing, 2004:402.)

other tumor types. The seizure can be either focal or generalized and may be associated with a postictal hemiparesis (Todd paralysis) or aphasia. Other focal signs associated with primary brain tumors include progressive hemiparesis.

Diagnostic Evaluation

The test of choice for diagnosis of a brain tumor is a contrast-enhanced MRI scan. CT is sometimes used because it is more widely available, lower in cost, and will detect over 90% of brain tumors. Contrast CT often shows a ring-enhancing lesion (see Figure 19-1), but ring enhancement can be seen with primary brain tumors, metastatic lesions (as in the figure), abscesses, and other inflammatory and rarely even vascular lesions. However, a CT scan can miss some structural lesions in the posterior fossa as well as low-grade tumors. A normal contrast-enhanced MRI of the head virtually rules out brain tumor.

LP for routine CSF analysis, as well as cytology, is sometimes performed to rule out meningeal involvement of metastatic tumors and as part of the evaluation for primary CNS lymphomas. If the patient has elevated ICP, however, LP is associated with risk of herniation and should be avoided.

CLASSIFICATION OF PRIMARY BRAIN TUMORS

The major categories of primary brain tumors are derived from the cell types present in the CNS that give rise to the neoplasm. The World Health Organization has presented a histologic classification of tumors of the CNS (Box 19-1). Some of the major types of brain tumors are discussed below and listed in Table 19-1.

BOX 19-1 HISTOLOGIC CLASSIFICATION OF TUMORS OF THE CENTRAL NERVOUS SYSTEM

Tumors of neuroepithelial tissue
  Astrocytic tumors
    Astrocytoma
    Anaplastic astrocytoma
    Glioblastoma multiforme
    Pilocytic astrocytoma
  Oligodendroglial tumors
    Oligodendroglioma
    Anaplastic oligodendroglioma
  Ependymal tumors
    Ependymoma
    Anaplastic ependymoma
  Choroid-plexus tumors
    Choroid-plexus papilloma
    Choroid-plexus carcinoma
  Embryonal tumors
    Medulloblastoma
    Primitive neuroectodermal tumor
Meningeal tumors
  Meningioma
  Hemangioblastoma
Primary central nervous system lymphoma
Germ-cell tumors
  Germinoma
  Choriocarcinoma
  Teratoma
Tumors of the sellar region
  Pituitary adenoma
  Craniopharyngioma
Metastatic tumors

Abridged from the World Health Organization classification.

TABLE 19-1

Common Primary Brain Tumors

Tumor	Typical Age of Presentation (yr)	Treatment	Median Survival (yr)
Glial tumors			
Astrocytomas			
Low-grade astrocytoma	20–40	Surgery or radiation	5–10
Glioblastoma multiforme	50–70	Surgery and radiation	1–2
Oligodendroglioma	30–40	Chemotherapy	10
Medulloblastoma	<15	Surgery and radiation	5–10
Meningioma	>50	Surgery	Normal (benign tumor)

GLIAL TUMORS

Glial tumors are divided into two major groups: astrocytic and oligodendroglial. Both can be either of low or high grade. Low-grade astrocytomas have a peak incidence in the third and fourth decade of life. New-onset seizure is the typical presentation, and MRI usually shows a nonenhancing lesion that is bright on T2-weighted images (Figure 19-2). If the tumor is in an area amenable to surgery, resection is usually performed. If resection is not possible due to the proximity to critical brain structures or large tumor size, radiation therapy is the treatment of choice. Median survival of patients with low-grade astrocytomas is approximately 5 years, although the range is broad and some patients can survive more than 10 years. Patients who die early usually have progression of their disease to high-grade malignant glioma.

The malignant astrocytomas are the most common glial tumors, and glioblastoma multiforme represents over 80% of the malignant gliomas. Glioblastoma usually affects patients in the sixth or seventh decade of life. MRI typically shows irregular contrast enhancement of the tumor, which is almost ring-like (Figure 19-3). The tumor involves the white matter and can spread across the corpus callosum, involving the other cerebral hemisphere. There is often associated edema, which can be severe enough to cause mass effect and herniation. Treatment involves surgical resection as the initial step. However, because the tumor is widely infiltrative, radiotherapy must be used as adjuvant treatment.

There is some controversy as to the effectiveness of chemotherapy, so it is usually reserved for salvage treatment. High-grade glial tumors sometimes respond to carmustine (also called BCNU), lomustine (CCNU), or procarbazine. Temozolomide is an orally administered alkylating agent that has been used in the treatment of high-grade gliomas that have not responded to other treatments. It has been shown to improve quality of life and slow the time to tumor progression. However, despite aggressive treatment, median survival is approximately 1 year for patients with glioblastoma multiforme and up to 3 years for

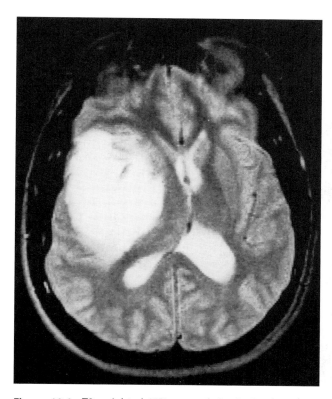

Figure 19-2 • T2-weighted MRI scan of the brain showing a large glioma characterized by high-intensity signal in the right hemisphere. The tumor is displacing and compressing the ventricular system.
(Reproduced with permission from Armstrong P, Wastie M, Rockall A. Diagnostic Imaging. 5th ed. Oxford: Blackwell Publishing, 2004:401.)

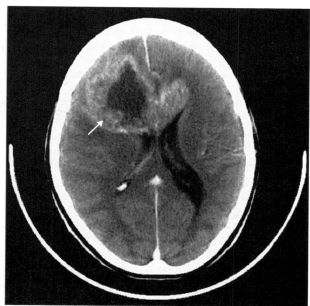

Figure 19-3 • Contrast-enhanced CT scan of the brain showing glioblastoma multiforme (arrow). Note the irregular enhancement pattern with a central area of necrosis. The tumor has also crossed the corpus callosum.
(Reproduced with permission from Patel P. Lecture Notes: Radiology. Oxford: Blackwell Publishing, 2005:268.)

patients with other malignant astrocytomas such as anaplastic astrocytomas.

Oligodendroglial tumors are tumors derived from oligodendrocytes. Like astrocytomas, they can be either low or high grade (anaplastic), which is of both prognostic and therapeutic importance. These tumors are often difficult to distinguish radiologically from astrocytomas. Treatment, however, is different, with chemotherapy being the mainstay for both low- and high-grade oligodendrogliomas. Median survival is approximately 10 years.

KEY POINTS

1. Glial tumors are either astrocytic or oligodendroglial.
2. Glioblastoma multiforme is the most common malignant glioma.
3. Treatment and prognosis depend on the grade of tumor.
4. A mnemonic for the differential diagnosis for ring-enhancing lesions on CT or MRI scans is **Dr. Gatt:**
   D: Demyelinating lesions (active)
   R: Resolving hematoma
   G: Granuloma
   A: Abscess
   T: Tumors, particulary metastasis, glioblastoma, and CNS lymphoma
   T: Toxoplasmosis

■ MEDULLOBLASTOMA

Epidemiology

Medulloblastoma is the most common malignant brain tumor of childhood and accounts for 25% of malignant primary brain tumors in children younger than 15 years.

Clinical Manifestations

The tumor arises from the cerebellum and therefore often presents with signs of increased ICP (headache, nausea, vomiting) when mass effect causes obstruction of the flow of CSF in the aqueduct of the brainstem. Because the tumor usually arises from the midline of the cerebellum, neurologic findings include truncal ataxia and unsteadiness of gait.

Diagnostic Evaluation

MRI or CT shows a contrast-enhancing tumor that is usually midline and often distorts or obliterates the fourth ventricle (Figure 19-4). Medulloblastoma has a high tendency to metastasize to other parts of the CNS, so once the diagnosis is made, contrast-enhanced imaging of the entire brain and spinal cord is necessary. The tumor may also metastasize outside of the nervous system, particularly to bone. Therefore a radionuclide bone scan and bone marrow aspirate should also be performed.

Treatment

Surgical resection is the first step in treatment. The goal is to remove as much tumor as possible without damaging the brainstem or causing permanent cranial nerve dysfunction. The next step is radiation therapy, and some centers also add chemotherapy. With treatment, the 5-year survival rate is approximately 50 to 75%, with the 10-year survival rate less than 50%.

KEY POINTS

1. Medulloblastoma is the most common malignant primary brain tumor of childhood.
2. Medulloblastoma arises from the cerebellum.
3. Medulloblastoma presents with increased ICP, ataxia, or both.
4. Contrast-enhanced imaging of the entire brain and spinal cord is indicated because medulloblastoma has a high tendency to metastasize to other parts of the CNS.

■ MENINGIOMA

Meningiomas are the most common benign brain tumor and the second most common primary brain tumor after the gliomas. They represent approximately 20% of the intracranial neoplasms. Meningiomas are derived from the cells that form the outer lining of the arachnoid granulations of the brain. Thus, as the name implies, they are derived from the meninges and, strictly speaking, not brain tumors.

Clinical Manifestations

Meningiomas can present with seizures, headaches, or focal neurologic deficits; they are more common in women and tend to occur in later life. However, there

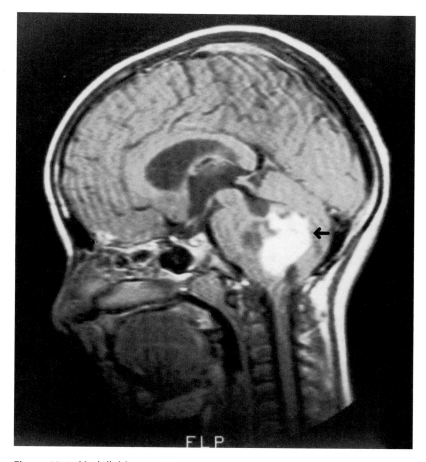

Figure 19-4 • Medulloblastoma (arrow) in a child as shown by sagittal MRI scan with contrast enhancement. Note that the fourth ventricle and middle portion of the cerebral aqueduct are obliterated, resulting in hydrocephalus, as illustrated by the dilated third and lateral ventricles.
(Reproduced with permission from Patel P. Lecture Notes: Radiology. Oxford: Blackwell Publishing, 2005:271.)

are many patients with asymptomatic meningiomas discovered with neuroimaging for unrelated reasons. Over 90% of meningiomas are supratentorial and can involve the falx, cerebral convexities, sphenoid wing, or olfactory groove. Therefore focal neurologic symptoms vary depending on the brain structures compressed by the meningioma.

Diagnostic Evaluation

Meningiomas can be diagnosed with either CT or MRI with contrast enhancement. On MRI, meningiomas can be missed with T1- and T2-weighted images because they are isointense or slightly hyperintense. However, they are brightly enhancing with contrast (Figure 19-5) and a "dural tail" at the margin of the tumor may be seen.

Treatment

Surgery is the primary treatment for meningiomas. However, asymptomatic meningiomas, especially those that are less than 2 cm in diameter without much associated edema, can be followed with annual CT scans with contrast. Even after complete resection, up to 20% recur within 10 years.

KEY POINTS

1. Meningiomas are the most common benign brain tumor.
2. Treatment is surgical for symptomatic lesions and observation for small asymptomatic lesions.

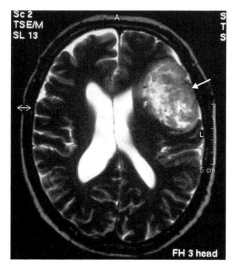

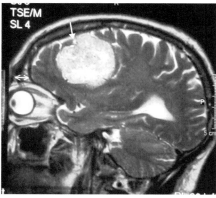

Figure 19-5 • Axial and sagittal MRI scans of the brain showing a brightly enhancing meningioma (arrows). On the sagittal view, the arrow tip is also pointing to the dural tail at the margin of the tumor.
(Reproduced with permission from Patel P. Lecture Notes: Radiology. Oxford: Blackwell Publishing, 2005:269.)

▪ PRIMARY CNS LYMPHOMA

Primary CNS lymphoma (PCNSL) is a diffuse non-Hodgkin's lymphoma. Some 98% of PCNSLs are B cell–derived. PCNSL formerly represented less than 1% of all primary brain tumors. However, over the last two decades, the reported incidence has tripled because of better detection methods and increased rates of acquired immunosuppression, especially the acquired immunodeficiency syndrome (AIDS), which increases the risk for PCNSL. However, for unclear reasons, the incidence of PCNSL has also increased among immunocompetent hosts.

Clinical Manifestations

The lesions are multifocal in approximately 40% of cases and are usually subcortical. The most common presenting symptoms are cognitive and behavioral changes, but hemiparesis, aphasia, or seizures can also occur. In immunocompetent hosts, the peak incidence is in the sixth and seventh decades of life.

Diagnostic Evaluation

Diagnosis is made with MRI, which shows the lymphoma to be located periventricularly with diffuse and homogenous enhancement. Stereotactic biopsy is usually required for definitive diagnosis. PCNSL can disseminate to the CSF in 25% of patients and to the eye in 20% of patients. Thus, LP for cytology and formal ophthalmologic evaluation must be performed.

Treatment

Unlike the case for other primary brain tumors, surgery plays no role in the treatment of PCNSL. Treatment is with chemotherapy, usually methotrexate, which can penetrate the blood-brain barrier. Chemotherapy is often combined with radiation, with a median survival of 3.5 years.

KEY POINTS

1. PCNSL has increased in frequency, largely due to the increased number of patients with AIDS.
2. PCNSL can spread to the CSF, eye, and bone.
3. PCNSL commonly presents with a change in mental status.
4. Treatment is chemotherapy with or without radiation.

▪ ACOUSTIC NEUROMA

Strictly speaking, acoustic neuroma is also not a primary brain tumor; it is a benign tumor of the eighth cranial nerve. It originates from the Schwann cell–glial cell junction of the vestibular portion of the nerve, so some authors have preferred to call the tumor **acoustic schwannoma** or **vestibular schwannoma.** These tumors account for 8% of all intracranial tumors and over 80% of all cerebellopontine angle tumors in adults. The tumors are typically unilateral except in cases of neurofibromatosis type 2, where they can be bilateral.

Clinical Manifestations

The most common symptom is unilateral hearing loss, not vertigo, though this is often suspected. Other symptoms include unilateral tinnitus or other cranial nerves dysfunction if the tumor becomes large enough to compress those nerves.

Diagnostic Evaluation

Audiometry is the best test for asymmetric unilateral sensorineural hearing loss. If imaging is warranted, MRI with contrast enhancement should be performed because the lesion enhances brightly with gadolinium.

Treatment

Because acoustic neuromas grow slowly, treatment options include observation, radiation therapy, and surgery. If the tumor is large, intervention should be considered because there is a risk for brainstem compression or hydrocephalus if the tumor continues to grow. Intervention should also be considered in patients with good hearing, because delay in treatment may result in hearing impairment.

KEY POINTS

1. Acoustic neuroma is a benign tumor.
2. It presents typically with unilateral hearing loss.
3. Acoustic neuroma can be bilateral in neurofibromatosis type 2.

■ PITUITARY ADENOMA

Pituitary adenomas are the most common pituitary tumors. They can present with either neurologic or endocrine manifestations. Neurologically, the most common symptom is headache; if the tumor continues to grow, it can compress the optic chiasm, located above the pituitary gland (Figure 19-6). This can result in bitemporal hemianopia because of the way that the visual fibers cross in the optic chiasm (see Chapter 4).

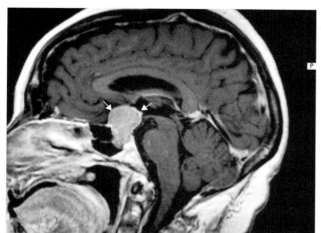

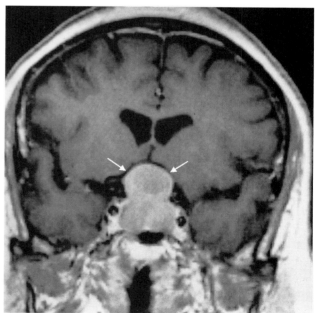

Figure 19-6 • Sagittal and coronal postcontrast MRI scans of the brain demonstrating a pituitary adenoma (arrows). Note that the tumor is anterior to the brainstem and extends upward, compressing the optic chiasm.
(Reproduced with permission from Armstrong P, Wastie M, Rockall A. Diagnostic Imaging. 5th ed. Oxford: Blackwell Publishing, 2004:406.)

Endocrine manifestations are either hypofunction or hyperfunction. The most common endocrine manifestation of pituitary adenoma is hypopituitarism, especially of the gonadotropin and growth hormone systems. Hyperfunction of the pituitary gland can result in oversecretion of prolactin, causing galactorrhea; growth hormone excess, causing either acromegaly or gigantism; or excess corticotropin, causing Cushing's disease.

Surgery through a transsphenoidal approach is usually the initial treatment. Also, in patients with prolactin-secreting adenomas, dopamine receptor agonists such as bromocriptine are used.

Chapter 20

Demyelinating Diseases of the Central Nervous System

■ MULTIPLE SCLEROSIS

Demyelinating diseases of the CNS are characterized by the pathologic hallmark of acquired loss of myelin with relative preservation of axons. The most common and best known of the CNS demyelinating diseases is MS. For many reasons MS is also one of the most feared diagnoses in neurology: it strikes young, healthy people in the prime of their lives, its course is marked by unpredictable relapses, almost any aspect of neurologic function may be affected, and the specter of lifelong disability requiring a wheelchair is a devastating one.

However, MS has a wide range of presentations and an equally wide range of prognoses; effective treatments aimed at both the underlying disease process and some specific complications are available. For the student, the study of demyelinating diseases provides an excellent opportunity to learn about dysfunction of different parts of the CNS and to master the wide variety of neurologic exam abnormalities that accompany these disorders.

Epidemiology

MS is a chronic neurologic disease that begins most commonly in young adulthood. The peak incidence of MS is between 20 and 30 years of age. Women are affected twice as often as men. Its prevalence in the northern United States is about 60 per 100,000. As discussed below, there are epidemiologic patterns to suggest both environmental and genetic influences.

Geographically, MS is more common in northern latitudes. The incidence in Scandinavian countries is higher than that in Italy, and the incidence in the northern United States is higher than that in the South. However, there are racial differences as well

(with a higher prevalence in white populations), and the implication of the geographic disparities is unclear. Interestingly, those who move from a low-risk to a high-risk geographic region or vice versa before the age of 15 adopt the risk of MS associated with their new home, while those who migrate after age 15 retain the risk associated with their childhood home. This supports the theory that a latent viral infection acquired in childhood may play a role in the pathogenesis of the disease.

There is strong evidence supporting a genetic predisposition to MS as well. For example, there is an increased incidence of MS in monozygotic twins compared with dizygotic twins, as well as an increased incidence in association with particular HLA alleles.

KEY POINTS

1. The peak incidence of MS occurs in young adulthood, between 20 and 30 years of age.
2. MS is more common in women and more common in whites.
3. The epidemiology of MS supports both environmental and genetic influences.

Clinical Manifestations

The neurologist's classic definition of MS is a disease marked by multiple white matter lesions separated in space and time. This means that multiple distinct areas of the CNS must be involved (rather than one area recurrently, for example), and that the disease must not be just a monophasic illness (with multiple areas affected only once simultaneously).

The clinical features are defined, as might be expected, by the location of the lesions. Thus, a right occipital lesion could result in a left homonymous hemianopia, while a right cervical spinal cord lesion may lead to an ipsilateral hemiparesis and loss of joint position sense with contralateral loss of pain and temperature sensation. Almost any neurologic symptom, in fact, can be produced by an MS lesion.

Common clinical features (Table 20-1) include corticospinal tract signs such as weakness and spasticity, cerebellar problems such as intention tremor and ataxia, sensory abnormalities such as paresthesias and loss of vibration and proprioception, and bladder dysfunction. Commonly, patients complain of fatigue. In later stages, cognitive and behavioral abnormalities and seizures may occur. A few particular syndromes characteristic of MS warrant further description.

Optic neuritis (ON) is a common initial presenting symptom of MS. (This fact reminds us that the optic nerve is actually an extension of the CNS rather than a true peripheral nerve.) ON is characterized by a painful loss of visual acuity in one eye. The vision may be blurry and there may be loss of color discrimination; severe episodes may lead to actual blindness. Pain may be predominant when the eye moves (i.e., when looking around). On exam there is loss of acuity and color vision, and the optic disc may be swollen, with indistinct margins (papilledema). A past history of ON is suggested by the presence of red desaturation (subtle loss of color appreciation), optic disc pallor or atrophy, and an RAPD (see Chapter 4).

Transverse myelitis describes an area of inflammatory demyelination in the spinal cord. Most commonly this is a partial lesion and does not mimic a complete spinal cord transection; rather, particular tracts may be interrupted at the level of the lesion in a patchy way. Thus there may be unilateral or bilateral weakness or sensory loss below the lesion. Bowel and bladder function may be lost. Reflexes may be exaggerated below the lesion, and Babinski signs may be present. Patients may report a band of tingling or pain around the torso at the level of the lesion.

Internuclear ophthalmoplegia (INO) is not a common finding in MS patients, but it is quite characteristic. The presence of an INO in a young person suggests few other diagnostic possibilities. An INO results from dysfunction of the MLF and leads to an inability to adduct one eye when looking toward the opposite side, with associated nystagmus of the abducting eye. Adduction of both eyes when observing a near target (convergence) is preserved.

Other clinical features characteristic of MS include **Lhermitte's sign**, a tingling, electric sensation down the spine when the patient flexes the neck, and a worsening of symptoms and signs in the heat, termed **Uhthoff's phenomenon.**

TABLE 20-1

Common Clinical Features of Multiple Sclerosis

Neurologic System	Clinical Sign or Symptom
Cranial nerves	Optic nerve dysfunction
	Visual acuity loss
	Red desaturation
	Papilledema or optic disc pallor
	Relative afferent pupillary defect (RAPD)
	Eye movement disorders
	Internuclear ophthalmoplegia
	Nystagmus
Motor system	Weakness
	Spasticity
	Reflex abnormalities
	Increased muscle stretch reflexes
	Babinski signs
	Clonus
Sensory system	Paresthesias
	Vibratory loss
	Joint position sense loss
	Lhermitte's sign
Cerebellar function	Ataxia
	Intention tremor
	Dysarthria
Autonomic system	Bladder dysfunction
Other	Fatigue
	Depression
	Uhthoff's phenomenon

KEY POINTS

1. MS is characterized by multiple lesions separated in space and time.
2. Almost any neurologic symptom can occur, depending on the location and burden of lesions.
3. Features characteristic of MS include ON, transverse myelitis, INO, Lhermitte's sign, and a worsening of symptoms in the heat.

Clinical Course and Prognosis

Most MS patients begin with a relapsing-remitting course (Figure 20-1), in which there are discrete episodes of neurologic dysfunction (relapses or "flares") that resolve after a period of time (usually weeks to months). Unfortunately, such a course usually evolves into one in which recovery from each relapse is incomplete and baseline functioning deteriorates (secondary progressive). Rarely, patients may have a relentlessly progressive course from the onset, either with superimposed relapses (progressive-relapsing) or without (primary progressive).

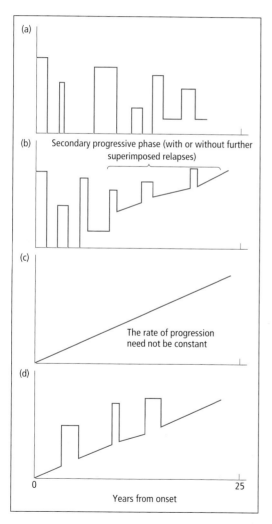

Figure 20-1 • Clinical course of multiple sclerosis: (a) relapsing-remitting, (b) secondary progressive, (c) primary progressive, (d) progressive-relapsing.
(Reproduced with permission from Ginsberg L. Lecture Notes Neurology. 8th ed. Oxford: Blackwell Publishing, 2005:131.)

To put the prognosis in broad terms, about one-third of MS patients lead lives of minimal disability and continue to work, about one-third have disability significant enough to prevent them from continuing at their jobs, and about one-third have severe disability, typically becoming wheelchair-bound. Features predicting a good prognosis include young age at onset, female sex, rapid remission of initial symptoms, mild relapses that leave little or no residual deficits, and a presentation with sensory symptoms or optic neuritis rather than motor symptoms.

KEY POINTS

1. Most MS patients have a relapsing-remitting course, which frequently evolves into a secondary progressive course.
2. Prognosis is quite variable and ranges from minimal to severe disability.

Diagnostic Evaluation

The diagnosis of MS begins with a thorough history and examination. In particular, patients often present with what appears to be a single episode of neurologic dysfunction, but upon further questioning may recall past episodes of seemingly unrelated neurologic symptoms that may in fact represent prior lesions separated in space and time. It is important to inquire specifically about past neurologic symptoms, particularly those that suggest optic neuritis, transverse myelitis, or other typical MS features. On exam, as well, evidence of old optic nerve or other neurologic lesions should be sought.

The two most useful laboratory studies are MRI and CSF analysis. On MRI, new MS lesions appear as discrete T2-hyperintense areas in the white matter of the brain or spinal cord. Ovoid lesions are classic. Fluid-attenuated inversion recovery (FLAIR) sequences also show these lesions particularly well (Figure 20-2). Acute lesions may not be evident on T1-weighted images but may enhance with gadolinium. Old, chronic MS lesions may become T1-hypointense, with a "black hole" appearance. MS lesions have a predilection for particular areas, including the periventricular white matter, juxtacortical regions, corpus callosum, and cerebellar peduncles. Sagittal images may demonstrate foci of demyelination spreading upward from the corpus callosum, termed **Dawson's fingers.**

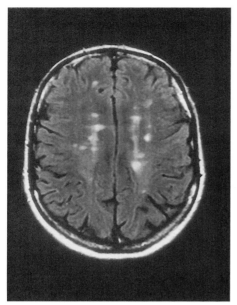

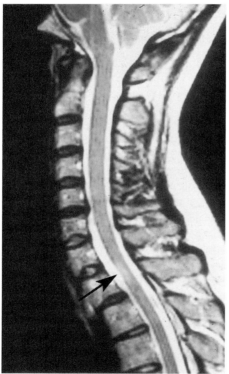

Figure 20-2 • MRI images of multiple sclerosis lesions. (Reproduced with permission from Ginsberg L. Lecture Notes Neurology. 8th ed. Oxford: Blackwell Publishing, 2005:133.)

The characteristic CSF finding is oligoclonal bands, found in more than 90% of MS patients at some point during their illness. These reflect intrathecal production of IgG antibodies by plasma cell clones. Although highly suggestive of MS, they can also be found in

other neurologic disorders. CSF studies during an acute relapse may show a moderate pleocytosis and elevated protein. Calculation of the IgG index, based on relative levels of IgG and albumin in the CSF and serum, can also suggest intrathecal antibody production.

Finally, visual evoked potentials can be used in suspected MS to document evidence of old optic neuritis. There is often an increased latency of the P100 wave on the affected side.

KEY POINTS

1. The diagnosis of MS begins with a thorough history and examination, particularly directed toward identifying past episodes of neurologic dysfunction.
2. MRI is the best imaging modality to detect both new and old MS lesions.
3. The characteristic CSF abnormality is the presence of oligoclonal bands.
4. Visual evoked potentials may provide evidence of old optic neuritis.

Pathology

The histologic appearance of an acute MS lesion is a sharply defined area of myelin loss with relative preservation of axons and associated signs of perivascular inflammation, including the presence of macrophages, lymphocytes, and plasma cells. Reactive astrocytes may be present. Chronic MS lesions are hypocellular and have extensive glial proliferation.

Treatment

Treatment for MS falls into three categories: acute therapies for relapses, chronic therapies that treat the underlying disease process, and symptomatic therapies that address the various complications of the disease.

Acute relapses of MS are most commonly treated with corticosteroids. A course of intravenous methylprednisolone followed by an oral prednisone taper is a common protocol. Although the effect of steroids on the long-term outcome is unclear, the duration of acute relapses is often shortened. A well-publicized trial demonstrated that intravenous steroids used to treat optic neuritis delayed but did not prevent the subsequent development of MS.

The therapies used in the chronic treatment of MS are immune-modulating agents (Table 20-2).

■ TABLE 20-2

Immune-Modulating Agents Used in the Treatment of Multiple Sclerosis

Drug	Administration	Side Effects
Interferon beta-1a (Avonex)	30 µg IM every week	Flu-like symptoms, anemia, depression, development of neutralizing antibodies
Interferon beta-1b (Betaseron)	250 µg SC every other day	Injection-site reactions, flu-like symptoms, depression, hematologic/liver abnormalities, development of neutralizing antibodies
Interferon beta-1b (Rebif)	44 µg SC three times a week	Flu-like symptoms, anemia, depression, development of neutralizing antibodies
Glatiramer acetate (Copaxone)	20 mg SC daily	Injection-site reactions, injection-related chest pain and shortness of breath

These include beta-1a interferon and beta-1b interferon, which are available in injection form and have been shown to decrease the rate of relapses, the burden of lesions seen on MRI, and the rate of accumulated disability. Both are currently used in relapsing-remitting and some secondary progressive patients. Side effects can include flu-like symptoms, depression, and injection-site reactions. It is important to check a CBC and liver function test routinely; interferons may cause leukopenia and reversible transaminitis. Patients who are doing poorly on interferons may have developed neutralizing antibodies to the interferons that reduce their effectiveness.

Glatiramer acetate is a polypeptide formulation injected subcutaneously that is also used in relapsing-remitting patients. Mitoxantrone, a chemotherapeutic agent that may be useful in patients with worsening MS, has dose-limiting cardiotoxicity as a potential drawback.

In patients who no longer respond to the above therapies, other immunosuppressive agents may be used, including azathioprine, cyclophosphamide, and methotrexate. Some use periodic pulses of corticosteroids. Of course these agents have a wide range of accompanying toxicities.

Several of the symptomatic complications that accompany MS have specific treatments. Spasticity can be managed with baclofen, diazepam, or tizanidine. Bladder dysfunction can be managed with anticholinergic agents (for urinary urgency) as well as intermittent self-catheterization. It is particularly important to address urinary problems so as to prevent recurrent infections, which can trigger MS relapses and lead to chronic renal disease. Unfortunately there are no effective treatments for tremor and ataxia, which are common disabling symptoms.

KEY POINTS

1. Acute MS relapses are treated with intravenous corticosteroids.
2. Interferons and glatiramer acetate are immune-modulating agents used to treat relapsing-remitting MS.
3. More toxic immunosuppressants are often used in refractory cases.
4. Symptomatic therapies include those for spasticity and bladder dysfunction.

■ ACUTE DISSEMINATED ENCEPHALOMYELITIS

Acute disseminated encephalomyelitis (ADEM) is a monophasic illness leading to areas of demyelination within the CNS, commonly following an antecedent viral infection or vaccination. ADEM may be difficult to distinguish from the initial presentation of MS.

Clinical and Radiologic Manifestations

As in MS, almost any neurologic symptom or sign can occur, depending on the location of the demyelinating lesions. In ADEM, the lesions are multiple and are frequently more patchy, bilateral, and confluent than in MS, where the lesions may be more discrete. ADEM lesions have a predilection for the posterior cerebral hemispheric white matter. Clinically, behavioral and cognitive abnormalities are often seen in ADEM, whereas they are uncommon until the late stages of MS. Radiologically, all areas of demyelination in ADEM appear acute and may enhance with gadolinium.

Diagnostic Evaluation

The diagnosis of ADEM may be suspected based on the clinical presentation and radiologic findings. CSF typically will show a lymphocytic pleocytosis (usually with more cells than seen in MS) and an elevated protein. Oligoclonal bands are rarely present. When the illness is indistinguishable clinically or radiologically from the initial episode of MS, definitive diagnosis of MS may not be possible unless or until a second episode of neurologic dysfunction occurs.

Prognosis and Treatment

By definition ADEM is a monophasic illness, and neurologic recovery is typically nearly complete. A course of intravenous corticosteroids is often administered to shorten the duration of the episode and lessen the severity of the symptoms.

■ LEUKOENCEPHALOPATHIES

Progressive multifocal leukoencephalopathy (PML) is characterized by dementia, focal cortical dysfunction, and cerebellar abnormalities. It is seen almost exclusively in patients with AIDS, leukemia, lymphoma, and other immunocompromised states. The JC virus is the causative agent and leads to demyelination by infecting oligodendrocytes. MRI characteristically shows multiple foci of white matter abnormalities, particularly in posterior regions. CSF analysis is usually normal. There are no effective treatments, and the prognosis is uniformly fatal.

Immunosuppressants such as tacrolimus and cyclosporine may cause a **post–organ transplant leukoencephalopathy**. Most commonly, these drugs produce an acute confusional state and cortical visual loss (blindness with preserved pupillary reactivity). MRI shows posterior white matter hyperintensities on T2-weighted images. The posterior leukoencephalopathy associated with these immunosuppressants can often be reversed by discontinuing or lowering the dose of the offending agent.

A sudden increase in blood pressure can cause **hypertensive leukoencephalopathy**. Patients present with an acute confusional state, seizures, headaches, and vomiting. Funduscopic examination shows papilledema with retinal hemorrhages and hard exudates. This syndrome may be accompanied by cardiac ischemia and hematuria. MRI shows T2-hyperintensities, usually in the parietal and occipital regions. Although completely reversible with appropriate antihypertensive treatment, hypertensive leukoencephalopathy can progress to coma or death.

Chapter 21

Infections of the Nervous System

Infections of the nervous system are common and often require urgent care. It is important for clinicians to be able to recognize them so that appropriate treatment can be initiated promptly. The major etiologic categories of infectious diseases are bacterial, viral, fungal, and parasitic.

▣ BACTERIAL MENINGITIS

Bacterial meningitis results from the inflammatory response to infection of the leptomeninges. Most cases of bacterial meningitis occur by hematogenous spread of a bacterial infection affecting the upper respiratory tract. Bacteria can also penetrate the subarachnoid space directly through skull or meningeal defects caused by trauma or surgery. Other potential sources are infections of parameningeal sites such as the ear, sinuses, and teeth (dental abscesses).

The most common symptoms of bacterial meningitis are fever, headache, confusion, and neck stiffness, but not all of these symptoms are always present. Diagnosis is made by examination of the cerebrospinal fluid (CSF) obtained by lumbar puncture (LP). If focal neurologic abnormalities are present on exam, brain CT or MRI should be done to identify a brain abscess or other mass lesion. CSF examination typically shows an elevated opening pressure (20 to 50 cm H_2O), elevated protein (100 to 500 mg/dL), decreased glucose concentration (<40% serum glucose), and pleocytosis (100 to 10,000 white cells/mL; normal is 5 cells or less) with a predominance of polymorphonuclear leukocytes. The CSF Gram stain is positive in 60 to 70% of cases, with positive CSF cultures in 75 to 80%.

The most common etiologic agents of bacterial meningitis are described in Table 21-1. In adults, *Streptococcus pneumoniae* accounts for one-third to one-half of all cases. *Haemophilus influenzae* meningitis in children has been reduced by 82% with preventive vaccination.

Treatment depends on the LP results and local antibiotic resistance patterns. If the LP and Gram stain are nondiagnostic or if LP is delayed, empiric antibiotic therapy should be started to treat the most common pathogens for a particular age group (see Table 21-1). The history and physical exam can help identify a particular pathogen. For example, *Neisseria meningitidis* can be associated with a petechial rash and can be responsible for epidemics in crowded living areas, such as those encountered by military recruits. Once the results from Gram stain or cultures are known, treatment can be tailored using antibiotics that have high penetrance into the CSF. Corticosteroids are often used as adjunctive treatment in children and have been shown to decrease the incidence of hearing loss and other neurologic sequelae. There are no data to support the use of corticosteroids in adults with bacterial meningitis. For prophylaxis after exposure to *Haemophilus* or *Meningococcus*, antibiotics are recommended: rifampicin 600 mg twice a day for 2 days or ciprofloxacin in a single 500-mg dose.

KEY POINTS

1. *S. pneumoniae* is the most common cause of bacterial meningitis in adults.
2. *N. meningitidis* can be responsible for epidemic meningitis in crowded conditions.
3. Meningitis is characterized by the triad of headache, fever, and nuchal rigidity.

TABLE 21-1

Common Etiologic Agents in Bacterial Meningitis

Age or Clinical Setting	Etiology	Empiric Treatment
Birth to 3 months	E. coli, group B streptococcus, L. monocytogenes	Ampicillin and broad-spectrum cephalosporin
3 months to 18 years	H. influenzae, N. meningitidis, and S. pneumoniae	Broad-spectrum cephalosporin*
18–50 years	S. pneumoniae and N. meningitidis	Broad-spectrum cephalosporin*
>50 years	S. pneumoniae, L. monocytogenes, and gram-negative rods	Ampicillin and broad-spectrum cephalosporin*
Head trauma or neurosurgical procedure	Staphylococci and gram-negative rods	Vancomycin and ceftazidime

*Add vancomycin if resistant pneumococcus is a significant local problem.

TUBERCULOSIS

Although tuberculosis (TB) is relatively uncommon in the United States, its incidence is 15 times greater in developing countries than in the United States. Approximately 1% of TB cases have a neurologic manifestation such as meningitis, a tuberculoma in the brain, or involvement of the spine (Pott's disease). TB meningitis is usually subacute to chronic in presentation but can begin acutely. In addition to the typical signs of meningitis, TB meningitis can present with cranial nerve palsies because inflammation and exudates often affect the base of the brain where the nerves exit the brainstem. Hydrocephalus is another complication of basilar meningitis. In addition, if the inflammation affects blood vessels, brain infarcts can occur.

CSF analysis typically shows an elevated protein, low glucose, and lymphocytic pleocytosis. CSF cultures can take 6 to 8 weeks to return and can be negative in one-third of cases. Thus, multiple spinal taps may be necessary; if suspicion is high enough, empiric treatment should be started. Diagnosis is confirmed by the demonstration of acid-fast bacilli in the CSF (fresh sample or after 4 to 6 weeks of culture). Most patients have extrameningeal tuberculosis, so a chest x-ray can be helpful, although pulmonary involvement is not invariable. Purified protein derivative (PPD) testing is positive in 50% of affected patients; it can be helpful if positive but does not exclude the disease if negative. CT or MRI with contrast enhancement can be helpful in demonstrating a tuberculoma in the brain or basilar inflammation characterized by enhancement of the basal meninges after contrast infusion.

Treatment for TB meningitis should include isoniazid, rifampin, ethambutol, and pyrazinamide in order to avoid drug resistance. In severe cases with focal neurologic deficits, corticosteroids are added. Vitamin B_6 should be given to prevent pyridoxine deficiency resulting from long-term use of isoniazid.

BRAIN ABSCESS

A brain abscess is a focal purulent process in the brain parenchyma. Abscesses usually arise from local spread of an infected contiguous site, such as the ear or sinuses, or hematogenous spread, especially from the lung. These abscesses tend to be solitary. If multiple brain abscesses are present, the cause is usually hematogenous spread from endocarditis or an immunocompromised state. Two-thirds of the responsible organisms are aerobic and one-third anaerobic. Around 30 to 60% of abscesses contain mixed flora.

Patients with brain abscess typically present with signs of a space-occupying lesion. Fever, neck stiffness, and an elevated peripheral white cell count are not common features of brain abscess, in contrast to the signs and symptoms of meningitis. Diagnosis is made by MRI or CT scan with contrast, which typically shows a ring-enhancing lesion with surrounding edema (Figure 21-1). Blood and CSF rarely disclose the causative organism. Because of risk of herniation (and low yield of identifying the infectious organism), LP is not indicated. For definitive diagnosis, surgical drainage with cultures is required.

Antibiotic therapy should be tailored to the specific culture and sensitivity results. If the cultures are negative (which can occur in 20% of patients), empiric antibiotic therapy should be aimed at broad coverage, because most abscesses contain multiple organisms. The usual empiric antibiotic regimen

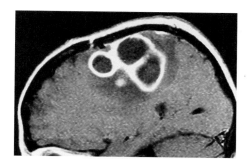

Figure 21-1 • Parasagittal MRI showing a multilocular brain abscess. The MRI was performed with a gadolinium and shows ring enhancement of the lesion with surrounding edema. (Reproduced with permission from Ginsberg L. Lecture Notes Neurology. 8th ed. Oxford: Blackwell Publishing, 2005:113.)

includes metronidazole for anaerobic coverage and either penicillin or a third-generation cephalosporin for coverage of streptococci and anaerobes. Surgical drainage of the abscess facilitates treatment, although antibiotics must be continued for 6 to 8 weeks.

KEY POINT

Brain abscess often appears as a ring-enhancing lesion on MRI or CT scan.

■ NEUROSYPHILIS

Syphilis is caused by the spirochete *Treponema pallidum* and is spread either sexually or vertically from mother to child. There are three stages of syphilis. Primary syphilis is characterized by painless chancres that can last 2 to 8 weeks after exposure. Typically, they appear within 3 weeks of infection. Secondary syphilis occurs 2 to 12 weeks after contact and can present with fever, malaise, and generalized lymphadenopathy. Neurologic complications occur in 1 to 2% of patients and most often consist of meningitis or cranial neuropathies, especially loss of hearing. This stage is followed by a latent period of months to many years.

In 30% of untreated patients, tertiary syphilis will develop. Manifestations include chronic syphilitic meningitis, which can be associated with brain infarcts due to associated arteritis. General paresis, another neurologic manifestation of tertiary syphilis, is caused by invasion of the brain by the spirochetes and results in Argyll Robertson pupils (small, irregu-

lar pupils that accommodate but do not react to light) and an encephalitis or dementia. Another manifestation of neurosyphilis is tabes dorsalis, characterized by a sensory ataxia with lightning-like pains (see Chapter 22). Patients typically have absent knee and ankle reflexes, impairment of proprioception because of posterior column dysfunction, and a positive Romberg sign. There can also be associated urinary or fecal incontinence. Charcot joints are caused by local tissue damage and trophic changes that occur when pain and temperature sensation is impaired.

Diagnosis is commonly made using treponemal and nontreponemal serologic tests. The fluorescent treponemal antibody (FTA) test is the most commonly used treponemal test. Nontreponemal tests include the rapid plasma reagin (RPR) and Venereal Disease Research Laboratory (VDRL) tests, which detect antibodies to membrane lipids of the treponemal spirochete. Because the nontreponemal tests are very sensitive but not very specific (i.e., they have a high false-positive rate), they are typically used as screening tests. If they are positive, the FTA can be performed to confirm infection. A negative FTA test virtually excludes neurosyphilis. If the test is positive in a patient with signs and symptoms of neurosyphilis, CSF analysis must be done to look for lymphocytic pleocytosis, increased protein, or a reactive CSF-VDRL test.

Treatment should be started in patients with a positive serum FTA and any of the above CSF abnormalities. High-dose intravenous penicillin G is the drug of choice.

KEY POINTS

1. Neurologic manifestations of syphilis can occur in secondary or tertiary syphilis.
2. Tabes dorsalis occurs in tertiary syphilis.
3. Serum VDRL is sensitive but not very specific; FTA is very specific for syphilis.

■ LYME DISEASE

Lyme disease is caused by the spirochete *Borrelia burgdorferi* and is transmitted by the deer tick. Lyme disease is the leading tick-borne disease in Europe and the United States. Clinical symptoms are varied and can involve multiple systems, including dermatologic, cardiac, rheumatologic, and neurologic systems. Neurologic manifestations include lymphocytic meningitis, cranial neuropathy (most commonly a unilateral or bilateral seventh nerve palsy), and painful inflammation of nerve roots.

Diagnosis is supported by erythema chronicum migrans, which is a gradually progressive circular rash with central clearing. The rash typically appears within 3 to 4 weeks of exposure in 60 to 80% of patients and can last days to weeks. Because of the small size of the deer tick species *Ixodes*, patients are often unaware of the tick exposure. Therefore a history of exposure can be helpful in making the diagnosis but is not necessary. Because some patients do not have all the above signs or symptoms, diagnosis often depends on serologic testing for antibody against *B. burgdorferi*. In order to prove infection of the nervous system, CSF (in addition to serum) must be obtained for antibody testing. A ratio of CSF to serum antibody greater than 1 indicates active CNS infection. Additionally, CSF may show a lymphocytic pleocytosis and mild elevation of protein.

For patients with severe symptoms, treatment is with intravenous antibiotics such as ceftriaxone. If symptoms are mild (i.e., facial weakness) oral antibiotics such as amoxicillin or doxycycline can be used.

KEY POINT

Lyme disease is caused by the spirochete *Borrelia burgdorferi*.

■ VIRAL INFECTIONS

Meningitis or encephalitis is the typical acute presentation of viral infections of the CNS. Viral meningitis is caused by the inflammatory response of leptomeningeal cells to viral infection. The clinical presentation can be identical to that of bacterial meningitis, with fever, headache, neck stiffness, nausea, and photophobia. If the infection involves the brain parenchyma itself, this is called **encephalitis;** when the meninges and brain are both involved, the term **meningoencephalitis** is used. Because the brain parenchyma itself is affected in encephalitis, the patient can have an altered level of consciousness, cognitive or behavioral abnormalities, focal neurologic deficits, or seizures.

The most common causes of epidemic viral meningitis and encephalitis are the enteroviruses, such as coxsackievirus and echovirus, and the arboviruses, such as eastern equine encephalitis, western equine encephalitis, Venezuelan equine encephalitis, St. Louis encephalitis, West Nile virus, and California encephalitis. Meningitis caused by enteroviruses and arboviruses is more common in the summer. Less common causes are herpes simplex virus (HSV), cytomegalovirus, Epstein-Barr virus, and varicella zoster virus.

LP should be performed for CSF analysis, which provides the best laboratory indication of a viral infection of the CNS or meninges (Table 21-2). In contrast to that of bacterial meningitis, the CSF profile for

■ TABLE 21-2

CSF Findings in Different Neurologic Infections

	Acute Bacterial Meningitis	Acute Viral Meningitis	Chronic Meningitis (bacterial and fungal)
White blood cells (normal <5/uL)	Very elevated (500–5,000) Mostly polymorphonuclear leukocytes	Moderately elevated (100–2,000) Predominantly lymphocytes.	Elevated (100–700) Predominantly lymphocytes
Protein (normal: 15–50 mg/dL)	Elevated (100–500 mg/dL)	Normal or mildly elevated	Markedly elevated (>100 mg/dL)
Glucose (normal range : 40–85 mg/dL)	Low (<40 mg/dL) or very low (can be <10 mg/dL)	Normal	Very low
Microscopic analysis	Positive	Negative (possible viral cultures and PCR)	Positive
Treatment	Antibiotics	Supportive (except herpesvirus treated with acyclovir)	Antibiotics and antifungals

viral meningitis shows a lymphocytic or monocytic pleocytosis, especially after 48 hours (neutrophils can be present initially), elevated protein, and a normal glucose level. The Gram stain will be negative, so viral meningitis is sometimes referred to as **aseptic meningitis**. It is often difficult to determine a specific viral etiology. Serologic and CSF viral cultures can aid the diagnosis, and newer techniques such as the polymerase chain reaction (PCR), which is available for several viruses, are often helpful. Diagnosis of viral meningitis is aided by imaging studies such as MRI, which can help exclude alternative diagnoses (such as a mass lesion) for the alteration in alertness, cognition, and behavior. In HSV infection, the MRI often shows contrast enhancement and edema of the temporal lobes. EEG can also be helpful and may show sharp-wave discharges in the temporal lobes in the case of HSV infection. Unfortunately, a definitive etiology is not found in many cases of meningitis or encephalitis.

Treatment for viral meningitis is mainly supportive, because there are no specific treatments for most viral infections. If HSV infection is suspected, however, treatment should begin promptly with intravenous acyclovir, even while tests are pending, because mortality is close to 70% in untreated cases.

Viral infections of the nervous system can also affect other sites, such as the spinal cord (myelitis), nerves (neuritis), nerve roots (radiculitis), and muscle (myositis). For example, herpes zoster (shingles) is a common manifestation of reactivated varicella zoster virus in the dorsal root ganglion. A sensation of burning pain is usually followed by eruption of a vesicular rash in a dermatomal pattern that most commonly involves the trunk or the face, particularly the first division of the fifth cranial nerve.

Treatment is typically supportive, with analgesics for pain. Oral acyclovir should be used when the infection involves the cornea or the ear, with hearing impairment and facial paralysis (Ramsay Hunt syndrome). Patients with herpes zoster who are immunocompromised should be treated with intravenous acyclovir. The role of corticosteroids is unclear at this time, but they may reduce pain early in the course of the illness.

KEY POINT

HSV meningitis is treated with acyclovir. Treatment for other viral causes of meningitis is typically supportive.

HUMAN IMMUNODEFICIENCY VIRUS

HIV is a retrovirus that can directly affect cells at any level of the nervous system and produce conditions like AIDS dementia complex and vacuolar myelopathy. HIV can cause peripheral nervous system disorders (see Chapter 23). In addition, the associated immunodeficiency provides the appropriate substrate for opportunistic infections of the CNS (toxoplasmosis, tuberculosis, cryptococcal meningitis, neurosyphilis, and cytomegalovirus encephalitis), other noninfectious conditions like CNS lymphoma and progressive multifocal leukoencephalopathy, and finally conditions related to the use of antiretroviral therapy.

Neurologic complications occur in more than 40% of patients with HIV. AIDS in the CNS is the "great imitator," producing symptoms and signs that can be confused with any other neurologic disorder. Occasionally neurologic symptoms are the first indication of HIV seroconversion; appropriate diagnostic testing will help to elucidate the true cause of a patient's symptoms. The history and clinical exam are important in establishing a diagnosis. Local neurologic symptoms usually indicate a space-occupying lesion, and opportunistic infection should be considered. Additional testing will include blood work, HIV serology, viral load, LP and CSF analysis, MRI of the brain and spine, and electrodiagnostic studies.

Since the introduction of very effective antiretroviral therapy, the incidence of opportunistic infections of the CNS has declined and survival has improved.

■ PROGRESSIVE MULTIFOCAL LEUKOENCEPHALOPATHY

Progressive multifocal leukoencephalopathy is a demyelinating disease caused by the JC virus. It is a rare disease but occurs more commonly in immunocompromised individuals such as those with Hodgkin's disease, other lymphomas, leukemia, or AIDS. Typically, there are multifocal areas of demyelination, more prominent in the subcortical white matter of the brain.

Clinically, onset of symptoms is subacute or chronic and can include focal signs such as hemiplegia or visual field abnormalities. Dementia can be present in the later stages. Definitive diagnosis is made by brain biopsy, but MRI can show nonenhancing patchy white matter abnormalities. CSF examination is usually normal. Currently, there is no specific treatment other than supportive management, and most patients die within 1 year.

KEY POINT

Progressive multifocal leukoencephalopathy is caused by the JC virus and is more common in immunocompromised individuals.

FUNGAL INFECTIONS

Fungal infections of the CNS tend to arise in immunocompromised patients. They have become more common recently because of the AIDS epidemic and newer immunosuppressive medical treatments. Fungi are eukaryotic organisms that reproduce by budding (yeasts) or by forming hyphae (molds). The most common fungi that cause CNS infections are *Cryptococcus neoformans* and *Coccidioides immitis*. Less common fungal infections of the CNS are due to *Histoplasma capsulatum* and *Candida* species, among others. Fungal infection can cause meningitis (acute, subacute, or chronic), granulomatous meningoencephalitis, abscess (solitary and multiple), granuloma, and infarcts of the brain.

Cryptococcus is the most common cause of fungal meningitis. Cryptococcosis can present with chronic headache, increased ICP, or cranial nerve signs. Infection occurs by inhalation of *Cryptococcus*, which is present in soil and pigeon excrement. CSF analysis demonstrates a lymphocytic pleocytosis, very low glucose, and an elevated protein level. The organism can be identified in the CSF with an India ink preparation, but false negatives can occur. In this case, the CSF can be tested for the cryptococcal antigen by latex agglutination; this test is highly sensitive and specific. Definitive diagnosis is made by a positive CSF culture. Treatment is with amphotericin B and flucytosine.

Coccidioides immitis is the second most common cause of fungal meningitis. Coccidioidomycosis is also caused by inhalation. Infections are more common in the southwestern United States and Mexico. Diagnosis is by CSF culture, with a CSF profile similar to that for cryptococcosis. Treatment is with intravenous and intrathecal amphotericin B.

KEY POINTS

1. *Cryptococcus* is the most common cause of fungal meningitis.
2. India ink preparation can help in diagnosing cryptococcosis.

TOXOPLASMOSIS

Toxoplasmosis is caused by the intracellular parasite *Toxoplasma gondii*. Cats are the definitive host for the parasite, but it can infect a variety of animals, including humans. Humans can be exposed to the parasite either through ingesting soil contaminated with cat feces or by consuming undercooked meat of infected animals. Once ingested, the cysts have a propensity to affect the CNS. Toxoplasmosis can also occur congenitally as one of the TORCH (toxoplasmosis, other agents, rubella, cytomegalovirus, herpes simplex) infections, which can be acquired in utero from the first trimester until delivery. In the adult population with AIDS, toxoplasmosis is the most common cause of an intracranial mass lesion. The clinical presentation is one of focal neurologic signs accompanied by fever, headache, and mental status changes.

CT or MRI with contrast shows a ring-enhancing lesion with mass effect; multiple lesions are usually present. The lesions are typically located in the basal ganglia or at the gray–white matter junction. Antibodies to *T. gondii* help support the diagnosis by proving prior exposure to the parasite. PCR analysis of CSF can also reveal the cause. In AIDS patients, diagnosis is often presumptive after an imaging study is obtained. Treatment with pyrimethamine, sulfadiazine, and folinic acid should be continued for 4 to 6 weeks, followed by lifelong maintenance therapy with the same medications to help prevent recurrence. If there is no clinical and radiologic improvement after 2 weeks, alternative diagnoses such as primary CNS lymphoma (see Chapter 19) should be considered. Brain biopsy may be needed to obtain a tissue diagnosis.

KEY POINTS

1. Fungal meningitis and toxoplasmosis are more common in immunocompromised patients.
2. Toxoplasmosis is the most common cause of a cerebral mass lesion in a patient with AIDS.

CYSTICERCOSIS

Cysticercosis is caused by the pork tapeworm *Taenia solium* when it forms cysts in tissues. Brain involvement is common and occurs in 50 to 70% of all cases. Cysticercosis is the most common parasitic infection of the CNS and is endemic to Central and South America and parts of Africa, Asia, and eastern Europe.

The most common presentations of cysticercosis are seizures, increased intracranial pressure with headache, and meningitis. CSF examination may be normal but can show pleocytosis (usually mononuclear), increased protein, and low glucose in cases where meningeal signs are present. Cysticercosis-specific IgG antibodies can also be detected in the CSF. CT or MRI helps make the diagnosis and can show ring-enhancing cystic lesions or small parenchymal calcifications representing calcified cysts.

Treatment involves symptomatic management using anticonvulsants to control seizures and shunting to control hydrocephalus if present. Albendazole is used to kill the parasite, and oral steroids are used sometimes to suppress the ensuing inflammatory reaction and edema.

KEY POINT

Cysticercosis is the most widespread parasitic infection of the CNS. It is occurs particularly often in Mexico, Central and South America, and Asia, where it represents the most common cause of new-onset seizures in the adult population.

22 Disorders of the Spinal Cord

Because the clinical presentations are diverse, spinal cord disorders can be challenging to the clinician. The diversity in presentation is due in part to the functional anatomy of the spinal cord, where sensory and motor systems are in proximity to one another. In order to understand the clinical manifestations of spinal cord disorders, one must understand the anatomy of the spinal cord.

◼ ANATOMY

The spinal cord is the caudal continuation of the lower brainstem. It begins at the foramen magnum and ends at the filum terminale. Below the T12 level, the spinal cord tapers rapidly, forming the conus medullaris, which signifies the end of the spinal cord at approximately the L1 level of the spine. The lumbar and sacral nerve roots must project downward before they can exit laterally at their appropriate levels. This collection of nerve roots is the cauda equina ("horse's tail").

The vascular supply to the spinal cord consists of a single anterior spinal artery and two posterior spinal arteries. The vertebral arteries each extend one branch downward and fuse to form the anterior spinal artery from above. The anterior spinal artery supplies blood to the anterior two-thirds of the spinal cord. The posterior spinal arteries, which also arise from the vertebral arteries above, supply blood to the posterior one-third of the spinal cord—that is, the dorsal columns. As the spinal arteries descend, they also receive blood from segmental arteries arising from the descending aorta. The most prominent of these is the artery of Adamkiewicz, which arises from the aorta and supplies the anterior spinal artery around the T8 level.

The spinal cord is divided grossly into gray and white matter. The gray matter contains the dorsal (posterior) and ventral (anterior) horns. The dorsal horn receives the dorsal root fibers of the sensory system, and the ventral horn contains the alpha motor neurons of the motor system. The intermediolateral cell column is located between the dorsal and ventral horns, extends from C8 to L1, and contains the preganglionic cell bodies for the sympathetic nervous system. The white matter in the spinal cord is composed of the myelinated axons of the motor and sensory systems.

Motor Pathways

In the spinal cord, the corticospinal tract begins at the junction of the medulla and the top of the spinal cord, just below the decussation of the medullary pyramids (Figure 22-1). Two main motor pathways are used for voluntary movement: the lateral corticospinal tract and the ventral corticospinal tract. The lateral corticospinal tract is the major motor pathway and is organized in a somatotopic fashion, with the fibers that innervate the motor neurons to the leg located laterally. Approximately 20% of the corticospinal fibers do not cross in the medulla. These fibers travel in the ventral corticospinal tract, cross in the spinal cord in the white matter anterior to the central canal, and then synapse on motor neurons in the ventral horn.

Clinical signs of corticospinal tract dysfunction include upper motor neuron (UMN) signs such as enhanced reflexes, increased tone, presence of extensor plantar response (Babinski sign), and weakness.

Other motor pathways exist, such as the rubrospinal and vestibulospinal tracts, but they are not as important clinically as the corticospinal tract for localizing lesions in the spinal cord.

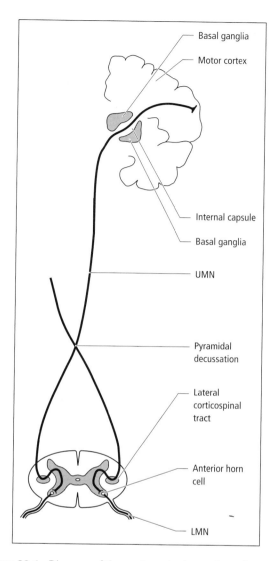

Figure 22-1 • Diagram of the corticospinal tract from the cortex to the ventral horn.
(Reproduced with permission from Ginsberg L. Lecture Notes Neurology. 8th ed. Oxford: Blackwell Publishing, 2005:37.)

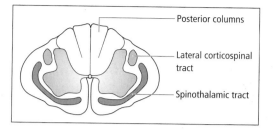

Figure 22-2 • Transverse section of the spinal cord showing the sensory pathways. The posterior columns relay information concerning proprioception and two-point discrimination. The spinothalamic tracts relay pain and temperature information.
(Reproduced with permission from Ginsberg L. Lecture Notes Neurology. 8th ed. Oxford: Blackwell Publishing, 2005:122.)

Sensory Pathways

The major sensory pathways in the spinal cord are the spinothalamic tract and the dorsal columns (Figure 22-2). Pain and temperature sensations are relayed to the brain by the spinothalamic tracts. First, painful stimuli are relayed to the spinal cord by small, thinly myelinated and unmyelinated fibers. The nerve fibers typically ascend two or three segments before synapsing in the dorsal horn. The fibers then cross to the other side of the cord in the anterior commissure and ascend in the lateral spinothalamic tract to the thalamus. Therefore a lesion in the spinothalamic tract (after it crosses) results in a loss of temperature and pain sensation on the opposite side of the body below the lesion. The spinothalamic tract is somatotopically organized, with the fibers innervating the sacrum and legs located laterally and the fibers innervating the arms located medially.

The dorsal columns relay information concerning joint position sense (proprioception) and two-point discrimination. Light touch is relayed by both the dorsal columns and the ventral spinothalamic tracts. Likewise, vibratory sense is probably relayed by several pathways in addition to the dorsal columns.

The dorsal columns are composed of two fiber tracts on each side of the spinal cord; the fasciculus gracilis relays information from the legs, whereas the fasciculus cuneatus relays information from the arms. These fiber tracts are organized somatotopically, with the leg fibers located medially because the incoming fibers from the arms push the fibers from the legs toward the middle of the cord.

The fibers in the dorsal columns do not synapse and cross the midline until they reach the gracile or cuneate nuclei in the medulla. Thus, a lesion of the spinal cord affecting the dorsal columns results in loss of joint position sense and fine two-point discrimination on the same side of the body as the lesion. Also, patients sometimes complain of tingling paresthesias or a band-like sensation in the extremities below the lesion.

SPINAL CORD SYNDROMES

Armed with knowledge of the anatomy of the spinal cord, one can localize lesions to the spinal cord and compare patterns of findings with known spinal cord syndromes in order to gain clues to the pathophysiology of the spinal lesion.

■ COMPLETE SPINAL CORD TRANSECTION

Complete transection of the spinal cord interrupts the sensory and motor pathways on both sides of the spinal cord. Causes of complete transection include trauma, cord compression from a large tumor, hematoma or abscess, and transverse myelitis. In the acute phase immediately following spinal transection, there is a period of "spinal shock," which can last days to weeks. During this period, reflexes and tone can be decreased or absent. After resolution of spinal shock, the reflexes become hyperexcitable, and tone increases to the point of spasticity, as expected. Because the entire cord is transected, there is complete loss of pain and temperature sense, joint position sense, and voluntary motor strength in all parts of the body below the lesion. This results in a sensory level where sensation is impaired below the lesion and preserved above the lesion (refer to Figure 6-3 for a dermatomal map). For example, a lesion involving the C2 cord level results in quadriplegia with sensory loss over the whole body and occiput of the head. Also, respiration is compromised, as the innervation of the diaphragm is supplied by the phrenic nerve, which arises from the C3, C4, and C5 nerve roots. Facial sensation is preserved because the trigeminal system (fifth cranial nerve) is intact. Spinal transection below T1 allows for complete use of the

arms with preservation of respiratory movements. Lesions of the lumbar and sacral cord result in varying degrees of paraplegia and sensory loss in the legs.

Useful landmarks that aid in the localization of the level of the lesion include the nipple line at T4 or T5 and the umbilicus at T10 or T11. Spinal transection at any level results in bladder and bowel dysfunction with concomitant loss of rectal sphincter tone. During spinal shock, the bladder initially becomes atonic, resulting in urinary retention. If the sacral spinal cord is intact, reflex emptying of the bladder occurs several weeks after the transection.

■ SPINAL CORD COMPRESSION

Cord compression from a mass such as a tumor, hematoma, epidural abscess, or herniated disc can present with the findings discussed above, but the severity of symptoms varies depending on the degree of compression. Cervical spondylosis, a degenerative condition of the spinal column, is common in older patients and may present with some of the features of spinal cord compression. On examination, one can find varying degrees of weakness in all four limbs in an UMN pattern (described in Chapter 5) as well as impairment of spinothalamic and dorsal column function. Treatment options for cervical spondylosis include wearing a soft cervical collar or surgical decompression.

Acute Cord Compression—A Neurologic Emergency

Acute spinal cord compression is a medical emergency. Delayed treatment can result in irreversible neurologic injury. Management entails stabilizing the patient and performing a thorough neurologic examination in order to localize the level of spinal injury. This allows one to focus either CT or MRI studies to the proper spinal level to determine the underlying lesion. The treatment for an epidural abscess includes intravenous antibiotics and surgical drainage. The treatment for spinal cord compression due to an epidural tumor includes adequate analgesia and corticosteroids. Patients with significant neurologic dysfunction should receive 100 mg of dexamethasone administered intravenously followed by 16 mg/day orally. Patients with pain and minimal neurologic signs can be given a lower initial dose of dexamethasone (10 mg IV) followed by 16 mg/day orally. The oral dose of dexamethasone should be tapered gradually once radiotherapy, the definitive treatment, is under way. Patients with small lesions and a normal neurologic exam may forego the use of corticosteroids.

BROWN-SÉQUARD SYNDROME

Brown-Séquard syndrome results from a unilateral lesion or hemisection of the spinal cord. Because only one-half of the spinal cord is affected, weakness is present only on the side of the body ipsilateral to the lesion. Additionally, there is loss of ipsilateral joint position sense and *contralateral* pain and temperature sensation below the lesion. The most common cause of Brown-Séquard syndrome is trauma, but spinal metastases causing cord compression can sometimes be responsible.

CENTRAL CORD SYNDROME

Lesions within the spinal cord itself (intramedullary) cause a central cord syndrome. The most common causes are tumors, syringomyelia, and hematomyelia. Syringomyelia (or syrinx) is a fluid-filled cavity in the spinal cord (Figure 22-3), while hematomyelia is a region of hemorrhage in the spinal cord. These lesions can occur anywhere in the spinal cord, but syringomyelia and hematomyelia occur more commonly in the cervical region. Syringomyelia is often associated with a type I Chiari malformation (see Figure 22-3), where the posterior fossa develops abnormally and the cerebellar tonsils are forced downward, which can exert pressure on the brainstem and upper cervical spinal cord. A type II Chiari malformation is often associated with a myelomeningocele (described later in this chapter) and results from downward herniation of not only the cerebellar tonsils but also the cerebellar vermis and fourth ventricle. In addition to syrinx formation, hydrocephalus is a common finding. Patients with a type II Chiari malformation often present soon after birth with signs and symptoms of hydrocephalus or brainstem dysfunction, such as choking or difficulty swallowing.

The typical scenario for a central cord syndrome occurs when the anterior commissure, which contains the crossing fibers of the spinothalamic tract, is disrupted. If the lesion is in the cervical cord, this results in loss of pain and temperature in a cape-like distribution because the crossing fibers from both arms are affected (Figure 22-4). Dorsal column function is usually spared.

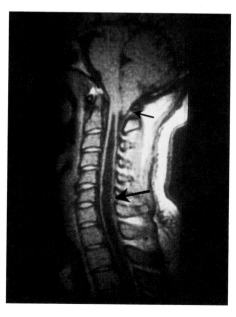

Figure 22-3 • Sagittal MRI scan of the spinal cord showing a hypointense region in the middle of the cord that represents a fluid-filled syrinx cavity (large black arrow). This syrinx is associated with a type I Chiari malformation characterized by the downward displacement of the cerebellar tonsils through the foramen magnum (small black arrow).
(Reproduced with permission from Ginsberg L. Lecture Notes Neurology. 8th ed. Oxford: Blackwell Publishing, 2005:123.)

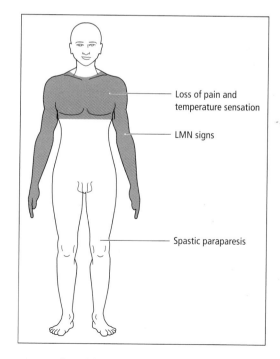

Figure 22-4 • Clinical features of syringomyelia.
(Reproduced with permission from Ginsberg L. Lecture Notes Neurology. 8th ed. Oxford: Blackwell Publishing, 2005:124.)

If an intramedullary lesion is large enough and extends into the anterior horn, segmental weakness can result because of involvement of the anterior horn cells. Additionally, if the lesion grows even larger, it can affect the spinothalamic tracts on both sides of the spinal cord. Because of the somatotopic organization of the spinothalamic tracts, with fibers from the sacrum located laterally, there can be sacral sparing because only the medial portions of the spinothalamic tract are compressed from the outwardly growing lesion. In lesions of this size, the corticospinal tracts are often involved bilaterally, resulting in weakness and spasticity below the lesion.

■ ANTERIOR SPINAL ARTERY SYNDROME

Because the single anterior spinal artery supplies blood to the anterior two-thirds of the spinal cord, compromise or occlusion of this artery due to thromboembolus, trauma, or mass lesion can result in infarction of the ventral (anterior) horns and the spinothalamic tracts. Corticospinal and spinothalamic dysfunction occurs below the site of infarction. Because the posterior spinal arteries supply the dorsal columns, joint position sense and two-point discrimination are unaffected.

■ DISEASES OF THE POSTERIOR AND LATERAL COLUMNS

Vitamin B_{12} deficiency results in combined dysfunction of the dorsal columns and corticospinal tracts, also referred to as subacute combined degeneration. This results in a spastic, ataxic gait. The spasticity is caused by corticospinal dysfunction, and the sensory ataxia by loss of proprioception from the dorsal column involvement.

Isolated dorsal column dysfunction can result from tabes dorsalis, a late complication of syphilis. The dorsal columns can degenerate to the point where the patient develops a sensory ataxia.

■ LESIONS OF THE CONUS MEDULLARIS AND CAUDA EQUINA

Pathologic lesions in the area of the cauda equina and conus medullaris cause similar symptoms due to involvement of multiple lumbar and sacral nerve roots. Typically, the patient has radicular pain, loss of sensation in the buttocks and legs, and leg weakness.

Lesions of the conus medullaris also typically cause more prominent symptoms of bowel, bladder, and sexual dysfunction.

■ CONGENITAL MALFORMATIONS OF THE SPINE

There are several congenital defects associated with the spine and spinal cord that result from failure of neural tube closure in the first trimester of gestation. The simplest is spina bifida occulta, which is characterized by a lack of vertebral arch closure with no other associated defect. This defect is typically localized to the L5–S1 region. Spina bifida cystica occurs when there is herniation of the dura and arachnoid through the vertebral arch defect. A myelomeningocele is herniation of the spinal cord and meninges through the veretebral arch defect. This is typically the most severe of the congenital malformations of the spine; symptoms are similar to those affecting the cauda equina, described above. These congenital defects may be detected in utero through the use of ultrasonography or by finding elevated levels of alpha-fetoprotein in maternal serum. The use of folic acid before conception greatly reduces the risk of defects in neural tube closure.

KEY POINTS

1. Spinal cord transection results in bilateral weakness and complete sensory loss below the lesion.
2. Spinal cord compression is a medical emergency requiring rapid evaluation and treatment.
3. "Spinal shock" is the acute phase of spinal cord transection; tone can be flaccid, with decreased reflexes.
4. Brown-Séquard syndrome is a hemisection of the cord with ipsilateral weakness and loss of proprioception and contralateral loss of pain and temperature sensation below the lesion.
5. Syringomyelia of the cervical spinal cord resulting in a cape-like distribution of pain and temperature loss is the classic example of a central cord syndrome.
6. Anterior spinal artery infarction results in bilateral weakness and loss of pain perception with sparing of dorsal column function.
7. Vitamin B_{12} deficiency results in subacute combined degeneration (involvement of dorsal columns and corticospinal tracts).
8. Tabes dorsalis is caused by late syphilis infection and results in impairment of dorsal column function.

MOTOR NEURON DISEASES

Motor neuron diseases (MNDs) are progressive and degenerative disorders characterized by the loss of motor neurons (upper, lower, or both). Common MNDs include amyotrophic lateral sclerosis (ALS), progressive muscular atrophy, and postpolio syndrome

■ AMYOTROPHIC LATERAL SCLEROSIS (LOU GEHRIG'S DISEASE)

The most important of the anterior horn cell disorders is ALS, or Lou Gehrig's disease, which has both upper and lower motor neuron signs because of involvement of the corticospinal tracts and motor neurons, respectively. ALS has its onset in middle and later life. Five percent of cases are familial in an automsomal dominant pattern (20% of these map to chromosome 21). Clinically, there are lower and upper motor neuron findings. Weakness, atrophy, and fasciculations are lower motor neuron signs, while hyperreflexia, clonus, spasticity, and the presence of a Babinski sign are upper motor neuron signs. These findings may coexist in the same limb. Weakness may commence in the legs, hands, proximal arms, or oropharynx (with dysarthria or dysphagia). Symptoms may include difficulty swallowing, limb weakness, slurred speech, impaired gait, facial weakness, and muscle cramps. Respiratory muscles may be affected in the later stages of these diseases. The cause(s) of most MNDs are not known, but environmental, toxic, viral, or genetic factors may be implicated.

The diagnosis is primarily clinical and the course of the disease relentless and progressive, without remission. Death typically results within 5 years. Electrodiagnostic studies can help confirm the diagnosis when they show active denervation in at least three body parts (e.g., limbs, cranial, and paraspinal muscles) and above the neck.

The major treatment is symptomatic and supportive. Riluzole is a glutamate inhibitor that prolongs life by 3 to 6 months but does not seem to improve function or quality of life.

■ SPINAL MUSCULAR ATROPHY

Spinal muscular atrophy (SMA) is a genetic MND caused by a progressive degeneration of motor neurons in the anterior horn of the spinal cord. The most common types of SMA are autosomal recessive disorders. Some include SMA I, or Werdnig-Hoffmann disease (usually present at birth and characterized by the inability to sit and death usually before age 2), SMA II (usually beginning between 3 and 15 months of age, with the ability to sit but not to walk), and SMA III, or Kugelberg-Welander disease, which appears between 2 and 17 years of age and includes abnormal walking; difficulty running, climbing steps, or rising from a chair; and slight tremor of the fingers. Finally, Kennedy's disease (progressive spinobulbar muscular atrophy), an X-linked recessive disorder, also affects the bulbar muscles and usually presents with dysphagia, dysarthria, weakness, and gynecomastia.

Poliomyelitis is an important cause of weakness, because the virus has a predilection for the anterior horn cells. Because of vaccination, this infection is now rare in developed countries.

KEY POINTS

1. ALS and polio are motor neuron diseases that affect the anterior horn cells.
2. ALS is characterized by upper motor neuron and lower motor neuron symptoms and signs in the same limbs.
3. EMG shows clear evidence of denervation.
4. Death usually occurs within 5 years.
5. Riluzole is the only treatment proven to prolong life marginally.
6. SMA affects lower motor neurons only.
7. Kennedy's disease is a lower motor neuron disorder characterized by bulbar muscle weakness (dysphagia and dysarthria), weakness, and gynecomastia.

The Peripheral Nervous System

The peripheral nervous system (PNS) consists of cranial nerves, spinal roots, peripheral nerves, neuromuscular junction, muscles, and autonomic ganglia. Afferent fibers connect the sensory receptors to the CNS, and efferent fibers connect the CNS to the effector (motor) apparatus. Three classically described pathologic changes affect peripheral nerve axons:

- **Wallerian degeneration:** After injury to axons and myelin, a distal disintegration of axon and myelin occurs.
- **Neuronal (or axonal) degeneration:** This develops after damage to the cell body of the neuron, resulting in the distal dying of the axon and subsequent loss of myelin.
- **Demyelination:** The myelin sheath is lost as a result of this process.

■ APPROACH TO PERIPHERAL NEUROPATHY

The goals in the evaluation of peripheral neuropathy (PN) are to localize the site of disease to the axon, myelin sheath, cell body, or vascular structures; identify the cause; and prescribe treatment when available.

Start by determining the types of symptoms (motor, sensory, autonomic, or mixed); the distribution of weakness (proximal or distal, symmetric or asymmetric); the nature and distribution of sensory involvement (small fiber, large fiber, or mixed); and the evolution of the condition (acute, subacute, or chronic) (Box 23-1).

The next step is to recognize a pattern of PN that will help to determine the etiology of the disease (Table 23-1). Finally, characterize the primary pathologic process by using electrodiagnostic studies, including nerve conduction studies and EMG.

BOX 23-1	APPROACH TO THE CLASSIFICATION OF PERIPHERAL NEUROPATHY

Functional involvement
  Motor
  Sensory
    Small fiber
    Large fiber
    Small and large fiber
  Autonomic
Anatomic distribution
  Asymmetric
  Symmetric
  Upper extremity
  Lower extremity
Temporal course
  Acute: GBS, porphyria, diphtheria, polio, toxins (thallium, lead, arsenic, Adriamycin), paraneoplastic, uremia, vasculitis
  Subacute: deficiency states (vitamins B_1 and B_{12}), toxins, uremia, diabetes, sarcoidosis, paraneoplastic, vasculitis, toxins, drugs
  Chronic: CIDP, diabetes, uremia
  Relapsing: CIDP
Pathologic mechanism
  Axonal
  Demyelination
  Combined neuropathy

GBS, Guillain-Barré syndrome; CIDP, chronic inflammatory demyelinating polyneuropathy.

KEY POINTS

1. The symptoms associated with involvement of small nerve fibers are neuropathic pain (described as aching, shooting, throbbing, or burning); temperature sensations; and autonomic dysfunction (cardiac arrhythmias, orthostatic hypotension, impotence, incontinence, and constipation).
2. The symptoms and signs associated with involvement of large fibers are loss of vibration and joint position sense, weakness, fasciculations, and loss of deep tendon reflexes.

INVESTIGATION OF THE PERIPHERAL NERVOUS SYSTEM

A logical and rational approach to the diagnosis of peripheral nervous system (PNS) disorders is fundamental. Tests are ordered sequentially, guided by the history, and clinical and electrodiagnostic findings. In general, first-line tests include a CBC, ESR, and rheumatoid profiles (for collagen disease, leukemia, vasculitis); renal and liver function tests (for uremic and hepatic disease); glucose and Hb-A1C levels (diabetes); vitamin B_{12} and folate levels (neuropathy with macrocytosis); thyroid function tests (hypothyroid neuropathy); serum protein electrophoresis and urine protein electrophoresis (dysproteinemias, monoclonal gammopathy, lymphoma, amyloidosis).

Second-line tests include urine porphobilinogen (acute intermittent porphyria); urine heavy metals such as lead, arsenic, and mercury; arsenic in hair and nails (arsenic neuropathy); hepatitis B antigen (Ag), antineutrophil cytoplasmic antibodies (Abs) (Wegener's granulomatosis); CT scan of the chest (cancer survey; carcinomatous neuropathy); CSF protein (Guillain-Barré syndrome, chronic inflammatory demyelinating polyneuropathy); CSF pleocytosis (Lyme disease, AIDS, paraneoplastic); serum HIV test (AIDS neuropathy); Lyme titers; anti-Hu Ab (paraneoplastic); anti-GM_1, MAG Ab (autoimmune neuropathy); and genetic testing for hereditary neuropathy.

Electrodiagnostic studies include nerve conduction studies and EMG. A nerve biopsy should be performed when indicated.

TABLE 23-1

Pattern-Recognition Approach to Peripheral Neuropathy

Pattern	Possible Causes
Symmetric proximal and distal weakness with sensory loss	GBS, CIDP
Symmetric distal weakness with sensory loss	Drug-induced, toxic, and metabolic neuropathies; hereditary neuropathies; amyloidosis
Asymmetric distal weakness with sensory loss	
Multiple nerves	Vasculitis; HNPP; infections such as leprosy, Lyme disease, sarcoidosis, and HIV
Single nerve	Compressive mononeuropathy and radiculopathy
Asymmetric distal weakness without sensory loss	Motor neuron disease, multifocal motor neuropathy
Asymmetric proximal and distal weakness with sensory loss	Polyradiculopathy or plexopathy, meningeal carcinomatosis or lymphomatosis, HNPP, hereditary neuropathies
Symmetric sensory loss without weakness	Cryptogenic sensory polyneuropathy; metabolic, drug-induced, or toxic neuropathies; leprosy
Asymmetric proprioceptive sensory loss without weakness	Sensory neuronopathies (ganglionopathies); consider paraneoplastic, Sjögren's syndrome, vitamin B_6 toxicity, HIV-related sensory neuronopathies, cis-platinum toxicity
Autonomic symptoms and signs	Diabetes mellitus, amyloidosis, GBS, vincristine, porphyria, HIV-related autonomic neuropathy, idiopathic pandysautonomia

GBS, Guillain-Barré syndrome; CIDP, chronic inflammatory demyelinating polyneuropathy; HNPP, hereditary neuropathy with liability to pressure palsy; HIV, human immunodeficiency virus.

Epidemiology

The prevalence of PN among patients with no recognized exposure to diseases or neurotoxic agents is 2%. Diabetes mellitus is the most common risk factor, followed by alcoholism, nonalcoholic liver disease, and malignancy. Among patients with one or two risk factors, the prevalence is 12 and 17%, respectively.

The most common causes of PN in the United States are hereditary (30%), followed by cryptogenic (23%), diabetes mellitus (15%), multifocal motor neuropathy (MMN), vitamin B_{12} deficiency, and drugs (Box 23-2).

IMMUNE-MEDIATED NEUROPATHIES

GUILLAIN-BARRÉ SYNDROME (ACUTE INFLAMMATORY DEMYELINATING POLYNEUROPATHY)

Epidemiology

There are 1 to 2 cases of Guillain-Barré syndrome (GBS) per 100,000 population per year. Males and females are at equal risk. Adults are more frequently affected than children. Of those affected, 5% will die of the illness, but more than 85% make an excellent recovery.

Pathogenesis

In 60–70% of patients, neurologic symptoms are preceded by an acute infection (usually respiratory or

TABLE 23-2

Root Syndromes

Segment	Sensation	Motor Deficit	Reflexes
Cervical			
C5	Pain in lateral shoulder; sensory loss over deltoid	Paresis of deltoid, supraspinatus, and biceps	Impairment of biceps reflex
C6	Radial side of the arm to thumb	Paresis of biceps and brachioradialis	Impairment or loss of biceps reflex
C7	Between 2nd and 4th finger	Triceps, wrist extensors and flexors, pectoralis major muscles	Impairment or loss of triceps reflex
Lumbosacral			
L3	Often none; sometimes medial thigh and knee	Quadriceps; adductor may be affected (differentiates from femoral neuropathy)	Loss of knee jerk; loss or impaired adductor reflex
L4	Medial leg below knee to medial malleolus	Quadriceps and anterior tibial muscles	Decreased knee jerk
L5	Dorsum of foot to great toe	Extensor hallucis longus, extensor digitorum longus, inversion and eversion of foot	None
S1	Lateral border of the foot	Plantar flexion, toe flexion	Decreased or absent ankle jerk

BOX 23-2 CLASSIFICATION OF PERIPHERAL NEUROPATHY BY ETIOLOGY

Immune-mediated neuropathies
  Guillain-Barré syndrome
  CIDP
  Multifocal motor neuropathy
  Neuropathy associated with monoclonal antibodies
  Immune-mediated ataxic neuropathies, including carcinomatous sensory neuropathy, sensory ganglionitis associated with Sjögren's syndrome, and idiopathic sensory ganglionitis
  Vasculitic neuropathies: Rheumatoid arthritis, Sjögren's, syndrome, hepatitis B, Lyme disease, HIV, etc.
Metabolic neuropathies
  Diabetic neuropathy
  Thyroid disease
  Hepatic neuropathy
  Uremic neuropathy
  Porphyric neuropathy (acute intermittent porphyria)
  Vitamin deficiency (B_1, B_6, B_{12})
  Critical illness neuropathy
Hereditary neuropathies
  Charcot-Marie-Tooth disease
  Amyloid neuropathies
  Hereditary neuropathy with liability to pressure palsy

Hereditary sensory and autonomic neuropathies
Neuropathy with leukodystrophy (metachromatic leukodystrophy, Krabbe's disease, adrenoleukoneuropathy)
Toxic neuropathies
  Metals: arsenic, lead, mercury, thallium
  Drugs: Vincristine, cisplatin, antiretrovirals
  Substance abuse: Alcohol, glue inhalation, nitrous oxide inhalation
  Industrial poisons: Acrylamide, carbon disulfide, cyanide, ethylene, hexacarbon, organophosphorous, trichloroethylene (trigeminal neuropathy)
Neuropathies associated with infections
  HIV
  Lyme neuropathy
  Leprosy (the most frequent infectious cause of neuropathy in the world)
  CMV and herpes
Entrapment and compressive neuropathies
  Upper extremity: Carpal tunnel syndrome or median neuropathy, ulnar neuropathy, radial neuropathy
  Lower extremity: Femoral and peroneal neuropathies, among others

CIDP, chronic inflammatory demyelinating polyneuropathy; HIV, human immunodeficiency virus; CMV, cytomegalovirus.

gastrointestinal). Some 25% of cases in the United States are preceded by infection with *Campylobacter jejuni* and others by a herpesvirus infection, most frequently cytomegalovirus or Epstein-Barr virus. Acute inflammatory demyelinating polyneuropathy (AIDP) is considered an autoimmune disease, with neural targets represented by gangliosides. Many antiganglioside antibodies are found in GBS, the most frequent being anti-GM_1, but anti-GD_{1a}, anti-GQ_{1b}, anti-GD_{1b}, and others are found as well.

Clinical Manifestations

GBS typically presents as a rapidly evolving, ascending areflexic motor paralysis with or without sensory disturbances. Initial symptoms often consist of tingling and pins-and-needles sensations in the feet, sometimes with lower back pain. Weakness evolves over hours to days, reaching its worst within 30 days (usually by 14 days). Bulbar weakness and respiratory muscle paralysis may occur. Tendon reflexes usually disappear after 3 days. Over 50% of patients develop facial weakness, and 10% have extraocular muscle paralysis. Pain is common. Autonomic dysfunction may be present, with orthostatic hypotension, transient hypertension, and cardiac arrhythmias.

The Miller-Fisher variant is characterized by gait ataxia, areflexia, and external ophthalmoplegia, usually without limb weakness. Nerve conduction studies are normal, and anti-GQ_{1b} Abs are positive in 90% of cases.

Diagnostic Evaluation

Albuminocytologic dissociation in the CSF (elevated protein but few or no cells) is characteristic. Usually the CSF protein rises after the first few days. Early electrodiagnostic findings may include prolonged distal latencies, variably prolonged or absent F waves, and possible conduction block. Early EMG changes include decreased motor unit recruitment. Routine laboratory evaluation should include CBC, ESR, liver function tests, and HIV test. The differential diagnosis includes spinal cord disease such as transverse myelitis and acute neuromuscular junction problems (myasthenia) or myopathy.

Treatment

Patients should be hospitalized. Monitoring should include frequent measurement of the forced vital capacity (FVC) and negative inspiratory pressure. An FVC below 15 mL/kg warrants transfer to the intensive care unit and likely intubation. Medical treatment includes intravenous immunoglobulin (IVIg) or plasmapheresis (equally effective). Intravenous steroids are not proven to be beneficial.

KEY POINTS

1. GBS is characterized by ascending paralysis and absent deep tendon reflexes.
2. CSF shows albuminocytologic dissociation: few cells and high protein.
3. Measurement of FVC is important in deciding whether the patient needs to be intubated (typically <15 mL/kg of body weight).
4. Treatment includes IVIg or plasmapheresis.

◼ CHRONIC INFLAMMATORY DEMYELINATING POLYNEUROPATHY

Chronic inflammatory demyelinating polyradiculoneuropathy (CIDP) is sometimes called chronic GBS. Although there are many similarities, the two conditions differ in time course and in response to steroids.

Epidemiology

CIDP may occur at any age, typically in adults between the ages of 40 and 60 years.

Clinical Manifestations

Patients experience a slowly evolving weakness beginning in the legs, with widespread areflexia and loss of vibratory sense (larger fiber). Weakness of neck flexors is often present. Painful paresthesias and other sensory symptoms can occur.

Diagnostic Evaluation

Diagnosis of chronic inflammatory demyelinating polyneuropathy is supported by clinical features, time course, relapses, prominent demyelinating features in nerve conduction studies, and CSF protein elevation. About 10% have associated systemic illness such as HIV infection, monoclonal gammopathy or Hodgkin's lymphoma.

Treatment

About 90% of CIDP improves with steroids, but 50% will relapse afterwards. Patients who do not respond to steroids may require plasmapheresis or intravenous immunoglobulin. Treatment is often required for years.

KEY POINTS

1. CIPD is a chronic, relapsing inflammatory polyradiculoneuropathy.
2. Weakness and areflexia are characteristic symptoms.
3. Treatment is with steroids. IVIg is also effective.

◼ MULTIFOCAL MOTOR NEUROPATHY

MMN is an uncommon disorder characterized by a pure motor multiple mononeuropathy. It can occur at any age. There is a slight male predominance. Evidence supports an immune-mediated mechanism.

Clinical Manifestations

Patients present with a slowly progressive, asymmetric, predominantly distal limb weakness that usually begins in the arms. Weakness develops in the distribution of individual nerves rather than following a spinal myotome; it can be severe in muscles with relatively normal bulk. Reflexes are spared in less affected muscles. Minor sensory symptoms are common. Objective sensory deficits, upper motor neuron findings, and cranial nerve findings are usually absent.

Diagnostic Evaluation

Diagnosis is made by clinical features plus electrodiagnostic studies demonstrating conduction block in motor nerves in areas not prone to compression. CSF protein is usually normal. Nerve biopsy is nonspecific. A very high IgM anti-GM_1 is found in 60 to 80% of patients with MMN. It is important to recognize and distinguish MMN from typical motor neuron disease because MMN responds to IVIg or immunosuppressive drug therapy such as cyclophosphamide.

■ NEUROPATHIES ASSOCIATED WITH MYELOMA AND OTHER MONOCLONAL GAMMOPATHIES

Approximately 10% of peripheral neuropathies are associated with serum monoclonal gammopathy (M protein) that reacts with myelin-associated glycoprotein (MAG). One-third of those patients have multiple myeloma, amyloidosis, macroglobulinemia, cryoglobulinemia, lymphoma, or leukemia.

Clinical Manifestations

These neuropathies develop as symmetric sensorimotor neuropathies that usually affect the legs more than the arms. This neuropathy causes prominent large-fiber sensory loss and sensory ataxia as well as weakness.

Diagnostic Evaluation

Electrodiagnostic studies show demyelination.

Treatment

Treatment depends on the cause. If the neuropathy is due to a plasmacytoma, excision and radiation of the tumor can be curative. In other cases, plasmapheresis may have some benefit.

METABOLIC NEUROPATHIES

■ DIABETIC POLYNEUROPATHY

Diabetic polyneuropathy is the most frequent form of diabetic neuropathy (Table 23-3) and is a common complication of diabetes mellitus; up to 60% of diabetic patients will develop neuropathy.

Epidemiology

The prevalence of diabetic neuropathy increases with the duration of diabetes; it usually develops after

■ TABLE 23-3

Diabetic Neuropathies

Type	Comments
Chronic progressive distal symmetric diabetic polyneuropathy	Mixed sensory-autonomic-motor polyneuropathy; variants include small-fiber (painful, usually spontaneous burning pain), large-fiber (ataxic), and autonomic
Diabetic proximal motor neuropathy (diabetic amyotrophy)	Severe thigh and back pain, followed within weeks by mild to severe hip and thigh muscle weakness with muscle atrophy; usually affects older type 2 diabetic patients
Acute axonal diabetic polyneuropathy (intensely painful acute or subacute progressive symmetric sensory axonal peripheral neuropathy)	Diabetic neuropathic cachexia (with worsening hyperglycemia); insulin neuritis (with improved hyperglycemia)
Diabetic mononeuropathy, radiculopathy, and polyradiculopathy	Can present with cranial neuropathy (third, fourth, and sixth nerves), multisegmental truncal radiculopathy, or limb mononeuropathy
Focal compression neuropathies associated with diabetes	Diabetic patients are more susceptible to compression neuropathies, such as median nerve at the wrist, ulnar nerve at the elbow, and peroneal nerve at the knee

5 to 10 years of the disease. Neuropathy can be present prior to overt diabetes and may be associated with impaired glucose tolerance. The pathogenesis of diabetic neuropathy is directly related to the prolonged effects of hyperglycemia.

Clinical Manifestations

Patients may report neuropathic pain and dysesthesias. More characteristic is a distal, symmetric, slowly progressive sensory loss in the lower extremities (stocking distribution, beginning with toes and feet before hands). Autonomic insufficiency can be an important feature. Weakness is a late feature.

Diagnostic Evaluation

Diagnosis is straightforward in established diabetes with typical clinical findings. It is an axonal polyneuropathy, usually involving small and large fibers.

Treatment

Glucose control is the best treatment. Symptomatic management of neuropathic pain includes the use of NSAIDs, tricyclic antidepressants, duloxetine, or anticonvulsants such as gabapentin, pregabalin, lamotrigine, and others.

KEY POINTS

1. Diabetic polyneuropathy is the most common and important of the diabetic neuropathies.
2. It usually involves small and large fibers.
3. The neuropathy is distal and symmetric, with a stocking-glove distribution.
4. Neuropathic pain may respond to anticonvulsants such as gabapentin.

■ OTHER METABOLIC NEUROPATHIES

Uremic Neuropathy

Uremic neuropathy is a symmetric, distally predominant sensorimotor axonal polyneuropathy. Foot drop and leg weakness are major manifestations.

Porphyric Neuropathy

Porphyric neuropathy is usually associated with acute intermittent porphyria. It is an acute or subacute sensorimotor axonal PN manifested by paresthesias and dysesthesias of the extremities sometimes with rapidly evolving weakness or paralysis (mimicking GBS), with areflexia and abdominal pain.

Critical Illness Neuropathies

Critical illness neuropathies develop in 50% of patients with severe medical illness who have been in the intensive care unit for more than 2 weeks. The etiology is unclear; often it may be related to an infection. Electrodiagnostic studies show an axonal neuropathy.

HEREDITARY NEUROPATHIES

Hereditary neuropathies are the most prevalent inherited neurologic disease and also the most common cause of polyneuropathy in patients referred to neurologic clinics in western countries.

Charcot-Marie-Tooth disease (CMT) is the most common inherited PN, with an estimated prevalence of 40 per 100,000 adults and 19 per 100,000 children. CMT typically presents in adolescence with symmetric, slowly progressive distal muscular atrophy of the legs and feet; in most cases, it eventually involves the hands. Hammer toes and pes cavus are common. The age of onset, severity, and rate of progression can vary, even within the same family.

KEY POINTS

1. CMT-2 is the only axonal motor neuropathy of the CMT family; the others are primarily demyelinating.
2. Hereditary sensory and autonomic neuropathy (HSAN) is a hereditary neuropathy that affects autonomic sensory or motor nerves.
3. There is no specific drug or gene therapy for hereditary neuropathies.

INFECTIOUS NEUROPATHIES

PN occurs in a number of infections, including viral, bacterial, parasitic, and prion disease. Most such peripheral neuropathies are beyond the scope of this chapter.

HIV NEUROPATHIES

HIV neuropathies include the following:

- **Distal sensory polyneuropathy:** occurs in more than 30% of patients with AIDS. It may be HIV-related, nucleoside treatment–related, or due to other neurotoxic medications.
- **Mononeuropathy and multiple mononeuropathies:** usually occur late in the illness, sometimes associated with superimposed infection (herpes, cytomegalovirus, hepatitis C, and syphilis), lymphomatous infiltration, or necrotizing vasculitis.
- **Acute inflammatory demyelinating polyneuropathy:** is similar to GBS and responsive to plasmapheresis and IVIg.
- **Lumbosacral polyradiculoneuropathy:** is uncommon but usually associated with cytomegalovirus infection. It is a devastating complication and presents as a rapidly progressive flaccid paraparesis, with sphincter dysfunction, perineal sensory loss, and lower limb areflexia.

NEUROPATHY OF LEPROSY

Leprosy is among the most common of all neuropathies in the world. It is caused by *Mycobacterium leprae* and characterized by sensory and motor involvement. It usually presents as a mononeuropathy multiplex or mononeuropathies with predilection for cooler areas such as distal limbs, nose, and ears. Deep tendon reflexes (DTRs) are usually preserved. There is often nerve hypertrophy, which can be palpated. Axonal damage, myelin changes, and nerve fiber loss are cardinal features of lepromatous leprosy.

ENTRAPMENT NEUROPATHIES

Entrapment neuropathies are a common group of mononeuropathies produced by nerve entrapment (pressure, stretch, friction, and so forth). They are reviewed in Table 23-4.

KEY POINTS

1. Leprosy is among the most common causes of neuropathy in the world.
2. HIV neuropathies are common.
3. Tips to remember about peripheral neuropathies are found in Table 23-5.

AUTONOMIC NEUROPATHIES

Autonomic neuropathies are a group of disorders that affect the sympathetic and parasympathetic nervous systems. Autonomic dysfunction may result from a lesion affecting one or more areas of the CNS or PNS and can be acquired or inherited. They can be primary or secondary—i.e., associated with another neuropathy or a systemic disorder.

Clinical Manifestations

Symptoms include orthostatic hypotension, diarrhea, constipation, early satiety, tachycardia or palpitation, blurred vision, urinary retention, and erectile dysfunction. **Pandysautonomia** refers to an acquired disorder, usually immune in nature, often following a viral infection, in which both the sympathetic and parasympathetic nervous systems are affected. Postural orthostatic tachycardia syndrome (POTS) occurs most commonly in women, with orthostatic light-headedness and near-syncopal episodes.

Autonomic neuropathy can be a prominent presentation in patients with diabetic neuropathy or a part of the more generalized polyneuropathy syndrome of diabetes. Autonomic neuropathy can also be seen in GBS, amyloid neuropathy, Chagas disease, paraneoplastic disorders, toxic and drug-induced neuropathies (from vincristine, cisplatin, acrylamide, amiodarone, etc.), and in systemic disorders like multiple system atrophy (MSA) and Lambert-Eaton myasthenic syndrome, and others.

Diagnostic Evaluation

Investigations include recording cardiovascular, sudomotor, gastrointestinal, genitourinary, respiratory, and pupillary autonomic functions. These include heart rate (R to R) variability with different maneuvers (deep breath, Valsalva, etc.), tilt-table testing, sudomotor responses [quantitative sudomotor axon reflex test (QSART)], and plasma and urinary catecholamines. The evaluation aims to assess the degree of autonomic system dysfunction with emphasis on localizing the site of the lesion. Additional testing will help to determine the cause of the dysfunction (primary or secondary).

Treatment

The prognosis and management of autonomic neuropathy depend on the diagnostic category and

■ TABLE 23-4

Entrapment Neuropathies

Nerve	Clinical features	Exam	Etiology
Upper extremity			
Median nerve: at the wrist is called carpal tunnel syndrome	Numbness or tingling involving one or more of the first four digits. Symptoms may awaken patient from sleep.	Weakness and atrophy of the thenar muscles, particularly APB. Decreased sensation in the volar aspect of the first three and a half digits. Tinel's and Phalen's signs may be present.	Compression of the median nerve at the wrist within the space known as the carpal tunnel.
Ulnar nerve: at the elbow	Paresthesias and pain in the fifth digit and the medial half of the fourth. Difficulty spreading the fingers.	Weakness and atrophy in the FDI and ADM.	Compression of the ulnar nerve in the cubital tunnel at the elbow.
Radial nerve	Wrist drop and sensory loss on the dorsal aspects of the hand.	Weakness includes triceps, brachioradialis, supinator, and wrist and finger extensors. The triceps is affected by axillary compression but spared by spiral groove compression. Weakness of wrist extensors causes wrist drop.	Compression of the radial nerve at the level of the axilla ("Saturday night palsy"); the spiral groove, or in the forearm (posterior interosseous neuropathy).
Lower extremity			
Meralgia paresthetica	Burning sensation and variable loss of sensation over the anterolateral thigh.	Area of sensory change over the lateral aspect of the thigh. Tender palpation of the inguinal ligament. No motor involvement.	Entrapment of the lateral femoral cutaneous nerve near the inguinal ligament.
Femoral neuropathy	Leg weakness on attempting to stand or walk. Pain in the anterior thigh is common.	Weakness of the quadriceps muscles, absent or diminished patellar reflex, and sensory loss over the anterior thigh—and, with saphenous nerve involvement, the medial leg/foot. Adductors intact (differentiates from an L2–3 radiculopathy).	Usually trauma from surgery, stretch injury (prolonged lithotomy position in childbirth), diabetes mellitus, and other inflammatory processes.
Peroneal neuropathy	Usually presents with foot drop with minimal sensory complaints.	Weakness of extensor hallucis longus, tibialis anterior, and the peroneal muscles (eversion of the foot); sensory loss over the dorsal part of the foot is mild.	Entrapment of the peroneal nerve between the neck of the fibula and the insertion of the peroneus longus muscle.

APB, abductor pollicis brevis; FDI, first dorsal interosseus; ADM, abductor digiti minimi.

TABLE 23-5

Tips to Remember in Peripheral Neuropathies

Type of Neuropathy	Tips
Neuropathies that may begin proximally	Sensory: porphyria, occasionally Charcot-Marie-Tooth and Tangier disease Motor: GBS, CIDP, diabetes
Neuropathies that may begin in the arms rather than the legs	Lead toxicity, leprosy, sarcoidosis, porphyria, entrapments, diabetes, vasculitic neuropathy, Tangier disease
Predominantly sensory neuropathies	Autoimmune: Miller-Fisher syndrome, IgM paraproteinemia, paraneoplastic, Sjögren's syndrome Toxic: pyridoxine and doxorubicin Infectious: diphtheria, HIV Nutritional: vitamin E deficiency
Painful neuropathies	Diabetic neuropathy, Fabry's disease, leprosy, alcoholic neuropathy, HSAN I, isoniazid, pellagra, paraneoplastic, infectious, vasculitic, HIV, inflammatory
Neuropathies that are predominantly motor	GBS, porphyria, and multifocal motor neuropathy
Neuropathy associated with cranial nerve involvement	Diphtheria, sarcoidosis, diabetes, GBS, Sjögren's syndrome, polyarteritis nodosa, Lyme disease, porphyria, Refsum's disease, syphilis, arsenic
Causes of mononeuritis multiplex	Trauma, diabetes, vasculitis, leprosy, HIV, Lyme, sarcoidosis, tumor infiltration, lymphoid granulomatosis, HNPP
Neuropathies associated with palpable peripheral nerves	CMT and Dejerine-Sottas, amyloidosis, Refsum's disease, leprosy, acromegaly, neurofibromatosis

primary cause if identified. Avoidance of exacerbating factors is recommended. Symptomatic therapy includes stockings (to avoid orthostatic hypotension); fludrocortisone (0.1 mg daily up to four times a day) to reduce salt loss; midodrine (10 mg two or three times daily) or phenylephrine for vasoconstriction; and prevention of postprandial hypotension and vasodilation.

Disorders of the Neuromuscular Junction and Skeletal Muscle

Myasthenia gravis (MG) and the Lambert-Eaton myasthenic syndrome (LEMS) are the two most common diseases of the NMJ (Table 24-1). Fatigable muscle weakness is the defining clinical feature of these disorders. In order to understand the clinical manifestations, pathophysiology, and approach to the treatment of these diseases, it is necessary to have some understanding of the anatomy and physiology of the NMJ. Nerve and muscle have both undergone structural and functional specialization at the NMJ, their point of contact. At the presynaptic bouton, secretory vesicles containing acetylcholine are concentrated at active zones formed by clusters of P/Q-type voltage-gated calcium channels. Across the synaptic cleft, the muscle membrane is thrown into folds at what is known as the **muscle endplate.** Acetylcholine receptors are clustered at the peaks of these folds. Depolarization of the nerve terminal, mediated by a sodium-dependent action potential, leads to activation of the voltage-gated calcium channels, which in turns leads to calcium influx into the presynaptic bouton. The rise in intracellular calcium triggers the release of acetylcholine via a process known as **exocytosis**, whereby the synaptic vesicles dock at the active zones and then fuse with the presynaptic membrane to release their contents into the synaptic cleft. The acetylcholine molecules diffuse across the cleft to bind to the acetylcholine receptors. This generates an inward sodium current through the acetylcholine-receptor ion pore, which leads to depolarization of the muscle endplate. This, in turn, triggers activation of the voltage-dependent sodium channels that line the troughs of the endplate membrane folds, resulting in muscle contraction. The action of acetylcholine is terminated when it is metabolized by acetylcholinesterase in the synaptic cleft.

■ MYASTHENIA GRAVIS

Acquired MG is an immunologic disorder in which antibodies are directed against the postsynaptic (muscle) nicotinic acetylcholine receptor (nAChR). Blockade and downregulation of these nAChRs reduces the probability that a nerve impulse will generate a muscle action potential.

Epidemiology

Acquired MG is the most common disorder of NMJ transmission. Its incidence is bimodal, with a peak in the second and third decades of life (during which women are more commonly affected) and a peak in the seventh and eighth decades (when it is more common in men). Earlier-onset MG is often associated with thymic hyperplasia, whereas thymoma is seen more commonly in the patients with later-onset disease.

Pathogenesis

In acquired MG, antibodies are directed against the postsynaptic nAChR. These antibodies directly block the binding of acetylcholine and lead to a complement-mediated attack and internalization of receptors. The result is distortion of the endplate with loss of the normal postjunctional folds and a reduction in the concentration of the receptors. Thus, even though acetylcholine is released normally from the presynaptic bouton, its effect at the endplate is reduced, with the result that the nerve impulse is less likely to generate a muscle action potential. This failure of neuromuscular transmission is what accounts for the weakness in patients with MG. Fatigability occurs because of depletion of presynaptic vesicles with sustained activity.

■ TABLE 24-1

Disorders of the Neuromuscular Junction and Skeletal Muscle

Disease	Clinical Phenotype	Dysfunctional Protein
Myasthenia gravis	Fatigable proximal muscle weakness; prominent ocular and bulbar involvement	Nicotinic acetylcholine receptor
Lambert-Eaton myasthenic syndrome	Fatigable proximal muscle weakness; ocular and bulbar involvement rare; prominent autonomic symptoms	P/Q-type voltage-gated calcium channel
Duchenne's and Becker's muscular dystrophy	Childhood onset of proximal muscle weakness, including neck flexors; no ocular or bulbar involvement	Dystrophin
Limb-girdle muscular dystrophy	Proximal muscle weakness; no ocular or bulbar involvement	Sarcoglycan and serveral others
Myotonic dystrophy	Distal muscle weakness and stiffness; myotonia; systemic features (ptosis, balding, etc.)	Dystrophica myotonica protein kinase (DMPK)
Emery-Dreifuss muscular dystrophy	Early onset of joint contractures; humeroperoneal pattern of muscle weakness	Emerin and lamin A/C
Hypokalemic periodic paralysis	Episodes of generalized weakness lasting hours to days	Skeletal muscle L-type voltage-gated calcium channel
Hyperkalemic periodic paralysis	Episodes of generalized weakness lasting minutes to hours	Voltage-gated sodium channel

Clinical Manifestations

Fatigable muscle weakness is characteristic. The specific symptoms depend on the distribution of this weakness. Ocular involvement is most common, manifesting as ptosis and diplopia. The pupils are never involved. Bulbar muscle weakness is next most frequent and manifests as dysarthria or dysphagia. Limb weakness is usually proximal and symmetric. Symptoms are typically worse with sustained activity or toward the end of the day. Examination is directed toward demonstrating weakness and fatigability. The patient should be asked to sustain a gaze or limb posture for a few minutes as well as following a brief period of exercise or repetitive muscle activity. DTRs are usually preserved or, if reduced, are in proportion to the degree of muscle weakness.

Most patients with MG have generalized disease, but as many as 15% may have involvement restricted to the ocular muscles. The sensitivity of the ancillary diagnostic tests depends on whether the disease is generalized or restricted.

Presentation with respiratory muscle weakness, termed **myasthenic crisis** constitutes a medical emergency. Respiratory muscle weakness may be present even in patients who do not appear short of breath, underscoring the importance of obtaining formal measures of pulmonary function—forced expiratory volume in 1 second (FEV_1) and negative inspiratory force (NIF)—in every patient with active disease. Myasthenic crisis should be distinguished from cholinergic crisis (a state of increased cholinergic drive due to overmedication with cholinesterase inhibitors). Apart from respiratory muscle weakness, cholinergic crisis is also characterized by the presence of increased bronchial secretions, salivation, diarrhea, nausea, vomiting, and diaphoresis.

Diagnostic Evaluation

The diagnosis of MG is primarily clinical, but support for the diagnosis may be obtained from various tests. Edrophonium chloride (Tensilon) is an antiacetylcholinesterase agent. It is administered intravenously and the patient observed for improvement in muscle strength. Antibodies against the nAChR may be detected in about 80% of patients with generalized MG and 55% of patients with ocular MG. Elevated titers confirm the diagnosis but negative titers do not exclude it. Seronegative MG is clinically indistinguishable from seropositive disease. Antibodies directed against MUSK (muscle-specific kinase) may be present in some patients with generalized seronegative disease. Repetitive nerve stimulation reveals a decremental response that is seen more commonly in proximal muscles. Single-fiber electromyography is the most sensitive clinical test of neuromuscular transmission. The characteristic finding in MG is increased jitter.

Treatment

Antiacetylcholinesterase drugs such as pyridostigmine inhibit the synaptic degradation of acetylcholine and thus prolong its effect. Although pyridostigmine provides adequate symptomatic therapy for many patients with MG, it does not affect the underlying immunopathology. Immune-modulating therapy thus serves as the mainstay for most patients with MG. There are few controlled trials of immunosuppressive therapy, but steroids, steroid-sparing agents such as azathioprine and cyclosporine, plasmapheresis, and intravenous immunoglobulin (IVIg) have all been used with some success. Plasmapheresis and IVIg provide rapid (but relatively short-lived) immunosuppression for patients with severe disease. Steroids and steroid-sparing agents are the mainstay for long-term immune therapy. The place and timing of thymectomy are not clear, but most would agree that it facilitates easier immunosuppression in young patients.

Patients who present with respiratory muscle weakness (myasthenic crisis) warrant admission to an intensive care unit, careful monitoring of respiratory function with intubation, and mechanical ventilation if necessary. Plasmapheresis or IVIg as well as high-dose steroids are appropriate under such circumstances, given their relatively rapid onset of action. Cholinesterase inhibitors are typically ineffective in patients with myasthenic crisis and should be discontinued (a practical measure that obviates the need to distinguish myasthenic from cholinergic crisis).

LAMBERT-EATON MYASTHENIC SYNDROME

Epidemiology

LEMS is an uncommon condition that is usually associated with an underlying small cell lung carcinoma. It is caused by antibodies directed against the presynaptic P/Q-type voltage-gated calcium channel. By reducing presynaptic calcium entry, these antibodies reduce the release of acetylcholine, leading to weakness.

Clinical Manifestations

Patients present with fatigable proximal weakness. DTRs are reduced or absent. In contrast to MG, bulbar and ocular symptoms are rare, but autonomic complaints (dry eyes, dry mouth, and impotence) are common. The characteristic finding is that of muscle facilitation: with brief intense exercise, muscle strength increases and reflexes may appear transiently. Fatigue develops with sustained activity.

Diagnostic Evaluation

The presence of elevated anti–voltage-gated calcium channel antibody titers together with an incremental response on repetitive nerve conduction studies helps to establish the diagnosis.

Treatment

The diagnosis of LEMS should prompt a thorough search for an underlying malignancy, even though a tumor is not always found. Initial therapy is directed at the underlying malignancy; in many patients, no further therapy is required. Steroids, azathioprine, IVIg, and plasmapheresis have all been used, but with less success than in MG.

KEY POINTS

1. MG is mediated by antibodies directed against the nAChR.
2. It presents with fatigable muscle weakness.
3. MG is treated with acetylcholinesterase inhibitors and steroids.

KEY POINTS

1. LEMS is mediated by anti–voltage-gated calcium channel antibodies.
2. It has a strong association with underlying small cell lung cancer.

■ SKELETAL MUSCLE DISORDERS

Disorders of skeletal muscle are a diverse group of conditions that do not lend themselves to easy classification. Discussion of these diseases is further complicated by the array of terminology used commonly. A few words of clarification may help. **Myopathy** is a nonspecific term used to refer to disorders of skeletal muscle. Muscular **dystrophy** refers to a group of hereditary conditions in which muscle biopsy demonstrates **dystrophic** changes (fiber splitting, increased connective tissues). **Myotonia** is a state of increased, sustained muscle contraction or impaired relaxation. The term **congenital** indicates onset of clinical disease in the early infantile period. **Myositis** implies an inflammatory process.

Broadly speaking, it is still useful to think of these disorders as inherited or acquired. The inherited disorders encompass the muscular dystrophies, the congenital myopathies, and the channelopathies as well as the metabolic and mitochondrial myopathies. The acquired disorders include the inflammatory myopathies, endocrine and drug- or toxin-induced myopathies, and a group of myopathies associated with other systemic illnesses. With recent advances in molecular genetics, there has been a shift toward thinking about and classifying at least the hereditary disorders on the basis of the underlying molecular defect. The approach adopted here is an attempt to synthesize clinical classification with newly acquired knowledge of the genetic basis of many of the inherited skeletal muscle disorders.

There is no single defining clinical feature of disorders of skeletal muscle. However, the selective involvement of particular groups of muscles (i.e., focal patterned weakness) is highly suggestive of a myopathic process. A detailed history and examination with particular attention to the age of onset, the presence of a family history, the nature of the symptoms and pattern of weakness as well as the tempo of the disease should allow a reasonable preliminary diagnosis to be made. Investigations like serum CK, EMG, and muscle biopsy should then lead to a definitive diagnosis in most cases.

The symptoms of muscle disease may be negative (weakness and fatigue) or positive (muscle pain, cramps, or stiffness). Weakness is the most common and important symptom; a detailed history of the sorts of activities with which the patient has difficulty provides a good indication of the pattern of weakness. Generalized fatigue or tiredness does not indicate a muscle disease, particularly when this is an isolated symptom. Muscle pain (myalgia) is a common symptom and also does not usually imply primary disease of muscle, particularly when it is an isolated symptom. Myalgias may be a feature of the inflammatory and metabolic myopathies. Patients with myotonia may complain of difficulty releasing a handgrip or of opening their eyes after squeezing them shut tightly.

The tempo of the symptoms is of major diagnostic importance. For example, acute or subacute onset of progressive weakness is a feature of some of the inflammatory myopathies, whereas chronic, slowly progressive (over years) weakness is most often encountered in the muscular dystrophies. Episodic weakness suggests one of the channelopathies or metabolic myopathies. The age of onset may also help point to a particular disease process. For example, among the dystrophies, the onset of Duchenne's muscular dystrophy (DMD) is usually around the age of 3, while many of the limb-girdle dystrophies begin only during adolescence. Of the inflammatory myopathies, dermatomyositis (DM) may occur at any age, but polymyositis is rare in children, and inclusion body myositis (IBM) usually affects the elderly. Finally, the family history may be very helpful, and the specific pattern of inheritance should be determined.

■ DYSTROPHINOPATHIES

DMD and Becker's muscular dystrophy (BMD) result from different mutations of the same gene, dystrophin, and are thus said to be **allelic.**

Clinical Manifestations

DMD and BMD should be thought of as a single disorder representing a spectrum of severity, with DMD more severe than BMD. Inheritance is X-linked, and onset is usually in childhood. The child may use an arm to push down on his thighs when arising from the floor (Gowers' sign), and there may be pseudohypertrophy of the calf muscles. Proximal muscle weakness, including neck flexors, predominates; there is usually sparing of ocular and bulbar muscles. DMD is relentlessly progressive, with the child becoming wheelchair-bound by the age of 10 or 12. Although primarily a disorder of skeletal muscle, cardiac and gastrointestinal smooth muscle involvement as well as CNS involvement are common. In DMD, death usually occurs around age 20 because of respiratory insufficiency and aspiration. Life expectancy is also reduced in BMD, but usually not so severely.

Diagnostic Evaluation

The CK level is typically markedly elevated in DMD and moderately so in BMD. A normal CK level provides strong presumptive evidence against the diagnosis. Muscle biopsy shows dystrophic features, with absent or reduced staining for dystrophin.

KEY POINTS

1. DMD and BMD are X-linked disorders that result from mutations in the dystrophin gene.
2. They present clinically as proximal muscle weakness in young boys.

■ LIMB-GIRDLE MUSCULAR DYSTROPHIES

The limb-girdle muscular dystrophies are a group of hereditary conditions in which the proximal muscles of the arms and legs are affected predominantly.

Clinical Manifestations

Most of these disorders are characterized by weakness of the limb-girdle muscles, with relative sparing of facial, extraocular, and pharyngeal musculature. Cardiomyopathy is less frequent than in the dystrophinopathies.

Classification

There are both autosomal dominant and recessive varieties. Some are due to mutations in proteins known as the sarcoglycans, which form part of the multimolecular dystrophin-associated glycoprotein complex.

Diagnostic Evaluation

CK level is usually elevated. The EMG is myopathic, and biopsy demonstrates nonspecific dystrophic changes. Immunohistochemistry with antibodies directed against the various sarcoglycan proteins may help to distinguish the different limb-girdle muscular dystrophies.

KEY POINTS

1. Limb-girdle muscular dystrophies are characterized clinically by shoulder and hip girdle weakness with relative sparing of extraocular, pharyngeal, and facial muscles.
2. They affect both boys and girls and may resemble the dystrophinopathies, requiring muscle biopsy for differentiation.

■ MYOTONIC DYSTROPHY

The classic form of myotonic dystrophy is the most common inherited skeletal muscle disorder affecting adults. Inheritance is autosomal dominant and the genetic defect is an unstable CTG expansion in the DMPK (dystrophia myotonica protein kinase) gene.

Clinical Manifestations

Myotonic dystrophy is a multisystem disease. Weakness and stiffness of distal muscles are usually the presenting symptoms in young adults. Action and percussion myotonia are often present. Proximal weakness develops later in the course of the disease. Systemic findings include cataracts, ptosis, arrhythmias, dysphagia (from esophageal myotonia), insulin resistance, testicular atrophy, and frontal balding. Neurobehavioral features (changes in affect, personality, and motivation) as well as cognitive dysfunction are also observed commonly.

Diagnostic Evaluation and Treatment

CK level is usually normal or only mildly elevated. EMG demonstrates myotonia. DNA testing for the CTG expansion is now available. Cardiac evaluation is important to screen for and prevent arrhythmias. There is no specific treatment for the muscle weakness, but drugs such as phenytoin and carbamazepine may reduce the myotonia. Management is otherwise supportive.

KEY POINTS

1. Myotonic dystrophy is the most common adult-onset muscular dystrophy.
2. It is a trinucleotide (CTG) repeat disorder.
3. Myotonic dystrophy presents with distal muscle weakness and myotonia.

■ EMERY-DREIFUSS MUSCULAR DYSTROPHY

Emery-Dreifuss muscular dystrophy is primarily caused by mutations in the **emerin** gene on the X chromosome. A rare autosomal dominant form of the disease results from mutations in the **lamin A** and **lamin C** genes on chromosome 1. **Emerin** is a trans (nuclear) membrane protein, and the lamin A and C genes also localize to the nuclear membrane.

Clinical Manifestations

This disorder is characterized by the early onset of joint contractures (predominantly affecting the elbows, ankles, and cervical spine), a slowly progressive humeroperoneal pattern of weakness and atrophy, and a cardiomyopathy that manifests as conduction abnormalities. The appearance of contractures prior to the onset of weakness and atrophy helps to distinguish this disorder from the other muscular dystrophies. The pattern of weakness is described as humeroperoneal because of early involvement of biceps, triceps, peroneal, and tibial muscles. Both tachy- and bradyarrhythmias may occur. Although female carriers do not develop weakness or atrophy, they are at risk for the cardiac complications.

Diagnostic Evaluation and Treatment

CK levels are typically mildly to moderately elevated. EMG is myopathic, and muscle biopsy usually demonstrates nonspecific dystrophic changes. The diagnosis may be confirmed by reduced or absent immunostaining for **emerin.** No specific treatment is available. Range-of-motion and stretching exercises may reduce the severity of contractures. Pacemaker placement may be lifesaving for patients with severe conduction abnormalities.

KEY POINTS

1. Mutations in the emerin and lamin A/C genes are responsible for Emery-Dreifuss muscular dystrophy.
2. Early contractures affecting the elbows, ankles, and cervical spine are characteristic.
3. Weakness occurs in a humeroperoneal distribution.
4. Cardiac conduction defects are an important cause of morbidity.

■ CHANNELOPATHIES

The channelopathies are a group of disorders characterized by ion channel dysfunction. The clinical manifestations are determined by the specific ion channel involved.

The periodic paralyses (PP) are autosomal dominant conditions that derive their designation from their cardinal manifestation, episodic muscle weakness. Attacks of weakness are usually associated with a change in serum potassium concentration; they are therefore classified accordingly into hypokalemic and hyperkalemic varieties. Hypokalemic PP is the result of a mutation in the pore-forming $\alpha 1S$-subunit of the skeletal muscle calcium channel that results in secondary dysfunction of the Na^+,K^+-ATPase. Hyperkalemic PP results from mutations in the skeletal muscle voltage-gated sodium channel.

KEY POINTS

1. The periodic paralyses are characterized by episodic muscle weakness.
2. They are caused by mutations in skeletal muscle membrane ion channels.

■ MITOCHONDRIAL MYOPATHIES

The mitochondrial myopathies are a heterogeneous group of disorders with systemic manifestations.

Inheritance

Mitochondrial DNA is entirely maternally inherited; this is therefore the usual mode of inheritance for mitochondrial disorders. Given that over 90% of mitochondrial proteins are encoded by nuclear genes, however, virtually all other patterns of inheritance may occur as well.

Clinical Manifestations

A number of characteristic syndromes have been identified. These include myoclonic epilepsy with ragged red fibers (MERRF); mitochondrial myopathy, encephalopathy, lactoacidosis, and stroke (MELAS); progressive external ophthalmoplegia (PEO); and the Kearns-Sayre syndrome.

Diagnostic Evaluation

There are no characteristic clinical or electrophysiologic findings in the mitochondrial myopathies, but a common finding is the co-occurrence of a myopathy and a peripheral neuropathy. Serum or CSF lactate and pyruvate are often increased. The histopathologic changes are also nonspecific and include the presence of ragged red fibers and variability of cytochrome oxidase staining.

KEY POINTS

1. The mitochondrial myopathies are clinically and genetically heterogeneous.
2. The myopathy is frequently accompanied by other systemic manifestations (e.g., seizure, stroke, migraine, diabetes).
3. Serum lactate and pyruvate are often increased.
4. Muscle biopsy may show ragged red fibers.

▇ DISTAL MYOPATHIES

The distal myopathies are a group of largely hereditary conditions in which muscle weakness at onset is predominantly distal. Distal muscle weakness, however, may occur atypically in acquired disorders such as polymyositis and inclusion body myositis, in which weakness is usually more proximal. Distal weakness may also occur in some of the other muscular dystrophies (e.g., fascioscapulohumeral, scapuloperoneal, and Emery-Dreifuss humeroperoneal).

▇ INFLAMMATORY MYOPATHIES

The noninfectious immune-mediated inflammatory myopathies include polymyositis (PM), dermatomyositis (DM), and inclusion body myositis (IBM).

Clinical Manifestations

PM and DM are characterized by proximal (usually symmetric) muscle weakness. Weakness in IBM is often asymmetric and may affect both proximal and distal muscles. Early selective involvement of forearm and finger flexors, as well as of knee extensors (quadriceps) and ankle extensors, should arouse suspicion of this diagnosis. Pharyngeal and neck flexor muscles may be affected, but facial and respiratory muscles are usually spared. IBM is often diagnosed only when patients thought to have PM fail to respond to steroids. DM is distinguishable by the associated purplish discoloration of the eyelids (heliotrope) and papular erythematous scaly lesions over the knuckles (Gottron patches).

These are systemic disorders, and extramuscular manifesations are not infrequent. Dysphagia is common and reflects oropharyngeal and esophageal muscle involvement. Cardiac manifestations include conduction defects, tachyarrhythmias, myocarditis, and congestive cardiac failure. Interstitial lung disease associated with the presence of anti-Jo-1 antibodies occurs in approximately 10% of patients. DM may occur in the context of systemic sclerosis or other mixed connective tissue disease, and there is an increased incidence of malignancy in patients with DM. In contrast to DM and IBM, PM is more often associated with other autoimmune diseases, including Crohn's disease, vasculitis, sarcoidosis, MG, and others.

Pathogenesis

DM is a microangiopathic disorder in which antibodies and complement are directed primarily against intramuscular blood vessels. Inflammation is due to muscle ischemia. PM and IBM are mediated by antigen-directed cytotoxic T-cell processes.

Diagnostic Evaluation

CK is elevated in more than 90% of patients with an inflammatory myopathy. While this is the most sensitive and specific marker for muscle breakdown, levels do not correlate with the degree of weakness. EMG demonstrates myopathic changes (often with accompanying denervation changes due to muscle fiber necrosis) and is useful in selecting a muscle for biopsy. The characteristic histologic abnormality in DM is perifasicular atrophy. Characteristic findings include fiber size variation, scattered necrotic and regenerating fibers, and endomysial inflammation with invasion of nonnecrotic muscle fibers with CD8+ T cells. The differing pathology in PM reflects the underlying pathophysiologic processes. The diagnosis of IBM requires the detection of red-ringed vacuoles and amyloid deposits.

Treatment

Corticosteroids are the mainstay of treatment in PM and DM, but they are of no benefit in IBM. IVIg has been shown beneficial in DM, but its role in PM is less clear. Plasmapheresis is probably not beneficial. Steroid-sparing agents such as azathioprine and methotrexate should be reserved for patients with refractory disease.

KEY POINTS

1. The inflammatory myopathies are characterized by muscle pain, weakness, and elevated CK level.
2. Proximal muscle involvement is found in PM and DM, but distal muscle weakness is more common in IBM.
3. PM and DM are steroid-responsive; IBM is resistant, but it may respond to IVIg.

■ ENDOCRINE AND DRUG- OR TOXIN-INDUCED MYOPATHIES

Thyrotoxic Myopathy

Although weakness is rarely the presenting complaint of patients with thyrotoxicosis, it is found on examination in many. Proximal muscle weakness and atrophy are usually the dominant clinical features, but rarely distal weakness may be the earliest manifestation. Bulbar and respiratory muscle involvement is uncommon. Reflexes may be brisk, reflecting shortened relaxation time. If Graves disease is the cause of thyrotoxicosis, the differential diagnosis of muscle weakness should include MG. The pathogenesis of thyrotoxic myopathy is unknown but may reflect enhanced muscle catabolism. CK level is typically normal, and EMG demonstrates myopathic units. Muscle strength will improve with treatment of the underlying thyrotoxic state, but beta blockers may improve strength acutely.

Hypothyroid Myopathy

Myopathic symptoms develop in about one-third of patients with hypothyroidism. The typical presentation is that of proximal muscle weakness, fatigue, myalgias, and cramps. Reflexes may demonstrate delayed relaxation. There may be an associated distal polyneuropathy. CK level is typically elevated (10 to 100 times normal). EMG shows nonspecific myopathic changes. Weakness usually improves following thyroid replacement, but recovery may lag behind a return to the euthyroid state.

Steroid Myopathy

Myopathy may result from increased glucocorticoids from either endogenous production or exogenous administration. The latter is more common, and although any synthetic glucocorticoid can cause myopathy, it is more common with the fluorinated compounds (e.g., triamcinolone and dexamethasone). Doses in excess of the equivalent of 30 mg of prednisone per day are associated with an increased risk of myopathy. The risk is reduced with alternate-day regimens. Typically, weakness begins after chronic administration of steroids, but it may occur within a few weeks. Weakness is predominantly proximal, with sparing of the ocular, bulbar, and facial muscles. CK level is usually normal. EMG is usually normal. Muscle biopsy typically demonstrates type II fiber atrophy, but this finding is nonspecific. Treatment requires a reduction in the steroid dose, switching to an alternate-day regimen or using a nonfluorinated compound.

Drug- or Toxin-Induced Myopathy

Many drugs and toxins have been implicated as causes of myopathy. Typically they produce a syndrome characterized by proximal myopathy and increased serum CK level. Some of the more commonly encountered drugs that induce myopathies are listed in Table 24-2.

KEY POINTS

1. Proximal muscle weakness is frequent in patients with either hypothyroidism or hyperthyroidism.
2. Proximal myopathy may result from excessive circulating steroids, either from increased endogenous production or exogenous administration.
3. CK level is usually normal in the metabolic myopathies except for hypothyroidism, in which it is typically elevated.

■ NEUROLEPTIC MALIGNANT SYNDROME

NMS is a disorder characterized by fever, depressed level of arousal, muscle rigidity, autonomic dysfunction and fever. It is most commonly encountered in the context of treatment with antipsychotics (haloperidol > chlorpromazine, fluphenazine > risperidone,

■ TABLE 24-2

Drug- or Toxin-Induced Myopathies

Disorder	Drug or Toxin	Clinical Syndrome
Necrotizing myopathy	HMG-CoA reductase inhibitors; cyclosporin; propofol; alcohol	Acute or insidious onset of proximal muscle weakness; CK level typically elevated
Steroid myopathy	Fluorinated glucocorticoids	Proximal muscle weakness; CK level usually normal
Mitochondrial myopathy	Zidovudine	Acute or insidious onset of proximal muscle weakness; CK level normal or only mildly increased
Inflammatory myopathy	Cimetidine; procainamide; L-dopa; phenytoin; lamotrigine; D-penicillamine	Acute onset of proximal muscle weakness; CK level typically increased
Critical illness myopathy	Corticosteroids plus neuromuscular blocking agents in patients with sepsis	Acute or subacute onset of generalized weakness; CK level may be normal or elevated

HMG-CoA, hydroxymethylglutaryl coenzyme A; CK, serum creatinine kinase.

olanzapine, clozapine, quetiapine) but may also occur with L-dopa withdrawal in patients with Parkinson's disease and in association with the use of tricyclic antidepressants, phenelzine, and metoclopramide. Although the etiology of this disorder is unclear, it has been suggested to result from central dopaminergic blockade. Management requires discontinuation of the offending drug, aggressive fluid resuscitation, and other supportive measures, usually in the context of an intensive care unit. Intravenous benzodiazepines, bromocriptine, amantadine, or dantrolene may be helpful.

Pediatric Neurology

Neurologic disorders in children are encountered commonly by pediatricians and general physicians. Many neurologic diseases that affect infants and children also affect adults, such as infection, epilepsy, inflammatory and demyelinating diseases, peripheral neuropathies, and myopathies; but some are characteristic of early ages, including developmental disorders, malformations, and genetically determined conditions. Seizures are among the most common neurologic problems in childhood (see Chapter 15).

The history is the most important component of the evaluation of a child with a neurologic problem. It shares the same principles as described for the adult history but also requires a complete review of the pregnancy, labor, and delivery, especially if a perinatal injury or congenital infection is suspected.

■ DEVELOPMENT AND MATURATION

One of the most important elements of the neurologic history is a developmental assessment of the child. The Denver Developmental Screening Test is an efficient and reliable method to assess achievement of developmental milestones. It evaluates four components of development: gross motor skills, fine motor adaptive skills, language, and personal-social interaction. Table 25-1 summarizes developmental milestones by age. This is based on averages and therefore can be used only with an understanding of the variability among children. Table 25-2 gives a brief description of primitive reflexes and their significance.

■ CEREBRAL PALSY

Cerebral palsy (CP) is a static disorder due to pre- or perinatal damage to cerebromotor pathways. It can be acquired or genetic. CP occurs in about 2.7 per 1,000 births. Risk factors for CP include hypoxic-ischemic insult to the brain in the perinatal period, prematurity, low birth weight, chorioamnionitis, prenatal viral infections, and prenatal strokes.

Classification

The most commonly used classification of CP is based on the distribution of the affected limbs:

- **Hemiparetic:** Weakness and spasticity are seen on one side of the body. Signs include fisting on the affected side, early hand preference, and increased reflexes with upgoing toes on the affected side.
- **Diparetic:** There is spasticity of all four limbs, affecting the legs more than the arms. The children are usually of normal intelligence and are less likely to have seizures than children with other forms of CP
- **Spastic quadriplegic:** All four limbs are affected. Seizures usually occur within the first 48 hours of life. The infant may show signs of cerebral hypotonia (see below).

Clinical Manifestations

CP may be diagnosed as early as the first week of life: infants may have flaccid weakness, asymmetric limb movements, or seizures. In older children, spasticity, dystonia, developmental delay, and drooling are common presentations.

Diagnostic Evaluation

The diagnosis of CP is based on the clinical symptoms and signs. The cause may not be determined, but the presence of a static (not worsening) disorder is suggestive. One must rule out other entities that

■ TABLE 25-1

Developmental Milestones

Age	Adaptive/Fine Motor Skills	Gross Motor Skills	Language	Personal/Social
1 month	Grasp reflex; hand fisted	Raises head slightly when prone	Facial response to sounds	Stares at face
2 months	Follows objects with eyes past midline	Lifts head from prone to 45 degrees	Coos	Smiles in response to others
4 months	Hands open; brings objects to mouth	Sits, head steady; rolls to supine	Laughs and squeals; turns toward voice	Smiles spontaneously
6 months	Palmar grasp of objects; starts transfer of objects	Sits independently; stands with hands held	Babbles (consonant sounds); mimics sounds	Reaches for toys; recognizes strangers
9 months	Pincer grasp; claps hands	Pulls to stand	Says "mama,""dada," nonspecifically; comprehends "no"; associates word and action ("bye-bye," "no," etc.)	Finger-feeds self; waves bye-bye
1 year	Helps to turn pages of book; tower of two blocks	Stands independently; walks with one hand held	2–4 words; follows command with gesture	Points to indicate wants
18 months	Turns pages of book; imitates vertical lines	Walks up steps	10–20 words; points to four body parts; obeys simple commands	Feeds self with spoon; uses cup
2 years	Solves single-piece puzzles	Jumps; kicks ball	Combines 2–3 words; uses "I" and "you"; 50–300 words	Removes coat; verbalizes wants
3 years	Copies circle; draws person with three body parts; imitates horizontal lines; towers of six cubes; draws circles	Throws ball overhand; walks up stairs, alternating feet	Gives full name, age, and sex; names two colors	Toilet trained; puts on shirt and knows front from back
4 years	Counts four objects; identifies some numbers and letters; uses scissors	Hops on one foot	Understands prepositions (under, on, behind, in front of); asks "how" and "why"	Dresses with little assistance; shoes on correct feet
5 years	Prints first name; counts 10 objects; draws triangle; draws person with several parts	Skips, alternating feet	Asks meaning of words; understands conjunctions and past tenses; knows colors	Ties shoes

■ **TABLE 25-2**

Primitive Reflexes

Reflex	Significance	Appears	Disappears
Moro	Elicited by head extension. Two phases: extension and abduction of arms and leg extension, followed by slower abductions of arms. Asymmetry indicates central nervous system disease such as hemiparesis, spinal cord lesion or brachial plexus injury.	Term newborns	3 months
Tonic neck	Turning head, arm and leg extended in the side toward the turn and flexion in the other side (fencing posture). If infant is unable to move out of posture, implies possible brain pathology.	1 month	5 months
Traction response	Lift baby by traction in both hands. Head lag after 6 months is pathologic and indicates hypotonia.	Birth	6 months
Parachute	Elicited by plunging suspended infant downward. Arms should thrust forward symmetrically as if breaking the fall. Also elicited with baby in sitting position and pushed forward. Arms should try to break the fall. Asymmetry suggests hemiparesis, spinal cord lesion, or brachial plexus pathology	6 months	Persists throughout life

may present with dystonia, ataxia, or spasticity but which progress with time (e.g., metabolic disorders, metachromatic leukodystrophy, and movement disorders such as levodopa-responsive dystonia). MRI is indicated only to exclude other structural causes such as tumor, stroke, or AVMs.

Treatment

In general, a multidisciplinary approach is necessary, with early infant stimulation, physical and occupational therapy, orthopedic and psychological evaluation, and speech therapy.

KEY POINTS

1. CP is a static disease; if the disease is progressing, it is not CP.
2. It occurs in almost 3 per 1,000 births.
3. The most common abnormality is spasticity.

■ MENTAL RETARDATION AND DEVELOPMENTAL DELAY

Mental retardation is the failure to develop normal mental capacities. It can be classified by the results of standard intelligence tests such as the Stanford-Binet IQ and the Wechsler Preschool and Primary Scale of Intelligence–Revised. Normal IQ is 100 with a standard deviation of 15. Mental retardation is classified as follows:

- Mild: IQ between 55 and 70
- Moderate: IQ between 40 and 55
- Severe: 25 to 40
- Profound: less than 25

There are many causes of mental retardation. Among them are prenatal and postnatal trauma (e.g., intracerebral hemorrhage and hypoxic-anoxic encephalopathy); congenital and postnatal infection (e.g., congenital rubella, syphilis, cytomegalovirus, toxoplasmosis, and HIV infection); chromosomal abnormalities (e.g., Down's syndrome, fragile X syndrome, Angelman's syndrome, Prader-Willi syndrome); chromosomal translocations (e.g., cri du chat syndrome); inherited metabolic disorders (e.g., hypothyroidism, galactosemia, Tay-Sachs disease); and toxic, nutritional, and environmental causes. Table 25-3 summarizes some chromosomal abnormalities associated with mental retardation.

Developmental delay is the failure to acquire age-appropriate cognitive, language, fine or gross motor skills, or social skills. The Denver Developmental Assessment is a standard test that can help establish

■ TABLE 25-3

Mental Retardation Syndromes Associated with Chromosomal Abnormalities

Condition	Epidemiology	Genetic Defect	Clinical Characteristics
Fragile X syndrome	Most common inherited form of MR; affects males more than females	Defect in the X chromosome; mutation in the 5' end of the gene with amplification of a CGG repeat (200 or more copies)	20% males are normal; 30% of carrier females are mildly affected; moderate mental retardation; behavioral problems; somatic abnormalities: long face, enlarged ears, and macro-orchidism
Prader-Willi syndrome	Uncommon inherited disorder	Absence of segment 11–13 on the long arm of the paternally derived chromosome 15	Mental retardation; decreased muscle tone; short stature; emotional lability and insatiable appetite (obesity)
Angelman's syndrome	Uncommon neurogenetic disorder	Deletion of segment 11–13 on the maternally derived chromosome 15	Mental retardation; abnormal gait; speech impairment; seizures; inappropriate happy behavior that includes laughing, smiling, and excitability ("happy puppet" syndrome)
Rett's syndrome	Progressive neurodevelopmental disorder; generally affects only females; most common cause of MR in women; incidence of 1 in 10,000 births	Causal gene is MeCP2, found in the long arm of chromosome X (X 28).	Normal development until 6–18 months; a first sign is hypotonia; autistic-like behavior; stereotyped hand movements (wringing and waving); lag in brain and head growth; gait abnormalities; seizures

MR, mental retardation.

the diagnosis. Many of the etiologies of developmental delay are similar to those responsible for mental retardation and include intrauterine toxins and infections, genetic abnormalities, migrational disorders, hypoxic-ischemic encephalopathy, and inborn errors of metabolism. Most often, though, no cause for developmental delay is found, in which case it is labeled idiopathic.

Treatment for both mental retardation and developmental delay includes referral to early intervention programs for special education and training.

KEY POINTS

1. Mental retardation implies a substantially below-average cognitive ability and adaptive behavior.
2. Developmental delay implies inability to achieve developmental milestones at the usual age. It is not synonymous with mental retardation.

■ AUTISTIC SPECTRUM DISORDERS

Autism is a developmental disorder of brain function. Usually, the etiology is unknown. Autism is the most common of the disorders that fall under the banner of **pervasive developmental disorder.**

Clinical Manifestations

Autism is characterized by a combination of social, behavioral, and language abnormalities with onset before age 3. Marked deficiencies in social and communication skills manifest as a lack of attachment to other members of the family and poor social interactions. A restricted range of behaviors, interests, and activities is demonstrated and may include repetitive and stereotyped behaviors such as toe walking, rocking, flapping, banging, and licking. Abnormal language features include echolalia and stereotyped speech.

Diagnostic Evaluation

The diagnosis is clinical. Differential diagnosis includes other causes of speech and language problems, such as deafness, mental retardation, and seizures (Landau-Kleffner syndrome). **Asperger's syndrome** can be considered a variant of autism characterized by social isolation and eccentric behavior with normal intelligence and language development.

Treatment

The treatment of autism includes support and behavior modification. No cures are available at present.

KEY POINT

Autism is characterized by a combination of social, behavioral, and language abnormalities.

■ DEVELOPMENTAL REGRESSION AND INHERITED NEURODEGENERATIVE DISORDERS

Developmental regression is defined as a loss of previously attained developmental milestones. It is often related to an inherited neurodegenerative disorder. It is one of the most distressing complaints confronted by pediatricians and neurologists. An extensive battery of diagnostic tests is the wrong approach. A complete history, physical and neurologic examination, and additional tests based on those findings are fundamental in reaching an accurate diagnosis. Always differentiate regression from developmental delay (see above). Table 25-4 shows common causes of progressive encephalopathy at different ages that can produce developmental delay or regression.

The inherited neurodegenerative diseases are classified according to the involved cellular element: the lysosome, peroxisome, mitochondria, Golgi apparatus, and cell membrane. Whatever the cellular and

---

■ TABLE 25-4

Causes of Progressive Encephalopathy

Onset before Age 2	Onset after Age 2
Mitochondrial disorders	AIDS
Hypothyroidism	Congenital syphilis
Neurocutaneous syndromes	Subacute sclerosing panencephalitis
Tuberous sclerosis complex	Enzymatic lysosomal disorders
Neurofibromatosis	Gaucher's disease
Gray matter disorders	Gangliosidosis
Infantile ceroid lipofuscinosis	Late-onset Krabbe's disease
Rett's syndrome	Metachromatic leukodystrophy
White matter disorders	Other gray matter disorders
Alexander's disease	Ceroid lipofuscinosis
Canavan's disease	Huntington's disease
Neonatal adrenoleukodystrophy	Mitochondrial disorders (MERRF)
Pelizaeus-Merzbacher disease (peroxisomal disorders)	Other white matter disorders
Disorders of amino acid metabolism	Adrenoleukodystrophy
Homocystinuria	Alexander's disease
Maple syrup urine disease	
Phenylketonuria	
Enzymatic disorders	
Gangliosidosis	
Gaucher's disease	
Krabbe's disease	
Mucopolysaccharidoses	
Metachromatic leukodystrophy	

AIDS, acquired immunodeficiency syndrome; MERRF, myoclonic epilepsy with ragged red fibers.

molecular mechanism responsible, it is possible to recognize common patterns of disease expression according to the age of onset, symptoms, and systems involved. The most common clinical features of neurometabolic diseases presenting in infancy and childhood are developmental delay or regression.

Lysosomal disorders are caused by genetic defects of lysosomal enzymes and cofactors that result in the accumulation of undegraded substrates in lysosomes. They are classified according to the accumulated material: sphingolipidoses, mucopolysaccharidoses, mucolipidoses, glycogen storage disease type II, sialidoses, and neuronal ceroid lipofuscinosis. Some of the most important characteristics of these clinical entities are reviewed in Table 25-5.

Peroxisomal disorders are a heterogeneous group of syndromes characterized by abnormalities in lipid metabolism. Multiple enzyme deficiencies have been characterized. They are rare. The most important are X-linked adrenoleukodystrophy and Zellweger's syndrome (see Table 25-5). Most of the degenerative diseases of infancy and childhood are not treatable. However, attempts to reach a final diagnosis are important in order to provide parents with genetic counseling, prognosis, and further management advice.

KEY POINTS

1. Neurodegenerative diseases involving the white matter include metachromatic leukodystrophy, Krabbe's disease, adrenoleukodystrophy, Pelizaeus-Merzbacher disease, Canavan disease, and Alexander's disease.
2. Peripheral nerve involvement is found in metachromatic leukodystrophy, Krabbe's disease, Canavan's disease, and adrenoleukodystrophy.
3. Congenital macular cherry-red spots (red color of the macula compared with a pale retina) are found in Tay-Sachs disease, Sandhoff's disease, Niemann-Pick disease, Gaucher's disease, metachromatic leukodystrophy, and sialidoses.

◾ NEUROCUTANEOUS DISORDERS

Neurocutaneous disorders (phakomatoses) are characterized by lesions in the CNS and PNS, skin, eyes, and other organs. A summary of neurocutaneous disorders and their clinical features is given in Table 25-6.

◾ THE HYPOTONIC INFANT

Hypotonia is a reduction in postural tone. It may be the manifestation of a CNS or PNS disorder or of both.

The most common cause of hypotonia is **cerebral hypotonia**, a static encephalopathy from pre- or perinatal brain injury. The most useful diagnostic finding in this group of disorders is not the hypotonia but the other signs of CNS dysfunction. Seizures, microcephaly, dysmorphic facies, and mental retardation point to the brain as the source of hypotonia. Usually, DTRs are increased and plantar reflexes are extensor.

Other causes of hypotonia include spinal cord disease (e.g., transection during breech presentation), anterior horn cell lesions (spinal muscular atrophy), neuromuscular junction abnormalities, and myopathies (congenital, metabolic, etc.). The physical exam and presence or absence of "central" signs may help to localize the site of disease.

KEY POINTS

1. Hypotonia can be central, peripheral, or both.
2. Cerebral hypotonia is usually associated with other signs of CNS dysfunction (seizures, developmental delay, etc.).
3. Infants with severe hypotonia but only marginal weakness usually do not have a disorder of the lower motor unit.

◾ ATTENTION DEFICIT–HYPERACTIVITY DISORDER

Clinical Manifestations

The essential features of attention deficit–hyperactivity disorder (ADHD) are inappropriate inattention, impulsivity, and hyperactivity for age. Children with the hyperactive-impulsive subtype are fidgety, leave their seats in the classroom, and have difficulty playing quietly. Children with the inattentive-distractible subtype do not pay close attention to details, have difficulty organizing tasks, and are forgetful in daily activities. There are many causes of ADHD, but most often there is a family history, implying a genetic etiology.

■ TABLE 25-5

Inherited Neurodegenerative Disorders

Disorder	Metabolic Defect	Chromosome and Inheritance	Notes
Tay-Sachs disease	Hexosaminidase A	15, autosomal recessive	Cherry-red spot. More common in Ashkenazi Jews.
Niemann-Pick disease	Sphingomyelinase	11, autosomal recessive	Cherry-red spot. More common in Ashkenazi Jews.
Gaucher's disease	Glucosylceramide ß-glucosidase	1, autosomal recessive	Cherry-red spot. Gaucher cells in bone marrow.
Krabbe's disease	Galactosylceramide ß-galactosidase	14, autosomal recessive	Globoid cells with peri-odic–acid Schiff (PAS)-positive granules.
Hurler's syndrome	α-L-iduronidase	4, autosomal recessive	Clouding of the cornea. Characteristic facies and dwarfism.
Hunter's syndrome	Iduronate sulfatase	X-linked	Hurler phenotype without corneal clouding.
Metachromatic leukodystrophy	Arylsulfatase A	22, autosomal recessive	Cherry-red spot. Demyelinating disorder. Can present as schizophrenia in adults. Positive urine sulfatides.
Adrenoleukodystrophy	Very long chain fatty acid oxidation	X-linked	White matter hyperintensity on MRI. May present as a neuropathy or myelopathy in adults.
Alexander's disease	Mitochondrial	11, autosomal recessive	Rosenthal fibers on biopsy. Macrocephaly. Dysmyelination of the CNS.
Canavan's disease	Aspartoacylase	Variety of mutations, autosomal recessive	Macrocephaly. Dysmyelination of the CNS.
Pelizaeus-Merzbacher disease	Proteolipid protein	X-linked	Pendular nystagmus. Dysmyelination of the CNS.
Leigh's disease	Mitochondrial	Autosomal recessive or X-linked	Bilateral putaminal hyperintensity on MRI.
Rett's syndrome	Methyl-CpG-binding protein-2	X-linked	Occurs exclusively in girls. Microcephaly, autism, and hand-wringing.
Neuronal ceroid lipo-fuscinosis	Excess lipofuscin storage	Variety of mutations, autosomal recessive	Dementia, myoclonus, ataxia, retinitis pigmentosa. Variety of forms with different ages of onsets and severities.

TABLE 25-6

Neurocutaneous Syndromes

	Inheritance	Neurologic Findings	Cutaneous Findings	Other Findings
Neurofibromatosis 1	Autosomal dominant; chromosome 17	Optic nerve gliomas	Café-au-lait spots, neurofibromas, axillary or inguinal freckles	Lisch nodules in the iris
Neurofibromatosis 2	Autosomal dominant; chromosome 22	Bilateral acoustic neuromas	Café-au-lait spots are less common than in NF-1	
Tuberous sclerosis	Autosomal dominant; TSC 1—chr 9, TSC 2—chr 16	Cortical tubers, subependymal nodules and astrocytomas, mental retardation, seizures	Adenoma sebaceum, ash-leaf spots, shagreen patches	Angiomyolipomas of kidneys, cardiac rhabdomyoma
Ataxia telangiectasia	Autosomal recessive; chromosome 11	Truncal ataxia, progressive dementia	Telangiectasias	Immunodeficiency and susceptibility to infections, leukemia, lymphoma
von Hippel Lindau	Autosomal dominant; chromosome 3	Cerebellar hemangioblastomas, ataxia		Renal lesions including hemangiomas and carcinomas, pheochromocytoma
Sturge Weber	Sporadic	Venous angioma of the pia mater, seizures, hemiparesis, mental retardation	Port-wine stain in the distribution of some divisions of the ophthalmic nerve	

Diagnostic Evaluation

A diagnosis is made by clinical history and neuropsychological screening tests. Children usually have normal IQs but low scores on tests of sustained attention. Imaging and laboratory tests are generally not helpful.

Treatment

The standard medical treatment of ADHD is with stimulant drugs like methylphenidate and dextroamphetamine. It is important to emphasize parent participation in the treatment program and behavioral modifications like goal setting, incentives, and punishments.

KEY POINTS

1. Children with ADHD usually have a positive family history for the disorder.
2. Stimulants like methylphenidate and dextroamphetamine are often effective treatments for ADHD.

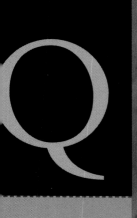

Questions

1. A 78-year-old woman with dementia and rigidity is hospitalized with dehydration. During her hospitalization, she becomes agitated and has prominent visual hallucinations. After a dose of haloperidol, she becomes very rigid and mute. The most likely type of dementia in this patient is:
   A. Alzheimer's disease (AD)
   B. Parkinson's disease (PD)
   C. Dementia with Lewy bodies
   D. Pick's disease
   E. Vascular dementia

2. A 32-year-old woman presents to the ER complaining of blurred vision and pain in the right eye. Your evaluation shows decreased visual acuity in the right eye that does not correct with pinhole testing. There is a relative afferent pupillary defect (RAPD) on the right, and testing of the right visual field shows a small central scotoma. The most likely localization of the lesion is the:
   A. Optic chiasm
   B. Optic nerve
   C. Optic tract
   D. Occipital cortex
   E. Optic radiations

3. In the course of evaluating an infant with developmental regression, a pediatric neurologist notes a cherry-red spot on funduscopic examination. Which of the following diagnoses is consistent with that finding?
   A. Alexander disease
   B. Hurler syndrome
   C. Krabbe disease
   D. Niemann-Pick disease
   E. Canavan disease

4. A 62-year-old woman presents with progressive distal symmetric paresthesias and dysesthesias, with preserved muscle strength. She smokes cigarettes. Your electrodiagnostic study indicates that this is likely a sensory neuronopathy. Which one of the following tests will help to find the possible etiology?

A. Anti-GM$_1$ antibodies
B. Anti-DNA antibodies
C. Anti-Hu antibodies
D. MRI of the spine
E. CT myelogram

5. A 40-year-old woman is evaluated in the ER after a motor vehicle accident resulting in left facial injuries. Examination after she recovers acutely demonstrates that her left seventh and eighth cranial nerves remain dysfunctional. Which of the following skull structures may have been affected by her injury?
   A. Cribriform plate
   B. Optic canal
   C. Superior orbital fissure
   D. Internal auditory meatus
   E. Jugular foramen

6. A 54-year-old woman was seen in the ER complaining of a severe headache. Head CT was normal, and an LP was performed. The opening pressure was 14 cm H_2O, and CSF analysis showed the following: 150 red blood cells, xanthochromic fluid, protein 55 (slightly increased), 15 white blood cells (90% lymphocytes), and normal glucose. Which of the following statements is true?
   A. The xanthochromia may have been caused by a traumatic tap.
   B. The lymphocytic pleocytosis indicates an active infectious process.
   C. Viral meningitis is unlikely because of the normal CSF glucose.
   D. The lymphocytic pleocytosis is likely reactive to the presence of blood within the CSF.
   E. The opening pressure is elevated and reflects pseudotumor cerebri.

7. A 29-year-old woman is brought into the ER in an unresponsive state. Her temperature is 37°C, heart rate 84 per minute, respirations 10, and blood pressure 152/84. On

examination, she withdraws to noxious stimulation only. Her right pupil is 10 mm and does not constrict to light. Her left pupil is 5 mm and reacts normally. Which of the following is clinically contraindicated?
A. Raising the head of the bed
B. Intravenous administration of mannitol
C. Hyperventilation
D. LP
E. Neurosurgical consultation

8. A patient presents with gradually worsening weakness of the proximal arm and leg muscles symmetrically over several months. On examination, neck flexors and extensors are found to be weak also. There is no muscle pain or tenderness. What is the most likely site of dysfunction in the nervous system?
A. Peripheral nerve
B. Brachial plexus
C. Spinal nerve root
D. Internal capsule
E. Muscle

9. An 8-year-old boy is brought to a child psychiatrist for evaluation of potential attention deficit–hyperactivity disorder. His mother states that his teachers have been concerned about his attention because they frequently have to repeat instructions to him. At home his brother has noticed that he will stare for several seconds at a time, during which he does not respond to questions. An EEG demonstrates a 3-Hz spike-and-wave pattern. Which of the following is the most appropriate treatment?
A. Methylphenidate (Ritalin)
B. Ethosuximide (Zarontin)
C. Clonidine (Catapres)
D. Fluoxetine (Prozac)
E. Carbamazepine (Tegretol)

10. A 28-year-old woman comes to the ER with a severe unilateral throbbing headache accompanied by photophobia and phonophobia. These headaches started in her teens and she has one every month. Which of the following medications is effective as abortive treatment?
A. Propranolol
B. Sumatriptan
C. Verapamil
D. Amitriptyline
E. Valproic acid

11. A 42-year-old man is brought to the neurologist for evaluation of a few months' history of personality changes. His family indicates that, over the previous year, he has made unusual movements with his hands, and he seems to have some memory difficulties. His father died in his fifties with a similar clinical syndrome, including prominent chorea

and dementia. The most likely genetic abnormality will be localized on chromosome:
A. 19
B. 6
C. 4
D. 11
E. 21

12. A 55-year-old woman with a history of ovarian cancer and moderate alcohol consumption is seen in the neurology ambulatory clinic with a 1-month history of progressive unsteadiness of gait and dysarthria. Examination confirms the presence of both gait and limb ataxia as well as nystagmus. These symptoms were fairly abrupt in onset, progressed over a period of a few weeks, and now appear to have stabilized, but there has been no sign of spontaneous improvement. Which of the following statements is correct?
A. The findings of gait ataxia, dysarthria, and nystagmus indicate diffuse involvement of the cerebellum and suggest that alcohol consumption is the likely cause.
B. The constellation of symptoms and their temporal evolution are most consistent with paraneoplastic cerebellar degeneration, a disorder associated with underlying gynecologic malignancy.
C. The constellation of symptoms and their temporal evolution are most consistent with paraneoplastic cerebellar degeneration (PCD), but ovarian cancer is an unusual cause of this syndrome.
D. The symptoms and signs indicate cerebellar hemispheric dysfunction and are most suggestive of a metastasis from the underlying ovarian cancer.
E. The sudden onset of symptoms and diffuse cerebellar involvement suggest midline cerebellar hemorrhage as the cause.

13. A 45-year-old man with multiple sclerosis (MS) comes to the neurology clinic complaining of urinary incontinence. He indicates that he experiences increased urgency and frequency of urination. The most likely urodynamic finding in this patient is:
A. An atonic bladder
B. A spastic bladder
C. Stress incontinence
D. Absence of abnormalities
E. Overflow incontinence

14. A 65-year-old man complains of a 3-month history of intermittent urinary incontinence. Urodynamic studies show an atonic bladder. Which of the following is most likely responsible for his problem?
A. Diabetes
B. Old stroke
C. Multiple sclerosis

D. Right parietal tumor

E. Pineal tumor

15. A 35-year-old man is seen in the neurology outpatient clinic with the complaint that his fingers occasionally "get stuck" when he tries to open jars. On examination you find subtle weakness of the fingers and toes as well as percussion myotonia. You suspect the diagnosis of myotonic dystrophy. Which of the following statements is true?

A. Myotonic dystrophy is a systemic disorder that may also cause cataracts, diabetes, mental retardation, and cardiac arrhythmias.

B. Myotonic dystrophy is primarily a disorder of skeletal muscle.

C. Myotonic dystrophy should not be considered in the differential diagnosis because it is an inherited disorder that typically manifests itself either at birth or early in life.

D. Myotonic dystrophy is an autosomal recessive disorder caused by a triplet expansion in the DMPK gene.

E. Electromyography is usually normal in myotonic dystrophy and genetic testing is essential to confirm the diagnosis.

16. An 18-year-old woman is brought to the neurology clinic by her mother, who explains that her daughter has been behaving strangely recently and appears to have paranoid delusions. She has a slight tremor of both hands and the examiner notes that there is a brownish discoloration of the cornea in the vicinity of the limbus. Laboratory studies show a mild transaminitis. Which of the following test results are most likely?

A. Increased serum copper and ceruloplasmin with decreased 24-hour urinary copper

B. Increased serum copper with decreased serum ceruloplasmin and increased 24-hour urinary copper

C. Decreased serum copper and ceruloplasmin and increased 24-hour urinary copper

D. Increased 24-hour urinary copper but decreased copper staining on liver biopsy

E. Increased serum copper and 24-hour urinary copper with decreased serum ceruloplasmin

17. A 40-year-old woman with SLE develops weakness of her right finger and wrist extensors and pain on the right dorsum of her hand several months after being diagnosed with left carpal tunnel syndrome and right sciatic neuropathy. What is the most likely diagnosis?

A. Mononeuropathy multiplex

B. Axonal polyneuropathy

C. Demyelinating polyneuropathy

D. Neuromuscular junction disease

E. Polyradiculopathy

18. A 70-year-old man develops the acute onset of an inability to speak. Examination reveals that he struggles to pronounce a complete word and cannot string words together. He is unable to repeat a sentence but can follow simple and multistep commands. What is the most likely diagnosis?

A. Global aphasia

B. Conduction aphasia

C. Broca aphasia

D. Wernicke aphasia

E. Transcortical motor aphasia

19. A 28-year-old woman is brought to the ER by her husband. In addition to having neck stiffness, she has had a fever for several days, has been somewhat confused, and has not been "acting like herself." LP shows 9 white blood cells with a lymphocytic predominance, 32 red blood cells, protein = 63, and glucose = 65. Gram stain is negative. What is the most likely diagnosis?

A. Bacterial meningitis

B. Viral meningitis

C. Fungal meningitis

D. Meningitis from tuberculosis

E. Subarachnoid hemorrhage

20. A healthy 32-year-old man is brought to the ER after he stopped speaking suddenly, fell to the ground, lost consciousness, and shook for 2 minutes. After the event, he was noted to have a tongue laceration and urinary incontinence. He has no history of similar events. His physical exam shows a mild right hemiparesis. Routine labs and a head CT are normal. An EEG performed the next day is normal. The normal EEG suggests that this man:

A. had a pseudoseizure and does not require anticonvulsants.

B. needs admission for long-term video-EEG monitoring.

C. probably had a seizure, and the normal EEG result is not surprising.

D. requires hyperventilation to elicit an absence seizure on EEG.

E. has actually had an ischemic stroke rather than a seizure.

21. Two days after coronary artery bypass surgery, a 62-year-old man with hypertension complains that "there is another man's arm in bed" with him. When asked to hold up his arms, the patient raises his right arm only. When asked about his left arm, he claims it is the examiner's or another patient's. What is the most likely diagnosis?

A. Right hemispheric stroke with neglect

B. Left hemispheric stroke with neglect

C. Conversion disorder

D. Adjustment disorder

E. Alien-limb phenomenon

22. A 35-year-old man with no known history of seizures is brought in by paramedics in status epilepticus. Which of the following medications is used as initial therapy for this condition?
    A. Benzodiazepines
    B. Barbiturates
    C. Propofol
    D. Carbamazepine
    E. Lamotrigine

23. A 34-year-old woman with multiple sclerosis develops double vision on looking to one side. Examination reveals normal eye movements except that, on attempted leftward conjugate gaze, the right eye does not adduct properly and the left eye has abducting nystagmus. What neuroanatomic structure is most likely affected?
    A. Internal capsule
    B. Oculomotor nucleus
    C. Spinal trigeminal nucleus (STN)
    D. Optic nerve
    E. Medial longitudinal fasciculus (MLF)

24. A 23-year-old woman presents with loss of vision in the right eye accompanied by slight pain in that eye over a period of 3 days. She has 20/200 acuity, red desaturation, and an afferent pupillary defect in the right eye. The remainder of her examination and MRI are normal. A diagnosis of optic neuritis is made. Which of the following is true about treatment?
    A. Interferon beta-1b will hasten recovery from this episode.
    B. Mitoxantrone is the most effective treatment.
    C. Medical treatment is not likely to help optic neuritis.
    D. Oral corticosteroids are preferred for the treatment of optic neuritis.
    E. Corticosteroids may delay the development of multiple sclerosis.

25. A 22-year-old right-handed woman develops horizontal diplopia acutely. Your evaluation shows normal right lateral gaze but difficulty with adduction of the right eye while looking to the left and nystagmus in the abducting left eye. What is the most likely anatomic localization?
    A. Left paramedian pontine reticular formation (PPRF) producing a right internuclear ophthalmoplegia (INO)
    B. Right PPRF producing a right one-and-a-half syndrome
    C. Right medial longitudinal fascicle (MLF) producing a right INO
    D. Left medial longitudinal fascicle producing a right INO
    E. Lateral geniculate nuclei

26. A 17-year-old girl is seen in the ambulatory neurology clinic with a 6-month history of tremor and ataxia. There is no family history of neurologic disease. On examination she is noted to have subtle chorea as well as a golden brown discoloration of the cornea. Which of the following diagnoses should you suspect?
    A. Sydenham's chorea
    B. Wilson's disease
    C. Huntington's chorea
    D. Gilles de la Tourette's syndrome
    E. Essential tremor

27. A 34-year-old man is seen in the neurology outpatient clinic with symptoms of headache and bilateral lower motor neuron (LMN) facial weakness. There is no history of a skin rash. Neurologic examination discloses a relative afferent papillary defect in the right eye as well as the bilateral facial weakness.
    A. Guillain-Barré syndrome (GBS) is the most likely diagnosis, and he should have an LP to help confirm the diagnosis.
    B. Lyme disease is the most likely diagnosis, and *Borrelia* serology should be sent to confirm the diagnosis.
    C. Sarcoidosis is likely the correct diagnosis, and appropriate investigations include MRI of the brain, LP and chest x-ray.
    D. Multiple sclerosis (MS) is most likely the correct diagnosis, as bilateral facial weakness and optic neuropathy are both common manifestations of this disease.
    E. Vasculitis, causing mononeuritis multiplex, is the most likely diagnosis, and so the patient should be referred for rheumatologic evaluation.

28. A 64-year-old man with a history of hypertension presents to the ER with the sudden onset of numbness of his left leg, arm, and face. His motor examination is normal. What is the most likely site of his lesion?
    A. Right thalamus
    B. Left thalamus
    C. Left postcentral gyrus
    D. Right precentral gyrus
    E. Right corona radiata

29. While playing baseball with some friends, a 15-year-old boy, who was not wearing a helmet, was hit accidentally on the side of the head with a ball. He was knocked unconscious briefly but recovered fully. Two hours later he became increasingly lethargic, so his parents brought him to the ER. When you evaluate the patient, he is barely arousable to your voice. He has mild weakness on the left side of his body, and his right pupil is slightly larger than the left pupil; the right pupil does not appear to react to light. What is the most likely cause of the patient's symptoms and signs?
    A. Concussion
    B. Epidural hematoma
    C. Diffuse axonal injury
    D. Ischemic infarct
    E. Drug intoxication

30. Which of the following syndromes or diseases could cause bilateral weakness and loss of pain and temperature sensation with preservation of joint position sense in both legs?
    A. Amyotrophic lateral sclerosis (ALS)
    B. Vitamin B_{12} deficiency
    C. Brown-Séquard syndrome
    D. Anterior spinal artery syndrome
    E. Tabes dorsalis

31. A 2-year-old child presents with new seizures. Her mother tells you that the child is not walking yet. He has a 5-year-old brother with a seizure disorder and mental retardation. On examination, using the Wood's lamp, you find hypomelanotic lesions. The most appropriate next test is:
    A. Skeletal surveillance
    B. Skin biopsy
    C. Head CT or MRI
    D. No need for further tests
    E. LP

32. A 3-year-old boy is brought to his pediatrician for evaluation of repetitive behaviors, delay of language development, and social isolation. He otherwise has normal motor development. Which of the following is a required feature of autism but not of Asperger syndrome?
    A. abnormal language development
    B. social isolation
    C. onset after age 3
    D. failure to meet milestones for gross motor development
    E. failure to meet milestones for fine motor development

33. A 62-year-old woman with a history of small cell lung carcinoma presents to the neurology clinic complaining of bilateral paresthesias of the lower extremities. She has no history of diabetes or family history of polyneuropathy. She describes severe pain in the soles of her feet when standing and has difficulty walking. On examination, there is severe pain to light touch over both soles. On your sensory examination description, you will state that this patient has:
    A. Hyperesthesia
    B. Paresthesia
    C. Allodynia
    D. Sensory loss
    E. Hypesthesia

34. A 38-year-old man presents to the ER complaining of mild headache. He had neck trauma a week earlier. The exam shows anisocoria, with the right pupil being 3 mm and the left 5 mm, both reactive to light. What other findings will help to localize the lesion?
    A. Look at the pupils in the dark and check tongue deviation.

B. Look for evidence of ptosis in the left eye and anhidrosis on the left face.
    C. Look for evidence of ptosis in the right eye and anhidrosis in the right face.
    D. Look for evidence of horizontal diplopia and a cut in the right visual field.
    E. Look for evidence of dysarthria and hemiparesis.

35. A 35-year-old woman presents to the ER reporting a few days of progressive ascending muscle weakness. She had a viral infection a few weeks earlier. On examination, you find diffuse weakness and areflexia. The most likely finding in the CSF is:
    A. High protein–high cell count
    B. High protein–low cell count
    C. Low protein–high cell count
    D. Low protein–low cell count
    E. Normal CSF

36. A 33-year-old man is seen in the ER for difficulty walking. He has paresthesias in his feet and left foot drop. Initial physical exam shows mild distal weakness in both legs with absent ankle jerks and reduced reflexes throughout. While the patient is waiting in the ER, his weakness worsens, involving the arms, but he has no difficulty breathing. You want to admit the patient to the intensive care unit. What will be your best argument to convince your ER attending to do so?
    A. Absence of upper extremity reflexes
    B. Decreased gag reflex
    C. A forced vital capacity FVC below 25 mL/kg
    D. The patient's weakness is worsening very quickly, and you fear that he may need mechanical ventilation
    E. You don't have an argument in this case

37. A 35-year-old man who is HIV-positive presents with radicular pain in the legs and associated bladder distention. The most likely agent responsible for these symptoms is:
    A. Cytomegalovirus
    B. *Clostridium*
    C. *Toxoplasma*
    D. *Cryptococcus*
    E. *Pneumocystis carinii*

38. A 45-year-old woman presents to the ER with "dizziness," by which she means that she feels a spinning sensation. The sensation is intermittent and seems to be exacerbated by head movement. She has some nausea with the episodes but otherwise has no other symptoms, such as double vision, weakness, hearing loss, tinnitus, or difficulty swallowing. What diagnosis is most likely?
    A. Vestibular neuronitis
    B. Ménière disease
    C. Brainstem infarction

D. Benign positional paroxysmal vertigo (BPPV)
E. Cerebellar infarction

39. A 32-year-old woman is seen in the neurology outpatient clinic with symptoms of diplopia and ptosis that fluctuate during the course of the day. Examination shows fatigable proximal weakness. You suspect that she has myasthenia gravis (MG). Which of the following statements concerning MG is true?
A. It is an autoimmune disorder caused by antibodies that are directed against presynaptic nicotinic acetylcholine receptors.
B. It is an autoimmune disorder caused by antibodies directed against postsynaptic muscarininc acetyl-choline receptors.
C. It is an autoimmune disorder caused by antibodies directed against presynaptic voltage-gated calcium channels.
D. It is an autoimmune disorder caused by antibodies directed against postsynaptic nicotinic acetylcholine receptors.
E. It is an autoimmune disorder caused by antibodies directed against the synaptic enzyme acetylcholinesterase.

40. A patient complains of difficulty chewing. On examination he is found to have decreased strength of his muscles of mastication. Which of the following cranial nerves is responsible for this motor function?
A. Trigeminal
B. Facial
C. Oculomotor
D. Glossopharyngeal
E. Hypoglossal

41. The following patients are being evaluated in a neurologic intensive care unit. For which one would the Glasgow Coma Scale (GCS) be used most commonly to follow his or her clinical status?
A. A 75-year-old man in coma after cardiac arrest
B. A 29-year-old woman with delirium after medication overdose
C. A 69-year-old woman with a thromboembolic stroke and Broca aphasia
D. A 20-year-old man who is unresponsive after head trauma
E. A 59-year-old man with subarachnoid hemorrhage after aneurysm rupture

42. A 68-year-old man taking warfarin falls while in the hospital, is found on the floor, and is difficult to rouse. He has a new right hemiparesis and an intracranial hemorrhage is suspected. What is the most appropriate initial radiologic study?
A. Head CT with contrast
B. Head CT without contrast

C. Skull x-ray
D. Cerebral angiography
E. Brain perfusion scan

43. A 75-year-old man presents to your office with a 1-month history of progressive pain in the left temporal area and pain in his jaw while eating. On laboratory testing, the patient is found to have an elevated ESR of 94. What is the treatment of choice?
A. Sumatriptan
B. Carbamazepine
C. Verapamil
D. Surgical resection of brain tumor
E. Prednisone

44. A 35-year-old man presents with his spouse to your office for difficulty concentrating. Further history also reveals that he has fallen asleep while driving as well as in the middle of important business meetings, despite sleeping at least 8 hours each night. He denies hallucinations or a history of his knees buckling while laughing. His wife reports that he snores loudly while sleeping. His examination is normal with the exception of moderate obesity. Which of the following tests would be most helpful in diagnosing this patient's disorder?
A. Multiple sleep latency test (MSLT)
B. EEG
C. MRI of the brain
D. LP
E. Polysomnography

45. A previously healthy 21-year-old presents to the ER after being involved in a high-speed motor vehicle accident. You note that the patient is unresponsive, makes no spontaneous movement, and has a dilated pupil on the right that is nonreactive to light. What is the best explanation for these signs?
A. Infarction of the left occipital lobe
B. Concussion from the motor vehicle accident
C. Uncal herniation
D. Cervical neck fracture
E. Diffuse axonal injury

46. An 84-year-old man is transferred from another hospital with a reported hypertensive hemorrhage. The films from that hospital are not available, and there are no further details. Which of the following is the most likely location of his hemorrhage?
A. Pons
B. Midbrain
C. Internal capsule
D. Frontal lobe
E. Corpus callosum

47. A 28-year-old man was recently diagnosed with obstructive sleep apnea. Of the following choices, which is the most appropriate treatment?
A. Pemoline
B. Methylphenidate
C. CPAP
D. Benzodiazepine
E. Clomipramine

48. A 45-year-old man with a prior history of migraine headaches with aura presents to the ER complaining of a progressive headache for the last month that is different from his usual migraine. There is no associated nausea or vomiting. His neurologic examination is completely normal. Your next step in management should be:
A. Brain imaging study
B. Abortive migraine treatment
C. Preventive migraine treatment
D. Reassurance and discharge home
E. Administration of pure oxygen

49. Which of the following features is most commonly associated with a pituitary adenoma?
A. Homonymous hemianopia
B. Bitemporal hemianopia
C. Ring enhancement on brain imaging with contrast
D. Seizures
E. Hemiparesis

50. A 24-year-old construction worker falls from a ladder and fractures his cervical spine with resulting signs of upper motor neuron (UMN) dysfunction. Which of the following signs is characteristic of an UMN lesion?
A. Hypotonia
B. Decreased reflexes
C. Flexor plantar response
D. Spasticity
E. Absent reflexes

51. A 67-year-old woman presents to the ER with a new onset of headache, nausea, vomiting, and unsteadiness of gait. Her history is significant for atrial fibrillation, for which she is chronically anticoagulated with warfarin. She also has a pacemaker in place. You are concerned about the possibility of a cerebellar hemorrhage. The imaging modality of choice is:
A. A CT scan, because this is the imaging modality most sensitive to the presence of acute intracranial blood.
B. An MRI, because blood in the posterior fossa will not be visualized on CT.
C. An MRI, because CT is contraindicated by the presence of a pacemaker.
D. A CT scan, because it provides the best images of the contents of the posterior fossa.

E. A CT scan, because this is the imaging modality most sensitive to the presence of acute intracranial blood.

52. A 22-year-old woman presents with acute bilateral facial nerve palsy and intermittent peripheral nerve symptoms for over 3 weeks. You find elevated Lyme titers in serum and CSF. What treatment would you choose first?
A. Oral doxycycline
B. Intravenous ceftriaxone
C. Oral amoxicillin
D. Oral amoxicillin and doxycycline
E. Fluconazole

53. A 58-year-old man is seen in the neurology ambulatory clinic with a 3-month history of right-sided resting tremor. On examination, he is noted to have mild masking of facial expression and there is diminished swing of the right arm when he walks. You suspect that he may have early idiopathic Parkinson's disease. Which of the following statements concerning this disorder is true?
A. Most cases are familial with mutations in the α-synuclein or parkin genes.
B. It is characterized by the death of dopaminergic neurons in the substantia nigra pars reticulata.
C. The four cardinal features of this disorder are tremor, rigidity, bradykinesia, and postural instability.
D. Impairment of vertical gaze is a common manifestation of this disorder.
E. Early falls are a common problem in this disorder.

54. A 5-year-old boy is seen in the pediatric neurology clinic. His motor milestones have been delayed, and examination discloses proximal muscle weakness with difficulty arising from the floor. There is pseudohypertrophy of his calf muscles. He has an older brother with Duchenne's muscular dystrophy (DMD) who is confined to a wheelchair. Which of the following statements concerning DMD is true?
A. It is an autosomal recessive disorder caused by mutation in the dystrophin gene.
B. It is an autosomal dominant disorder caused by mutation in the dystrophin gene.
C. DMD and limb-girdle muscular dystrophy are allelic disorders, both being due to mutations in the dystrophin gene.
D. It is a disorder caused by mutation in the dystrophin gene, which is located on the X chromosome.
E. DMD and Becker's muscular dystrophy are allelic disorders, due to mutations in the dystrophin gene on chromosome 4.

55. A 9-year-old boy presents with difficulty walking. Neurologic examination demonstrates, among other

things, that he performs rapid alternating movements poorly, with a lack of proper rhythm and coordination. This finding, called dysdiadochokinesis, is most typically associated with dysfunction of which of the following brain structures?

A. Basal ganglia
B. Medulla
C. Cerebellum
D. Parietal lobe
E. Thalamus

56. An ischemic stroke involving the right side of the pons could lead to which of the following patterns of weakness?

A. Left facial weakness and right body weakness
B. Right facial weakness and left body weakness
C. Right facial weakness and right body weakness
D. Left arm weakness and right leg weakness
E. Right arm weakness and left leg weakness

57. A 27-year-old woman with complex partial seizures is well controlled on carbamazepine. Which of the following is a characteristic side effect of this medication?

A. Thrombocytopenia
B. Agitation
C. Diabetes insipidus
D. Nephrolithiasis
E. Hyponatremia

58. A 53-year-old construction worker is brought to the ER with a severe, sudden-onset headache accompanied by vomiting. A CT scan of his head demonstrates a subarachnoid hemorrhage. Which of the following is a common cause of subarachnoid hemorrhage?

A. Tearing of bridging veins
B. Laceration of the middle meningeal artery
C. Aneurysmal rupture
D. Amyloid angiopathy
E. Arteriovenous malformation rupture

59. A 45-year-old woman has an MRI scan of the brain for evaluation of progressive headaches. The MRI scan shows a lesion that enhances in a homogenous manner with contrast administration. Which of the following lesions is most likely to account for the appearance of the MRI scan?

A. Glioblastoma multiforme
B. Meningioma
C. Brain abscess
D. Toxoplasmosis
E. Granuloma

60. A 75-year-old man is brought to the ER after having lost consciousness briefly in his bathroom. By the time he arrives he is feeling fine and is able to give a clear account of what happened. He recalls walking to the bathroom to urinate. Shortly thereafter he became light-headed and felt as if his vision were graying out. These symptoms lasted for about 30 seconds. The next thing he recalls is awakening on his bathroom floor. His wife notes that he was unconscious only briefly. Which of the following descriptions pertinent to this clinical scenario is correct?

A. The symptoms of light-headedness and graying out of vision are atypical symptoms described by patients with syncope.
B. He has micturition syncope.
C. Orthostatic hypotension is the likely explanation for his syncopal episode.
D. Vasovagal syncope is the likely explanation for his syncopal episode.
E. Vestibular neuronitis is the likely explanation for his symptoms.

61. A 36-year-old man comes to the ER with a 4-day history of fever and a generalized unwitnessed seizure 2 hours earlier. MRI of the brain with gadolinium shows contrast enhancement of both temporal lobes and, in a nontraumatic tap, 10,000 RBCs and 15 white blood cells. What is the most likely organism responsible for this clinical picture?

A. Enterovirus
B. *Streptococcus* species
C. *Cryptococcus neoformans*
D. Herpes simplex virus (HSV-1)
E. *Meningococcus*

62. A 55-year-old woman comes to the neurology clinic complaining of numbness in the last two fingers of her right hand; it tends to worsen at night. On examination, you find a positive Tinel sign at the right elbow (percussion of the ulnar nerve at the right elbow produces a tingling sensation in the last two fingers of the right hand). You are convinced that this is an ulnar neuropathy at the right elbow and perform electrodiagnostic studies. Why do you think that this is a peripheral nerve problem?

A. The acuteness of presentation
B. The physical examination findings
C. The symptoms described by the patient
D. You don't think this is a peripheral nerve problem
E. There is no CNS complaint

63. A 25-year-old man is now comatose after suffering blunt-force trauma to the head. On the basis of the clinical history, neurologic exam, and head CT scan, he is diagnosed with an epidural hematoma. Of the following choices, which is the best treatment option?

A. Neurosurgical decompression
B. Hyperventilation
C. Administration of mannitol

D. Conservative management with close monitoring of vital signs and neurologic status

E. Administration of tissue plasminogen activator

64. A 19-year-old man is admitted to a neurology service with an episode of transverse myelitis. Workup includes an MRI of his head and LP. Which of the following distinguishes acute disseminated encephalomyelitis (ADEM) from multiple sclerosis (MS)?

A. Presence of oligoclonal bands in the CSF

B. Pleocytosis with neutrophilic predominance

C. Monophasic course

D. Multiple lesions on MRI

E. A positive family history of ADEM

65. A 55-year-old man with type 2 diabetes presents with a 5-week history of pain in his right knee, followed by weakness and atrophy of his right quadriceps Exam shows weakness of the right quadriceps and iliopsoas muscles and an absent right knee jerk. This presentation is most characteristic of what?

A. Diabetic distal symmetric polyneuropathy

B. Proximal diabetic neuropathy or diabetic amyotrophy

C. Mononeuropathy multiplex

D. Stroke

E. These conditions are not seen in diabetics

66. A 17-year-old man is accidentally hit on the left side of the head with a baseball bat while playing a game with some friends. He loses consciousness and is taken to an emergency room. A head CT scan showed a lenticular shaped hyperdensity in the epidural space over the left temporal region that is exerting some mild mass effect on the brain. Which of the following mechanisms best explains the patient's head CT scan results?

A. Tearing of bridging veins

B. Laceration of the middle meningeal artery

C. Impact of the brain over bony prominences of the skull

D. Rotational acceleration and deceleration of the head

E. Rupture of a cerebral aneurysm

67. A 56-year-old woman is referred to the neurology clinic by her optometrist, who noted that she had limited movement of her eyes. The patient herself notes only that she has fallen a few times in recent months. Examination confirms that there is marked limitation of vertical eye movements (both up and down gaze). There is mild rigidity in both arms and legs but no tremor. Her postural reflexes are poor. Which of the following is the most likely diagnosis?

A. Parkinson's disease (PD)

B. Progressive supranuclear palsy (PSP)

C. Corticobasal ganglionic degeneration

D. Miller-Fisher syndrome (MFS)

E. Chronic progressive external ophthalmoplegia (PEO)

68. A 65-year-old obese woman is referred to the neurology clinic with complaints of burning pain in both feet, which has been present for several months. You suspect that she may have a small fiber peripheral neuropathy. The most likely findings on examination are:

A. Symmetric weakness and atrophy of intrinsic muscles of the feet with loss of ankle reflexes

B. Symmetric stocking pattern diminution of pinprick and temperature sensation

C. Symmetric stocking pattern diminution of vibration and joint position sense with absent ankle reflexes

D. Symmetric stocking pattern diminution of all sensory modalities with absent DTRs in the arms and legs

E. Symmetric stocking pattern diminution of vibration and joint position sense with retained ankle reflexes

69. A 45-year-old man presents with a several-month history of weakness in his lower and upper extremities. On examination, in addition to weakness in multiple muscle groups, he demonstrates atrophy, hyperreflexia, spasticity of the legs, and bilateral Babinski signs. Fasciculations in multiple muscles are also noted. His sensation to pain, temperature, and joint position sense appear intact. What is his most likely diagnosis?

A. Amyotrophic lateral sclerosis (ALS)

B. Vitamin B_{12} deficiency

C. Anterior spinal artery syndrome

D. Central cord syndrome

E. Brown-Séquard syndrome

70. A 25-year-old man presents to your office with excessive daytime sleepiness, visual hallucinations while falling asleep, and a history of transiently losing tone in his extremities and falling to the ground when he is angry or laughing. Of the following choices, what would be his single best treatment option?

A. Pemoline

B. Venlafaxine

C. Clomipramine

D. CPAP

E. Methylphenidate

71. A 54-year old man is seen in the neurology clinic with complaints of resting tremor of the left hand and a general feeling of slowing down. As an example he explains that it takes him at least 20 minutes to get dressed in the morning. You suspect that he has idiopathic Parkinson's disease (PD). If you are correct, examination would be most likely to show which of the following combinations of physical signs?

A. Asymmetric rest tremor, asymmetric rigidity, and poor postural reflexes

B. Symmetric rest tremor, asymmetric rigidity, and poor postural reflexes

C. Asymmetric rest tremor, symmetric rigidity, and poor postural reflexes

D. Symmetric rest tremor and rigidity and poor postural reflexes

E. Asymmetric rest tremor, symmetric rigidity, and impairment of vertical gaze

72. A 55-year-old man with a history of hypertension is seen in the ER with complaints of clumsiness and incoordination; these began 2 days earlier and have increased in severity. He also reports double vision on lateral gaze, which resolves when one eye is covered. He is awake, alert, and oriented. Examination shows restricted eye movements in all directions, with eye abduction in both directions most limited. DTRs are absent, and there is impaired joint position sense. The most likely diagnosis is:

A. Brainstem stroke

B. Cerebellar infarction with compression of the brainstem

C. Miller-Fisher syndrome (MFS)

D. Myasthenia gravis (MG)

E. Alcoholic cerebellar degeneration

73. A 44-year-old woman presents to the ER complaining of urinary incontinence and lower back pain. What will be the most useful next diagnostic procedure to try in the effort to find the etiology of her problem?

A. Urodynamic studies

B. Blood testing including glucose level

C. MRI of the spine

D. Post-void residual

E. LP

74. A 48-year-old woman reports recurrent episodes of stabbing unilateral pain associated with tearing and conjunctival injection. Which of the following is characteristic of chronic paroxysmal hemicrania as opposed to cluster headache?

A. Unilateral pain

B. Conjunctival injection

C. Male predominance

D. Indomethacin responsivity

E. Headache duration of hours

75. A 75-year-old right-handed man with hypertension, diabetes, and hypercholesterolemia is seen in the ER. His family explains that he has had difficulty doing things around the house for the last few days. The patient himself admits that he has found it difficult to get dressed and to prepare his breakfast, but he feels healthy otherwise. On examination his speech is fluent, and he is able to name objects and repeat short phrases without difficulty. He is, however, unable to mimic certain activities described by the examiner, although seems to have no difficulty understanding what it is that he is supposed to do.

A. He likely has a form of Wernicke aphasia due to a lesion in the left superior temporal lobe.

B. He likely has a form of apraxia due to a lesion in the right frontal lobe.

C. He likely has a form of Wernicke aphasia due to a lesion in the left inferior frontal lobe.

D. He likely has a form of apraxia due to a lesion in the right parietal lobe.

E. He likely has a form of apraxia due to a lesion in the left frontal or parietal lobe.

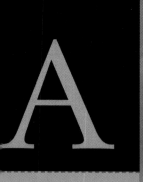

Answers

1. C	26. B	51. A
2. B	27. C	52. B
3. D	28. A	53. C
4. C	29. B	54. D
5. D	30. D	55. C
6. D	31. C	56. B
7. D	32. A	57. E
8. E	33. C	58. C
9. B	34. C	59. B
10. B	35. B	60. B
11. C	36. D	61. D
12. B	37. A	62. B
13. B	38. D	63. A
14. A	39. D	64. C
15. A	40. A	65. B
16. B	41. D	66. B
17. A	42. B	67. B
18. C	43. E	68. B
19. B	44. E	69. A
20. C	45. C	70. E
21. A	46. A	71. A
22. A	47. C	72. C
23. E	48. A	73. C
24. E	49. B	74. D
25. C	50. D	75. E

1. C (Chapter 12)

The presence of visual hallucinations is an early symptom of dementia with Lewy bodies (DLB). Other characteristics include cognitive decline, fluctuations of alertness, extrapyramidal symptoms, and an extraordinary sensitivity to neuroleptics. Visual hallucinations and sensitivity to neuroleptics are not early signs of AD, PD, Pick's disease, or vascular dementia.

2. B (Chapter 4)

Decreased visual acuity that does not correct with pinhole testing, an RAPD, and a central scotoma are characteristic of optic nerve disease. A lesion affecting the optic chiasm will produce a bitemporal heteronymous hemianopia. If a lesion affects the optic tract, the optic radiations (in both temporal and parietal areas) or the occipital cortex (unilaterally), it will produce a homonymous hemianopia; that in the occipital cortex may be "macular sparing."

3. D (Chapter 25)

Niemann-Pick disease, Gaucher disease, and Tay-Sachs disease are all associated with cherry-red spots in the macula. Niemann-Pick disease is an autosomal recessive disorder caused by sphingomyelinase deficiency. Alexander disease and Canavan disease are dysmyelinating disorders with prominent macrocephaly but not cherry-red spots. The classic ophthalmologic finding of Hurler syndrome is clouding of the cornea rather than a cherry-red spot in the macula. Krabbe disease is an autosomal recessive disorder caused by galacto-sylceramide ß-galactosidase deficiency. It does not produce a cherry-red spot in the macula.

4. C (Chapter 23)

One possible etiology of sensory neuronopathies is a paraneoplastic disorder, in particular small cell lung cancer. This is generally associated with positive anti-Hu antibodies (anti-neuronal antibodies) and can also be associated with paraneoplastic encephalomyelitis, ataxia, and autonomic neuropathy. Anti-GM$_1$ has been associated with multifocal motor neuropathy with conduction block. MRI of the spine would not help at this stage. Other causes of sensory neuronopathy include Sjögren syndrome, pyridoxine intoxication, and chemotherapy (cisplatin). Chest CT to search for occult malignancy is also recommended.

5. D (Chapter 1)

Each cranial nerve courses through a particular foramen, or opening, in the skull. Skull base fractures and other such injuries can result in damage to these structures and injury to the associated cranial nerves. The seventh (facial) and eighth (vestibulocochlear) nerves both course through the internal auditory meatus, which may have been damaged in this woman's case.

6. D (Chapter 2)

This woman has had a subarachnoid hemorrhage. Bleeding into the subarachnoid (CSF) space typically initiates an inflammatory response, one manifestation of which is a lymphocytic pleocytosis. Xanthochromia is the result of breakdown of blood within the subarachnoid space. Its presence in a bloody CSF sample helps to distinguish intrathecal hemorrhage from a traumatic tap. The CSF glucose is typically normal in both subarachnoid hemorrhage and viral meningitis. It is frequently low in bacterial, mycobacterial, and carcinomatous meningitis. An opening pressure of 14 cm H$_2$O is within the normal range of 6 to 15 cm H$_2$O.

7. D (Chapter 3)

This patient's clinical presentation suggests increased intracranial pressure (ICP) from a right hemispheric lesion. The "blown" right pupil suggests that herniation of the right hemisphere has compressed the right oculomotor nerve. Choices A through C are all measures that acutely decrease ICP, while neurosurgery may be needed as a more definitive intervention. Performing an LP in this situation could be dangerous and could actually precipitate worsening herniation.

8. E (Chapter 5)

Symmetric proximal weakness usually suggests a primary muscle problem, as does weakness of neck flexors and extensors. The absence of muscle pain and tenderness does not argue against a primary muscle pathology. The other listed choices would not usually result in this pattern of weakness.

9. B (Chapter 15)

This child likely has absence seizures, which are frequently diagnosed after a teacher or parent notices inattention, "daydreaming," or staring episodes. Absence seizures last a few seconds each, can occur many times a day, and have a classic EEG appearance. Ethosuximide and valproic acid are typical drugs of choice.

10. B (Chapter 10)

This woman is suffering from a migraine headache. Sumatriptan is effective as abortive treatment. The other medications are effective in decreasing the severity and frequency of attacks and are used as preventive therapy.

11. C (Chapter 12)

This case represents an early onset of dementia with associated personality changes and movement disorder (chorea)—the classic triad of HD. HD is linked to chromosome 4p16.3, also known as the HD gene, encoding for a protein called huntingtin. The mutation produces an unstable CAG repeat sequence with more than 40 repeats. HD is not linked to the other chromosomes listed.

12. B (Chapter 8)

PCD is typically a pancerebellar syndrome with clinical manifestations including ataxia, dysarthria, and nystagmus. The underlying malignancy is typically a gynecologic one or breast cancer. The temporal evolution is typically that of acute or subacute onset with fairly rapid progression over weeks to months, followed by stabilization. Metastatic cerebellar disease would more likely affect a cerebellar hemisphere and produce lateralized cerebellar dysfunction. Alcoholic cerebellar degeneration typically affects the vermis, and the characteristic manifestation is that of a gait ataxia. Stroke (ischemic or hemorrhagic), although abrupt in onset, would not be expected to progress over a period of weeks to months.

13. B (Chapter 9)

MS characteristically produces an upper motor neuron bladder or spastic bladder with increased frequency and urgency. Stress incontinence is an involuntary loss of urine during coughing, sneezing, laughing, or other physical activities that increase intra-abdominal pressure. An atonic bladder is characterized by overflow incontinence and increased capacity and compliance.

14. A (Chapter 9)

Atonic bladder implies an LMN lesion at the level of the conus medullaris, cauda equina, sacral plexus, or peripheral nerves. It is characterized by overflow incontinence and increased capacity and compliance. Diabetes is the only one in the group able to produce that type of lesion.

15. A (Chapter 24)

Myotonic dystrophy is a multisystem disorder that may also cause frontal balding, diabetes, and gastrointestinal symptoms. It is the most common adult-onset muscular dystrophy. It is inherited in an autosomal dominant fashion and is caused by a triplet repeat expansion in the DMPK gene. EMG typically shows myotonic discharges.

16. B (Chapter 16)

She likely has Wilson disease, an autosomal dominant disorder of copper metabolism that presents with neuropsychiatric symptoms as well as a movement disorder. The pigment changes in the cornea are Kayser-Fleischer rings and are characteristic of Wilson disease.

17. A (Chapter 5)

The patient's current symptoms are suggestive of a right radial neuropathy. Multiple sequential mononeuropathies, each affecting a single peripheral nerve, are known as mononeuropathy multiplex. Pain is a typical feature. Patients with rheumatologic conditions are susceptible; vasculitis may be involved.

18. C (Chapter 11)

Broca aphasia is characterized by effortful nonfluent speech and an inability to repeat, with relatively preserved comprehension. Transcortical motor aphasia is similar but features preserved repetition.

19. B (Chapter 21)

Along with the clinical picture, a CSF profile of lymphocytic pleocytosis, elevated protein, normal glucose, and a negative Gram stain point to a viral or aseptic meningitis. The clinical presentations of problems A through D could appear very similar, but the CSF analysis is crucial in identifying the responsible organism. Bacterial meningitis tends to produce a granulocytic pleocytosis. Fungal meningitis is usually associated with hypoglycorrhacia (defined as a CSF-serum glucose ratio below 0.4). Subarachnoid hemorrhage characteristically produces a large number of RBCs (thousands).

20. C (Chapter 2)

About 50% of patients with epilepsy have normal routine EEGs. A seizure is a clinical diagnosis, and this patient's convincing story supersedes the negative EEG. Long-term video-EEG monitoring is not required to prove the diagnosis of seizure. While hyperventilation can help to elicit absence seizure activity on EEG, his history and age make an absence seizure unlikely. Although an ischemic stroke can precipitate a seizure, this man's history is most suggestive of seizure. The right hemiparesis is more likely a Todd paralysis rather than an ischemic stroke.

21. A (Chapter 11)

This patient exhibits a form of neglect, in which he does not recognize his left arm as his. Right frontal or parietal lesions are the most common etiology. In the alien-limb phenomenon, patients retain awareness of the limb but feel that it is not under their control.

22. A (Chapter 15)

Benzodiazepines are the first agents used in the treatment algorithm for status epilepticus. Typically, phenytoin and then phenobarbital are used subsequently. Propofol is used if status epilepticus becomes refractory, while carbamazepine and lamotrigine are antiepileptic drugs that are not available in parenteral form.

23. E (Chapter 20)

The clinical description is of an internuclear ophthalmoplegia (INO). This is an uncommon but characteristic feature of MS and is due to demyelination affecting the MLF.

24. E (Chapter 20)

Intravenous corticosteroids may delay but not prevent the development of MS in a patient with optic neuritis. They are preferred to oral corticosteroids. Inteferon beta-1b and mitoxantrone are used for MS but not in the treatment of isolated optic neuritis.

25. C (Chapter 4)

Lesions of the MLF produce an INO. The clinical characteristics of a right INO include inability to adduct the right eye in left lateral gaze plus nystagmus of the abducting left eye. Adduction during convergence is maintained because this action does not depend on the MLF. "One-and-a-half syndrome" occurs as a consequence of a lesion involving the PPRF or sixth-nerve nucleus and the adjacent ipsilateral MLF. This produces an ipsilateral gaze palsy and INO on the contralateral side; the only eye movement present in the lateral plane is abduction of the contralateral eye.

26. B (Chapter 12)

The corneal discoloration represents a Kayser-Fleischer ring, which is characteristic of Wilson disease. The diagnosis should be confirmed with tests of serum copper and ceruloplasmin as well as a 24-hour urinary copper determination. Sydenham chorea is a poststreptococcal immunologic disorder, and HD is a neurodegenerative disorder characterized by chorea and dementia. Kayser-Fleischer rings are not present in either of these latter conditions. Tourette syndrome is a genetic disorder characterized by motor and vocal tics. Chorea is not a feature of this syndrome. Similarly, essential tremor is not characterized by ataxia or chorea.

27. C (Chapter 18)

Sarcoidosis is one of the most common causes of bilateral LMN facial weakness. It is also an important cause of a lymphocytic meningitis (hence the headache) and may cause a variety of other cranial neuropathies, including optic neuropathy (hence the relative afferent papillary defect). MS is another important cause of optic neuritis, but bilateral facial weakness would be unusual. GBS may cause bilateral facial weakness but typically in the context of areflexia and generalized weakness; the relative afferent papillary defect would be unusual. Lyme disease may cause bilateral facial weakness similarly (although unilateral facial weakness would be more common); the afferent papillary defect would not be expected. Vasculitis is an extremely unusual cause of bilateral facial weakness.

28. A (Chapter 14)

Because of the sudden onset of symptoms along with the patient's stroke risk factors, he most probably has had a pure sensory stroke. The most likely lesion is in the contralateral thalamus, because the sensory pathways cross prior to synapsing in the thalamus. The left postcentral gyrus is on the wrong side to explain the patient's deficit. Also, it is unusual to have sensory loss of the face, arm, and leg equally from a stroke affecting the postcentral gyrus. This is because the middle cerebral artery provides blood to the face and arm regions of the cortex, while the anterior cerebral artery supplies blood to the leg region. The precentral gyrus is predominantly involved in motor pathways and not the sensory system. A lesion of the right corona radiata would be expected to cause a left hemiparesis rather than left hemisensory loss.

29. B (Chapter 17)

The middle meningeal artery travels between the skull and the dura. When this vessel is damaged (typically due to trauma resulting in a skull fracture that lacerates that artery), blood accumulates in the epidural space, resulting in an epidural hematoma. Patients often have a brief episode of loss of consciousness at the time of trauma, followed by a lucid interval and then clinical deterioration as the bleeding continues. Diagnosis and treatment constitute an emergency, because the blood will continue to collect and may cause brain herniation if untreated.

Diffuse axonal injury or an ischemic infarct would be expected to have a sudden onset without a progressive decline in function. Likewise, a concussion should not cause progressive neurologic decline and, like drug intoxication, would not result in the physical signs seen in this case.

30. D (Chapter 22)

ALS is a motor neuron disease with involvement of the lower motor neurons and corticospinal tracts. Weakness, muscle atrophy, and muscle fasciculations are prominent features. Sensory findings are not typical of ALS. Vitamin B_{12} deficiency classically results in degeneration of the dorsal columns and corticospinal tracts. Therefore joint position sense loss and weakness are typical features, whereas pain and temperature are spared. Brown-Séquard syndrome results from hemisection of the spinal cord. The classic features are ipsilateral weakness and loss of joint position sense with contralateral loss of pain and temperature sensation below the lesion. Tabes dorsalis is a late complication of neurosyphilis and is characterized by isolated dorsal column dysfunction resulting in loss of joint position sense. Anterior spinal artery syndrome usually results from infarction of the anterior spinal artery, causing ischemia to the anterior two-thirds of the spinal cord. Therefore dorsal columns are spared but weakness and loss of pain and temperature sensation result because of involvement of the ventral horns and spinothalamic tracts.

31. C (Chapter 25)

This patient meets the diagnostic criteria for tuberous sclerosis complex (TSC). A head CT or MRI may identify cortical tubers, subependymal giant cell astrocytomas, or other lesions. The other tests do not help in the evaluation of TSC.

32. A (Chapter 25)

A diagnosis of autism requires a combination of social, behavioral, and language abnormalities with onset before age 3. Asperger syndrome shares social isolation and eccentric behavior with autism. Language is normal in Asperger syndrome. Neither gross nor fine motor delay is a required feature of either condition.

33. C (Chapter 6)

Allodynia is pain provoked by normally innocuous stimuli; hyperesthesia is increased sensitivity to sensory stimuli, and paresthesias are abnormal spontaneous sensations. "Hypesthesia" refers to decreased sensation.

34. C (Chapter 4)

This patient appears to have a Horner's syndrome on the right, likely produced by a carotid dissection as a consequence of neck trauma. Horner's syndrome is characterized by unilateral miosis, ptosis, and (sometimes) ipsilateral facial anhidrosis as a result of impaired sympathetic innervation. Examine the pupils in the dark (turn the lights off and look at the pupils during the first 5 to 10 seconds). A dilation lag in the small pupil and anisocoria greater in darkness means a sympathetic defect in the smaller pupil and will help with the diagnosis.

35. B (Chapter 23)

This patient appears to have a Guillain-Barré syndrome. Albuminocytologic dissociation means high protein with almost no cells in the CSF, which is characteristic of this syndrome. Immediately after the onset of weakness, however (the first 3 to 4 days), the CSF could be completely normal. Additional studies to corroborate the diagnosis include nerve conduction studies and EMG to demonstrate slowing of conduction velocities, prolongation of F-wave latency, and possible conduction block.

36. D (Chapter 23)

This patient appears to have acute ascending weakness with loss of reflexes characteristic of Guillain-Barré syndrome or acute inflammatory demyelinating polyradiculoneuropathy. His exam worsens while in the ER, and that should be an indication that he is deteriorating quickly and needs to be admitted to the ICU for close observation. An FVC below 15 mL/kg is an indication for intubation and mechanical ventilation.

37. A (Chapter 23)

Cytomegalovirus (CMV) infection is the most common cause of polyradiculitis or cauda equina syndrome in an immunocompromised individual. The other agents do not affect the nerve roots or cauda equina primarily. Cytomegalovirus polyradiculitis occurs in about 2% of AIDS cases and is characterized by the subacute onset of a flaccid paraparesis, sacral pain, paresthesias, and sphincter dysfunction. PCR evaluation of the CSF for CMV can provide a definitive diagnosis. Treatment is with ganciclovir or foscarnet or, in severe cases, both drugs.

38. D (Chapter 7)

Her symptoms consist of a feeling of movement—which is vertigo. The intermittent nature of her vertigo, the exacerbation with head movement, and the absence of brainstem signs are consistent with BPPV. In order to confirm the diagnosis, one can perform the Dix-Hallpike maneuver at the bedside. Brainstem and cerebellar infarctions rarely present with isolated vertigo, and Ménière's disease is characterized by hearing loss and tinnitus along with episodic vertigo.

39. D (Chapter 24)

The primary antigenic target in autoimmune MG is the postsynaptic acetylcholine receptor. Presynaptic voltage-gated calcium channels are the target of the Lambert-Eaton myasthenic syndrome.

40. A (Chapter 1)

The trigeminal nerve is responsible for the muscles of mastication. The facial nerve innervates the muscles of facial expression, the oculomotor nerve subserves eye movements, the glossopharyngeal nerve innervates some pharyngeal muscles, and the hypoglossal nerve moves the tongue.

41. D (Chapter 3)

The GCS—which provides a composite assessment of unresponsive patients based on their eye movements, motor function, and language ability—is typically used for patients after head trauma. It has prognostic value for head-injured patients and is easy for nonphysicians to use.

42. B (Chapter 3)

A noncontrast head CT is the imaging study of choice in suspected intracranial hemorrhage. This allows for the easiest delineation of acute blood, which should appear hyperdense (bright) on this study. Head CT with contrast, skull x-ray, and brain perfusion scan do not help to identify acute blood. Cerebral angiography would be indicated only if a ruptured aneurysm or other vascular anomaly were suspected as the cause of an intracranial hemorrhage.

43. E (Chapter 10)

The patient's clinical presentation is typical for temporal arteritis: age over 50, pain over the temporal arteries, jaw claudication, and an elevated ESR. Definitive diagnosis is made by temporal artery biopsy. Treatment with prednisone for several months must be initiated early, because involvement of the ophthalmic artery can lead to blindness if diagnosis and treatment are delayed.

44. E (Chapter 13)

The patient's history and obesity are most consistent with a diagnosis of obstructive sleep apnea. While narcolepsy is also associated with excessive daytime sleepiness, patients typically have associated hypnagogic hallucinations or cataplexy, which are absent in this patient. Therefore, polysomnography is the test that would be most helpful in confirming the diagnosis. The MSLT is useful for diagnosing narcolepsy while MRI of the brain, LP, and EEG would be of no diagnostic value in this patient.

45. C (Chapter 17)

Uncal herniation results from mass lesions of the middle cranial fossa. This patient most likely has a hemorrhage in the middle cranial fossa from head trauma. If large enough, the mass lesion causes displacement of the medial portion of the temporal lobe (uncus) downward over the tentorium cerebelli. This typically results in compression of the brainstem and entrapment of the third cranial nerve. This compression can cause coma due to disruption of the ascending arousal system from the brainstem. It causes an ipsilateral dilated pupil due to compression of the parasympathetic nerve fibers (traveling with the third cranial nerve) that normally cause pupillary constriction. Diffuse axonal injury can result in coma but would not be expected to be responsible for a unilateral dilated pupil that is nonreactive to light.

46. A (Chapter 14)

Intracerebral hemorrhages caused by hypertension are most often found in the basal ganglia, thalamus, pons, and cerebellum, in order of decreasing frequency.

47. C (Chapter 13)

Pemoline and methylphenidate are stimulants used for the treatment of narcolepsy. Clomipramine is a tricyclic antidepressant used for the treatment of cataplexy. Because obstructive sleep apnea is characterized by repetitive episodes of upper airway obstruction during sleep, treatment is often with CPAP, which helps maintain airway patency during sleep. Alcohol and sedating drugs such as benzodiazepines can decrease upper airway tone, resulting in worsened symptoms. Last, obesity is a risk factor for obstructive sleep apnea, so weight loss may prove beneficial in obese patients.

48. A (Chapter 19)

A headache that is either different from the normal pattern or progressive deserves to be investigated further with a brain imaging study. Slowly progressive brain tumors can be associated with a normal neurologic exam or minor abnormalities. Nausea and vomiting need not be present, especially in the early stages of a tumor. Administration of pure oxygen is an effective treatment for cluster headaches, but the patient's description is not consistent with this diagnosis.

49. B (Chapter 19)

Seizures or hemiparesis are not usual features of pituitary adenoma. Varying degrees of bitemporal hemianopia (a visual field deficit in the temporal visual fields bilaterally) may be caused by compression of the optic chiasm. A homonymous hemianopia results from dysfunction of the optic radiations or visual cortex posterior to the chiasm. On brain imaging with contrast, pituitary adenomas usually enhance in a homogenous manner and do not typically exhibit ring enhancement.

50. D (Chapter 22)

Signs of UMN or corticospinal tract dysfunction include hypertonia, spasticity, increased reflexes, and an extensor plantar response (Babinski sign). Signs of lower motor neuron (LMN) dysfunction include hypotonia, decreased or absent reflexes, and a flexor plantar response (downgoing toe). Weakness may be present with either UMN or LMN dysfunction.

51. A (Chapter 2)

CT is the imaging modality of choice for demonstrating acute intracranial bleeding. While it is true that MRI provides better visualization of the contents of the posterior fossa, a cerebellar hemorrhage usually will be visible on CT. Patients with pacemakers and other implanted metal objects cannot undergo MRI. Although MRI with diffusion-weighted imaging is the most sensitive modality for ischemic stroke, a susceptibility-weighted MRI sequence is preferred for detecting intracranial blood.

52. B (Chapter 21)

In the presence of severe Lyme disease with CNS involvement, as in this case, intravenous antibiotics followed by oral therapy comprise the first choice. Here, intravenous ceftriaxone is the first choice. The combination of oral amoxicillin and doxycycline is the most common treatment for uncomplicated Lyme disease. Fluconazole is an antifungal and has no value in the treatment of *Borrelia burgdorferi* infection.

53. C (Chapter 12)

Pathologically, PD is characterized by progressive death of dopaminergic neurons of the substantia nigra pars compacta. Most cases of PD are sporadic, but there are reports of familial cases in which mutations in the parkin and α-synuclein genes have been described. Impairment of vertical gaze is a common feature of progressive supranuclear palsy (PSP), a neurodegenerative disorder that is also characterized by parkinsonian features. Despite the gait manifestations of PD, early falls are actually uncommon (but are common in PSP).

54. D (Chapter 24)

DMD and BMD are allelic disorders due to mutations in the dystrophin gene, located on the X chromosome. The inheritance pattern is X-linked. The limb-girdle muscular dystrophies are a heterogeneous group of disorders, some with autosomal dominant and some with autosomal recessive inheritance. Mutations in a wide variety of genes have been reported in patients with limb-girdle muscular dystrophy, including the sarcoglycan genes.

55. C (Chapter 1)

The cerebellum is the primary brain structure involved in coordination, although other components of the motor pathways are involved as well. Testing for rapid alternating movements is part of the coordination exam. The other choices listed have little or no primary role in coordination.

56. B (Chapter 5)

"Crossed signs" can occur with unilateral lesions in the pons if descending motor fibers heading for the ipsilateral facial nucleus are affected, with the descending fibers heading for the contralateral spinal cord. With right pontine lesions, the right face and left body could be weak.

57. E (Chapter 15)

Characteristic side effects of carbamazepine include hyponatremia, agranulocytosis, and the risk for Stevens-Johnson syndrome. Except for the hyponatremia, these side effects are rare.

58. C (Chapters 14 and 17)

Tearing of bridging veins produces a subdural hematoma. Laceration of the middle meningeal artery causes an epidural hematoma. Amyloid angiopathy is a cause of lobar hemorrhage in the elderly. Although arteriovenous malformation (AVM) rupture is a cause of subarachnoid hemorrhage, aneurysmal rupture is a more common cause.

59. B (Chapter 19)

Meningiomas enhance in a bright and mainly homogeneous manner. Certain tumors (particularly glioblastoma multiforme and metastatic lesions), brain abscesses, toxoplasmosis, granulomas, and active demyelinating lesions typically show ring enhancement after contrast administration. While lymphomas can enhance in a homogeneous manner, they can also be ring-enhancing.

60. B (Chapter 7)

Micturition syncope is a form of reflex or neurogenic syncope that involves the triggering of cardioinhibitory and/or vasodepressor responses. The symptoms of light-headedness and graying of vision are typically reported by patients with syncope. Other symptoms might include a heavy feeling at the base of the neck, buckling at the knees, and tinnitus. Although orthostatic hypotension is a common cause of syncope, the occurrence of syncope after micturition, rather than upon standing, suggests that this is not the cause in this case. Vasovagal syncope is another common cause of syncope but typically occurs in the setting of acute pain or with a strong emotional response. Vestibular neuronitis is characterized by vertigo, and there is no associated loss of consciousness.

61. D (Chapter 21)

In HSV infection, the MRI often shows contrast enhancement and edema of the temporal lobes. An EEG can also be helpful and may show sharp-wave discharges in the temporal lobes. Treatment for viral meningitis is mainly supportive, because there are no specific treatments for most viral infections. If HSV infection is suspected, however, treatment should begin promptly with intravenous acyclovir even while tests are pending, because mortality is close to 70% in untreated cases.

62. B (Chapter 23)

Physical examination is the most important information to define symptoms as belonging to the peripheral nervous system (PNS). Sensory symptoms can have a central or peripheral origin. The acuteness of the presentation does not help localization in this case. Paresthesias may be seen in both PNS and CNS dysfunction.

63. A (Chapter 17)

Neurosurgical decompression is the treatment of choice for an epidural hematoma that has resulted in uncal herniation. This is a neurosurgical emergency, so conservative management would only result in further neurologic decline. While hyperventilation and administration of mannitol may help to decrease intracranial pressure, these are temporizing measures; neurosurgical decompression is necessary to remove the accumulating blood. Because the patient has a hemorrhage, tissue plasminogen activator, which is used in acute ischemic strokes, would be contraindicated.

64. C (Chapter 20)

ADEM is a monophasic demyelinating illness. MS is characterized by multiple white matter lesions separated in space and time and is therefore not monophasic. Oligoclonal bands in the CSF are more common in MS than in ADEM. The pleocytosis of ADEM is lymphocytic. Both MS and ADEM can produce multiple lesions on MRI. ADEM is acquired and commonly occurs after viral infections or vaccinations. A positive family history is more likely to be relevant for a patient with MS.

65. B (Chapter 23)

This is a common presentation of proximal diabetic neuropathy, also known as diabetic amyotrophy. It represents a form of polyradiculoneuropathy that has a predilection for the lumbosacral plexus and in general tends to recover spontaneously over months to years. The etiology is likely different from the more common distal symmetric polyneuropathy seen in diabetes.

66. B (Chapter 17)

The patient's symptoms and head CT findings are consistent with an epidural hematoma, which results from laceration of the middle meningeal artery. The classical head CT finding of an epidural hematoma is a hyperdense region with a biconvex or lenticular shape. Tearing of bridging veins results in a subdural hematoma. Impact of the brain over the bony prominences of the skull results in cerebral contusions. On head CT, these areas appear as hyperdensities within the brain parenchyma and not in the epidural or subdural spaces. Diffuse axonal injury results from rotational acceleration and deceleration of the head and can be associated with either a normal head CT scan or hemorrhages within the deep white matter of the brain. Lastly, rupture of a cerebral aneurysm results in subarachnoid hemorrhage and not an epidural hematoma.

67. B (Chapter 16)

Progressive supranuclear palsy is a disorder characterized by parkinsonism, supranuclear impairment of eye movements (vertical gaze typically affected more prominently than horizontal gaze), and impaired postural reflexes. Corticobasal ganglionic degeneration and PD may also cause rigidity and poor postural reflexes, but are not typically associated with eye movement abnormalities. The MFS and chronic PEO are both associated with eye movement abnormalities, but these disorders affect the external ocular muscles rather than the supranuclear gaze centers and are not associated with extrapyramidal features.

68. B (Chapter 18)

Small-fiber neuropathy typically produces symptoms of neuropathic pain, and examination discloses impaired temperature and pinprick sensation. Other sensory modalities are mediated by large fibers. Weakness and atrophy reflect involvement of motor fibers rather than small-fiber sensory function.

69. A (Chapter 22)

The patient exhibits both upper motor neuron signs (hyperreflexia, spasticity, and Babinski signs) and lower motor neuron signs (atrophy and fasciculations), which are the hallmark of ALS. Weakness can occur with either lower motor neuron (LMN) or upper motor neuron (UMN) dysfunction. None of the other options listed would cause widespread findings in both. Vitamin B_{12} deficiency classically results in degeneration of the dorsal columns (loss of joint position sense) and corticospinal tracts (UMN signs). Anterior spinal artery syndrome usually results from infarction of the anterior spinal artery, causing ischemia to the anterior two-thirds of the spinal cord. Therefore dorsal columns are spared, but weakness and loss of pain and temperature sensation result because of involvement of the ventral horns and spinothalamic tracts. Central cord syndrome is most common in the cervical cord and typically results in loss of pain and temperature sensation in a cape-like distribution. Brown-Séquard syndrome results from hemisection of the spinal cord. The classic features are ipsilateral weakness and loss of joint position sense with contralateral loss of pain and temperature sensation below the lesion.

70. E (Chapter 13)

The patient's history of excessive daytime sleepiness, visual hallucinations while falling asleep (hypnagogic hallucinations), and transient loss of tone triggered by emotional states (cataplexy) is characteristic of narcolepsy. Of the choices listed, methylphenidate is the best option, as it will treat the excessive daytime sleepiness and cataplexy. Clomipramine and venlafaxine are primarily effective for treating the cataplexy but will not improve the patient's daytime sleepiness. CPAP is a treatment for obstructive sleep apnea. Pemoline is an effective medication, but due to possible hepatic toxicity, it is usually reserved for use when other medications have failed.

71. A (Chapter 16)

The extrapyramidal features of idiopathic PD are typically asymmetric. Postural reflexes may be impaired in a number of extrapyramidal disorders including idiopathic PD. Impaired vertical gaze is more typical of progressive supranuclear palsy than of idiopathic PD.

72. C (Chapter 8)

MFS is a disorder characterized by ataxia, ophthalmoplegia, and areflexia. It is considered a variant of the Guillain-Barré syndrome and is associated with the finding of anti-GQ1b antibodies in the serum. Stroke (involving either the brainstem or cerebellum) should be sudden in onset and typically would not be expected to progress over a period of several days. Ophthalmoplegia may be seen in both MG and the MFS, but areflexia is not a feature of MG. Alcoholic cerebellar degeneration may be associated with a peripheral neuropathy and loss of joint position sense and deep tendon reflexes but should not produce ophthalmoplegia (unless associated with Wernicke encephalopathy, in which case confusion should also be present).

73. C (Chapter 9)

Acute urinary incontinence is an emergency. MRI of the spine will help to determine whether an acute lesion is responsible for the incontinence (cauda equina or conus medullaris syndrome, spinal cord compression, etc.). Determination of the PVR would not help in this situation, and urodynamic studies are not indicated in the acute setting. Lumbar puncture is not indicated in this situation.

74. D (Chapter 10)

Both chronic paroxysmal hemicrania and cluster headache are unilateral and can produce conjunctival injection. Chronic paroxysmal headache is more common in women, whereas cluster headache is more common in men. Response to indomethacin is seen in chronic paroxysmal hemicrania but not in cluster headache. Episodes of chronic paroxysmal hemicrania typically last for 20 minutes rather than hours.

75. E (Chapter 11)

Although the patient's symptoms are somewhat nonspecific, examination shows that he has normal language function but with inability to perform certain actions described by the examiner. "Apraxia" refers to the inability to perform a learned motor task and it is typically caused by lesions in either the frontal or parietal lobe of the dominant hemisphere.

Appendix: Evidence-Based Resources

Chapter 2

Hasbun R, Abrahams J, Jekel J, Quagliarello VJ. Computed tomography of the head before lumbar puncture in adults with suspected meningitis. N Engl J Med 2001;345:1727–1733.

Kidwell CS, Chalela JA, Saver JL, et al. Comparison of MRI and CT for detection of acute intracerebral hemorrhage. JAMA 2004;292:1823–1830.

Warach S, Chien D, Li W, Ronthal M, Edelman RR. Fast magnetic resonance diffusion-weighted imaging of acute human stroke. Neurology 1992;42:1717–1723.

Young GR, Humphrey PR, Shaw MD, Nixon TE, Smith ET. Comparison of magnetic resonance angiography, duplex ultrasound, and digital subtraction angiography in assessment of extracranial internal carotid artery stenosis. J Neurol Neurosurg Psychiatry 1994;57:1466–1478.

Chapter 3

Booth CM, Boone RH, Tomlinson G, Detsky AS. Is this patient dead, vegetative, or severely neurologically impaired? Assessing outcome for comatose survivors of cardiac arrest. JAMA 2004;291:870–879.

Malik K, Hess DC. Evaluating the comatose patient. Rapid neurologic assessment is key to appropriate management. Postgrad Med 2002;111:38–50.

Wijdicks EF. The diagnosis of brain death. N Engl J Med 2001;344:1215–1221.

Chapter 4

Corbett JJ. The bedside and office neuro-ophthalmology examination. Semin Neurol 2003;23:63–76.

Lueck CJ, Gilmour DF, McIlwaine GG. Neuro-ophthalmology: examination and investigation. J Neurol Neurosurg Psychiatry 2004;75(suppl 4): iv, 2–11.

Newman NJ. Neuro-ophthalmology and systemic disease—Part I. An annual review (1994). J Neuroophthalmol 1995;15:109–121.

Newman NJ. Neuro-ophthalmology and systemic disease—Part II. An annual review (1994). J Neuroophthalmol 1995;15:241–253.

Chapter 6

Cervero F. Spinal cord mechanisms of hyperalgesia and allodynia: role of peripheral input from nociceptors. Prog Brain Res 1996;113:413–422.

Landy S, Rice K, Lobo B. Central sensitisation and cutaneous allodynia in migraine: implications for treatment. CNS Drugs 2004;18:337–342.

Chapter 7

Baloh RW. Clinical practice. Vestibular neuritis. N Engl J Med 2003;348:1027–1032.

Furman JM, Cass SP. Benign paroxysmal positional vertigo. N Engl J Med 1999;341:1590–1596.

Grubb BP. Neurocardiogenic syncope. N Engl J Med 2005;352:1004–1010.

Hilton M, Pinder D. The Epley (canalith repositioning) manoeuvre for benign paroxysmal positional vertigo. Cochrane Database Syst Rev 2004;(2):CD003162.

Chapter 8

Albin RL. Dominant ataxias and Friedreich ataxia: an update. Curr Opin Neurol 2003;16:507–514.

Rubino FA. Gait disorders. Neurologist 2002;8:254–262.

Shams'ili S, Grefkens J, de Leeuw B, van den Bent M, Hooijkaas H, van der Holt B, Vecht C, Sillevis Smitt P. Paraneoplastic cerebellar degeneration associated with antineuronal antibodies: analysis of 50 patients. Brain 2003;126:1409–1418.

Chapter 9

Agarwal P, Rosenberg ML. Neurological evaluation of urinary incontinence in the female patient. Neurologist 2003;9:110–117.

Delancey JO, Ashton-Miller JA. Pathophysiology of adult urinary incontinence. Gastroenterology 2004;126(suppl 1):S23–S32.

Payne CK. Epidemiology, pathophysiology, and evaluation of urinary incontinence and overactive bladder. Urology 1998;51(suppl 2A):3–10.

Thomas DR. Pharmacologic management of urinary incontinence. Clin Geriatr Med 2004;20:511–523, vii–viii.

Chapter 10
Edlow JA, Caplan LR. Avoiding pitfalls in the diagnosis of subarachnoid hemorrhage. N Engl J Med 2000;342:29–36.

Headache Classification Subcommittee of the International Headache Society. The International Classification of Headache Disorders: 2nd edition. Cephalalgia 2004;24(suppl 1):9–160.

Lipton RB, Bigal ME, Goadsby PJ. Double-blind clinical trials of oral triptans vs. other classes of acute migraine medication— a review. Cephalalgia 2004;24:321–332.

Purdy RA, Kirby S. Headaches and brain tumors. Neurol Clin 2004;22:39–53.

Chapter 11
Damasio AR. Aphasia. N Engl J Med 1992;326:531–539.

Gernsbacher MA, Kaschak MP. Neuroimaging studies of language production and comprehension. Annu Rev Psychol 2003;54:91–114.

McClain M, Foundas A. Apraxia. Curr Neurol Neurosci Rep 2004;4:471–476.

Parton A, Malhotra P, Hussain M. Hemispatial neglect. J Neurol Neurosurg Psychiatry 2004;75:13–21.

Chapter 12
Cummings JL. Alzheimer's disease. N Engl J Med 2004;351:56–67.

Knopman DS, Boeve BF, Petersen RC. Essentials of the proper diagnoses of mild cognitive impairment, dementia, and major subtypes of dementia. Mayo Clin Proc 2003;78:1290–308.

Ritchie K, Lovestone S. The dementias. Lancet 2002;360: 1759–1766.

Chapter 13
Malhotra A, White DP. Obstructive sleep apnoea. Lancet 2002;360:237–245.

Scammell TE. The neurobiology, diagnosis, and treatment of narcolepsy. Ann Neurol 2003;53:154–166.

Chapter 14
Alamowitch S, Eliasziw M, Algra A, Meldrum H, Barnett HJ—the North American Symptomatic Carotid Endarterectomy Trial (NASCET) Group. Risk, causes, and prevention of ischaemic stroke in elderly patients with symptomatic internal-carotid-artery stenosis. Lancet 2001;357:1154–1160.

Mohr JP, Thompson JL, Lazar RM, et al. A comparison of warfarin and aspirin for the prevention of recurrent ischemic stroke. N Engl J Med 2001;345:1444–1451.

Sacco RL. Risk factors for TIA and TIA as a risk factor for stroke. Neurology 2004;62(suppl 6):S7–S11.

Tissue plasminogen activator for acute ischemic stroke. The National Institute of Neurological Disorders and Stroke rt-PA Stroke Study Group. N Engl J Med 1995;333:1581–1587.

Chapter 15
Chang BS, Lowenstein DH. Mechanisms of disease: epilepsy. N Engl J Med 2003;349:1257–1266.

Nguyen DK, Spencer SS. Recent advances in the treatment of epilepsy. Arch Neurol 2003;60:929–935.

Schachter SC. Seizure disorders. Primary Care 2004;31:85–94.

Chapter 16
Dalakas MC, Fujii M, Li M, McElroy B. The clinical spectrum of anti-GAD antibody-positive patients with stiff-person syndrome. Neurology 2000;55:1531–1535.

Management of Parkinson's disease: an evidence-based review. Movement Disorders 2002;17(suppl 4):S1–166 (no authors listed).

The Parkinson Study Group. Levodopa and the progression of Parkinson's disease. N Engl J Med 2005; 351:2498–2508.

Chapter 17
Harris OA, Colford JM, Good MC, Matz PG. The role of hypothermia in the management of severe brain injury: a meta-analysis. Arch Neurol 2002;59:1077–1083.

Shackford SR, Wald SI, Ross SE, et al. The clinical utility of computed tomographic scanning and neurologic examination in the management of patients with minor head injuries. J Trauma 1992;33:385–394.

Chapter 18
Hoitsma E, Faber CG, Drent M, Sharma OP. Neurosarcoidosis: a clinical dilemma. The Lancet Neurol 2004;3:397–407.

Martin RJ. Central pontine and extrapontine myelinolysis: the osmotic demyelination syndromes. J Neurol Neurosurg Psychiatry 2005;75(suppl 3):22–28.

McIntosh C, Chick J. Alcohol and the nervous system. J Neurol Neurosurg Psychiatry 2004;75:(suppl 3):16–21.

Moore PM, Richardson B. Neurology of the vasculitides and connective tissue diseases. J Neurol Neurosurg Psychiatry 1998;65:10–22.

Watkins PJ, Thomas PK. Diabetes mellitus and the nervous system. J Neurol Neurosurg Psychiatry 1998;65:620–632.

Chapter 19
Hentschel SJ, Lang FF. Current surgical management of glioblastoma. Cancer J 2003;9:113–125.

Soffietti R, Ruda R, Mutani R. Management of brain metastases. J Neurol 2002;249:1357–1369.

Chapter 20
Bergamaschi R, Ghezzi A. Devic's neuromyelitis optica: clinical features and prognostic factors. Neurol Sci 2004;25(suppl 4): S364–S367.

Calabresi PA. Diagnosis and management of multiple sclerosis. Am Fam Physician 2004;70:1935–1944.

Filippini G, Munari L, Incorvaia B, Ebers GC, Polman C, D'Amico R, Rice GP. Interferons in relapsing remitting multiple sclerosis: a systematic review. Lancet 2003;361:545–552.

Frohman EM. Multiple sclerosis. Med Clin North Am 2003;87: 867–897.

Garg RK. Posterior leukoencephalopathy syndrome. Postgrad Med J 2001;77:24–28.

Chapter 21
Hussein AS, Shafran SD. Acute bacterial meningitis in adults. A 12-year review. Medicine 2000;79:360–368.

Schmutzhard E. Viral infections of the CNS with special emphasis on herpes simplex infections. J Neurol 2001;248:469–477.

van de Beek D, de Gans J, McIntyre P, Prasad K. Steroids in adults with acute bacterial meningitis: a systematic review. Lancet Infect Dis 2004;4:139–143.

Chapter 22
Bensimon G, Lacomblez L, Meininger V. A controlled trial of riluzole in amyotrophic lateral scelrosis. ALS/Riluzole Study Group. N Engl J Med 1994;330:585–591.

Lacomblez L, Bensimon G, Leigh PN, Guillet P, Meininger V. Dose-ranging study of riluzole in amyotrophic lateral sclerosis. ALS/Riluzole Study Group II. Lancet 1996;347(9013): 1425–1431.

Lacomblez L, Bensimon G, Leigh PN, Guillet P, Powe L, Durrleman S, Delumeau JC, Meininger V. A confirmatory dose-ranging study of riluzole in ALS. ALS/Riluzole Study Group II. Neurology 1996;47(suppl 4):S242–250.

Chapter 23
Koller HB, Kieseier C, Jander S, Hartung HP. Chronic inflammatory demyelinating polyneuropathy. N Engl J Med 2005;352: 1343–1356.

Kornberg AJ, Pestronk A. Antibody-associated polyneuropathy syndromes: principles and treatment. Semin Neurol 2003;23:181–190.

Verma S, Estanislao L, Simpson D. HIV-associated neuropathic pain: epidemiology, pathophysiology and management. CNS Drugs 2005;19:325–334.

Chapter 24
Dalakas MC, Hohlfeld R. Polymyositis and dermatomyositis. Lancet 2003;362:971–982.
Emery AE. The muscular dystrophies. Lancet 2002;359:687–695.

Newsom-Davis J. Therapy in myasthenia gravis and Lambert-Eaton myasthenic syndrome. Semin Neurol 2003; 23:191–198.

Sanders DB. Lambert-Eaton myasthenic syndrome: diagnosis and treatment. Ann N Y Acad Sci 2003;998:500–508.

Vincent A, Palace J, Hilton-Jones D. Myasthenia gravis. Lancet 2001;357:2122–2128.

Chapter 25
Online: Mendelian Inheritance in Man: http://www.ncbi.nlm.nih.gov/entrez/query.fcgi?db=OMIM

Nissenkorn A, Michelson M, Ben-Zeev B, Lerman-Sagie T. Inborn errors of metabolism: a cause of abnormal brain development. Neurology 2001;56:1265–1272.

Palmer FB. Strategies for the early diagnosis of cerebral palsy. J Pediatr 2004;145:S8–S11.

Rappley MD. Clinical practice. Attention deficit–hyperactivity disorder. N Engl J Med 2005;352:165–173.

Spence SJ, Sharifi P, Wiznitzer M. Autism spectrum disorder: screening, diagnosis, and medical evaluation. Semin Pediatr Neurol 2004;11:186–195.

Wenger DA, Coppola S, Liu SL. Insights into the diagnosis and treatment of lysosomal storage diseases. Arch Neurol 2003;60:322–328.

Index

Index note: page references with a *b*, *f*, or *t* indicate a box, figure, or table on the designated page; page references in **bold** indicate a discussion of the subject in the Questions and Answers section.

Abducens nerve (CN VI), 4, 5*t*, 32–33, 35

Abducens palsy, 33, 34

Abductor pollicis brevis, 6*f*

Absence epilepsy, 105*t*

Absence seizures, 16, 103, 103*f*, **184, 194**

Acalculia, 77, 78

Accessory nerve (CN XI), 5, 5*t*

Acoustic neuroma, 135

Acoustic schwannoma, 135

Acquired immune deficiency syndrome (AIDS)
>as cause of progressive encephalopathy, 179*t*
>CSF findings of conditions with, 11*t*
>dementia associated with, 82*b*
>neurologic infections associated with, 147–149
>PN associated with, 157*t*
>as risk for PCNSL, 134

Acrobatic psychogenic gait, 60

Acromegaly
>PN associated with, 165*t*
>related to pituitary tumors, 136

Acrylamide poisoning, PN associated with, 159*b*, 163

Action dystonia, 115

Action tremor, 113, 113*b*

Acute axonal diabetic polyneuropathy, 161*t*

Acute confusional state, 25–26, 81

Acute disseminated encephalomyelitis (ADEM)
>CSF findings associated with, 11*t*
>monophasic course of, 141–142, **191, 199**

Acute dystonic reactions, 111

Acute inflammatory demyelinating poly-radiculoneuropathy (AIDP), 158, 159, 163

Acute intracranial hemorrhage, 23*b*

Acute ischemic stroke, 23*b*

Acute spinal cord compression, 152–153

Acute subdural hematoma, 119, 119*f*

Adamkiewicz, artery of, 150, 154

Addison's disease, dementia associated with, 82*b*

Adductor reflexes, 8

Adie's pupil, 30, 31

Adrenal insufficiency, 24*b*

Adrenoleukodystrophy, 179*t*

Adrenoleukoneuropathy, 159*b*

Adventitious movements, in motor examinations, 6

Age, CSF findings associated with, 11*t*

Agnosia
>evaluation of, 78
>prosopagnosia in, 78
>visual agnosia in, 78

Agraphia, 77, 78

Akathisia, movement disorder of, 111

Akinetic-rigid gait, 59, 59*t*

Alcoholic cerebellar degeneration, ataxia associated with, 57, 57*b/t*

Alcohol use/abuse
>acute intoxication or withdrawal with, 126*t*
>as cause of altered consciousness, 24*b*
>as cause of chorea, 114*b*
>as cause of new-onset seizures, 104
>cerebellar degeneration associated with, 126, 126*t*, 127, 127*t*
>effects on the nervous system, 126, 126*t*, 127, 127*t*
>Peripheral neuropathy associated with, 157*t*, 158, 159*b*, 165*t*
>tremor related to, 113*b*
>vitamin deficiencies associated with, 126, 127, 127*t*

Alexander's disease, as cause of progressive encephalopathy, 179*t*, 180, 181*t*

Alexia without agraphia, 77

Allelic mutation, 169

Allodynia, 49, **187, 196**

Alpha waves, in EEG, 15, 15*f*, 16

Altered consciousness
>clinical approach to, 20, 20*f*, 21, 22, 22*f/t*
>defined, 20
>differential dx for, 22–23, 23*b*
>diffuse causes of, 23, 24*b*
>reversible etiologies of, 20*f*
>structural causes of, 23*b*

Alternate cover test, 34

Alzheimer's disease (AD)
>clinical manifestations of, 83
>dementia associated with, 82, 82*b*, 83–84
>etiology and risk factors for, 82–83
>pathology and epidemiology of, 82, 83

Ambulation
>abnormalities of, 8–9
>arm swing with, 8
>difficulty initiating, 8–9, 59

Amino acid metabolism disorders, as cause of progressive encephalopathy, 179*t*

Aminoaciduria, ataxia associated with, 57*b*

Amyloid-beta protein precursor (AbPP), 83

Amyloidosis
>Peripheral neuropathy associated with, 157, 157*t*, 158, 159*b*, 161, 164
>urinary incontinence associated with, 62*f*, 64

Amyloid precursor protein (APP), 83

Amyotrophic lateral sclerosis (ALS)
>as cause of dementia, 82*b*
>as differential dx for spinal cord disorders, 43
>presentation and clinical course of, 155, **191, 200**

Anaplastic astrocytoma, 130*b*

Anaplastic ependymoma, 130*b*

Anaplastic oligodendroglioma, 130*b/t*, 132

Aneurysm, of right middle cerebral artery, 13*f*

Aneurysmal subarachnoid hemorrhage, 71

Angelman's syndrome, mental retardation associated with, 177

Angiography, cerebral, 13, 13f

Angiotensin converting enzyme (ACE), 124

Anisocoria, 27, 29–31, 31b, **187, 196–197**

Ankle, reflexes associated with, 7, 7f, 8, 41t

Anomia, 74, 76t

Anosognosia, 80

Anoxia, as cause of dystonia, 115

Anterior cerebral artery, 94f, 100

Anterior choroidal artery, 95f

Anterior communicating artery, 95f, 100, 100f

Anterior inferior cerebellar artery (AICA), 94, 94f, 95f

Anterior ischemic optic neuropathy (AION)
    optic disc abnormality with, 31, 32t
    vision loss caused by, 29b, 30t

Anterior spinal artery, 95f

Anterior spinal artery syndrome, 154, **187, 196**

Anterolateral system, 46, 47f

Antidromic study, 16

Antiepileptic drugs (AEDs), 106, 107t, **190, 199**

Antinuclear antibody (ANA), 127

Antiphospholipid syndrome (APS), 128

Antiretrovirals, PN associated with, 159b

Anxiety, as cause of myoclonus, 115b

Aphasia
    Broca's aphasia in, 74–75, 75f/t, **185, 195**
    conduction aphasia in, 76–77
    defining and diagnosing, 74–75, 75f/t, 76, 76t
    as differential dx for acute confusion, 26
    focal sign of, 23
    global aphasia in, 77
    perisylvian aphasia in, 77
    subcortical aphasia in, 77
    transcortical aphasia in, 77
    transcortical sensory aphasia in, 77
    types of, 74–75, 75f/t, 76, 76t, 77
    Wernicke's aphasia in, 75, 75f/t, 76

Apraxia
    defining and diagnosing, 77–78
    etiologies of, 78
    types of, 77, **192, 200**

Arbovirus, in viral meningitis or encephalitis, 146

Areflexia, associated with cerebellar ataxia, 57t

Argyll Robertson pupils, 31, 145

Argyrophilic round intraneuronal inclusions (Pick bodies), 87

Arithmetic skills, 94f

Arsenic neuropathy, 157, 159b, 165t

Arteriovenous malformation (AVM)
    as differential dx for CP, 177
    presentation of, 30t, 101
    as risk for cerebral hemorrhage, 100, 101

Artery of Adamkiewicz, 150, 154

Aseptic meningitis, 147, **185, 195**

Asperger's syndrome, 179, **187, 196**

Astasia-abasia gait, 60

Astrocytic tumors of the brain, classification of, 130, 130b/t, 131

Ataxia
    associated with vitamin deficiencies, 127, 127t
    classification of, 56, 57b
    defined, 56
    evaluating patients with, 56, 56b, 57, 57b/t, 58
    gait deficits associated with, 8
    from hemispheric lesions, 56
    related to subacute combined degeneration, 154
    from vermal lesions, 56
    See also Gait disorders

Ataxia-telangiectasia, as neurocutaneous syndrome, 57b, 182t

Atherosclerosis, as risk factor for vascular dementia, 85

Atonic bladder, 63, 63t, 65t, **184, 195**

Atonic seizure, 104

Attention
    acute confusional state of, 25–26
    in neurologic examinations, 4
    in patient with neglect, 79, 79f

Attention-deficit-hyperactivity disorder (ADHD), 180, 182

Attenuation, 11

Autism, 178–179, **187, 196**

Autoimmune neuropathy, 157

Autonomic failure, syncope with, 54–55

Autonomic neuropathy, 125b, 163, 165

Autosomal dominant spinocerebellar degeneration, 57b, 58

Autosomal recessive cerebellar degenerative disorders, 57b

Axillary nerve
    shoulder abduction associated with, 6f
    testing of, 40t

Axonal disease, NCS and EMG findings with, 16, 16t, 17, 17t

Axonal polyneuropathy, associated with thyroid disease, 128t

Babinski sign, 2, **191, 200**
    associated with spinal cord disorders, 43
    in coma/altered consciousness evaluations, 22
    focal sign of, 23
    with MS, 138t
    reflexes associated with, 8

Bacterial infections
    CSF findings associated with, 11t
    of the nervous system, 143–144, 144t, 146t

Bacterial meningitis
    altered consciousness with, 21, 24b
    CSF findings associated with, 11t
    etiologic agents of, 143, 144t
    symptoms and diagnosis of, 143

Ballism, movement disorders of, 114

Banging, associated with autism, 178

Basilar artery, 94, 94f, 95, 95f, 96, 100f

Battle's sign, 118

Becker muscular dystrophy (BMD), 167t, 169–170

Behçet's disease, 123t

Benign positional paroxysmal vertigo (BPPV), 53, 53b, **187–188**

Benign rolandic epilepsy, 105t

Beta waves, in EEG, 15, 15f

Biceps muscle
    elbow extension associated with, 6f
    reflex associated with, 7, 7f, 8, 41t

Bitemporal hemianopia, associated with pituitary tumors, 136, **189, 198**

Bladder incontinence
    associated with neurosyphilis, 145
    associated with transverse myelitis, 138, 138t
    See also Urinary incontinence

Blood patch, 11, 72

Blood vessels, as pain-sensitive structures, 67

Borrelia burgdorferi, 145–146, **198**

Botulism, INO associated with, 33

Bowel incontinence
    associated with neurosyphilis, 145
    associated with spinal disorders, 43
    associated with transverse myelitis, 138, 138t

Boxer's encephalopathy, 82b

Brachial plexus
    disorders of, 40t, 42, 42f, 43
    injury of, 2

Brachioradialis muscle, 41t

Brain
abscess in, 23*b*, 144–145, 145*f*
cerebral hemorrhages in, 100, 100*f*, 101
congenital vascular anomalies of, 101
metabolism of, 14
Brain death, criteria for, 25
Brain infarct, fungal infections as cause of, 148
Brain ischemia
by decreased systemic perfusion, 96
by embolism, 95–96
left hemisphere lesion as, 96
mechanisms of, 95–96
by thrombosis, 95
Brainstem
differential dx for lesions in, 45
disorders of, 43, 44*f*, 45, 45*f*
functioning of, 21–22, 22*f*
infarct of, 52, 53*b*
sensory changes with disorders in, 50*t*, 51
symmetrical/asymmetrical reflexes of, 23
Brain tumors
altered consciousness associated with, 23*b*
clinical presentation of, 129, 129*f*, 130
diagnostic evaluation of, 129*f*, 130, 131*f*
metastatic, 129, 129*f*, 130, 130*b*
primary, 120, 120*t*, 129, 130, 130*t*
treatment of, 132, 134
Broca's aphasia, 74–75, 75*f/t*, **185, 195**
Broca's area, 75*f*
Brodmann's area, 27
Brown-Séquard syndrome, 153

C5
elbow flexion associated with, 6*f*
reflexes associated with, 7, 7*f*, 8
shoulder abduction associated with, 6*f*
C6
elbow flexion associated with, 6*f*
reflexes associated with, 7, 7*f*, 8
wrist extension associated with, 6*f*
C7
elbow extension associated with, 6*f*
finger extension associated with, 6*f*
reflexes associated with, 7, 7*f*, 8
wrist extension associated with, 6*f*
wrist flexion associated with, 6*f*
C8
finger flexion associated with, 6*f*
wrist flexion associated with, 6*f*

California encephalitis, 146
Caloric testing, 34–35
in brainstem function, 21, 22*t*
performing test for, 22*t*
Campylobacter jejuni, incidence of GBS related to, 159
Canavan's disease, progressive encephalopathy associated with, 179*t*, 180, 181*t*
Candida, in CNS fungal infections, 148
Capillary telangiectasia, 101
Carbon disulfide poisoning, PN associated with, 159*b*
Carbon monoxide
as cause of altered consciousness, 24*b*
as cause of chorea, 114*b*
Carcinomatous meningitis, altered consciousness associated with, 24*b*
Carcinomatous sensory neuropathy, 159*b*
Cardiac arrest, as cause of altered consciousness, 24*b*, 25
Cardiac disorders, associated with inflammatory myopathies, 170, 172
Carotid artery
aneurysm of, 29*b*
MRA of, 14
Carotid endarterectomy, 98
Carotid sinus hypersensitivity, 54*t*
Carpal tunnel syndrome, 2, 159*b*
Cataplexy, 90, **200**
Cauda equina, 150, 154
Caudate infarction/hemorrhage, as cause of chorea, 114*b*
Cavernous angioma, 101
Central cord syndrome, 49, 153, 153*f*, 154
Central herniation, 121
Central nystagmus, 36*t*
Central sleep apnea, 128*t*
Central vertigo, 52, 53*b*
Cerebellar ataxia
associated with thyroid disease, 128*t*
symptoms/signs associated with, 56, 56*b*
Cerebellar degeneration
associated with alcohol use/abuse, 126, 126*t*
ataxia associated with, 57*b/t*
Cerebellar hemorrhage
ataxia associated with, 56, 57*b/t*
imaging studies of, **189, 198**
Cerebellar tonsils, 153, 153*f*

Cerebellar vermis, 153
Cerebellitis, postinfectious, 57, 57*b/t*
Cerebellum
ascending and descending tracts of, 94*f*
functions of, 56
infarct of, 52, 53*b*, 56, 57*b/t*
pathways to and from, 94*f*
signs/symptoms of disease of, 56, 56*b*, **189–190, 198**
tremor associated with outflow tract disorder of, 113*b*
Cerebral angiography, 13, 13*f*
Cerebral artery aneurysm, 13*f*
Cerebral artery stroke, 2
Cerebral hemispheres
differential dx for lesions in, 45
disorders of, 43, 44*f*, 45, 45*f*
homunculus of the motor strip in, 43, 45, 45*f*
Cerebral hemorrhage
intraparenchymal hemorrhage as form of, 98*f*, 100–101
subarachnoid hemorrhages (SAH) in, 11*t*, 21, 24*b*, 71, 100, 100*f*, 120, 120*f*, **183, 190, 194, 199**
Cerebral hypotonia, 180
Cerebral palsy (CP)
classification of, 175
differential dx for, 177
diparetic, 175
hemiparetic, 175
presentation and diagnosis of, 175, 177
spastic quadriplegic, 175
urinary incontinence associated with, 62*f*
Cerebrospinal fluid (CSF)
analysis of, 10–11, 11*t*
findings of neurologic infections, 146*t*, **187, 197**
leakage with head trauma, 118
on MRI imaging, 12
production and volume of, 10
Cerebrovascular disease, 62*f*, 63–64
Cervical spondylosis
left hand weakness with, 2
urinary incontinence associated with, 62*f*
Chagas disease, autonomic neuropathy associated with, 163
Channelopathies, 167*t*, 171
Charcot joints, 145
Charcot-Marie-Tooth (CMT)
as differential dx for peripheral nerve disorders, 41
hereditary, 159*b*, 162, 165*t*

Cherry red spots, macular, 180, **183, 193**

Cheyne-Stokes respirations, 121

Chiari malformation, type I and II, 153, 153f

Chiasm, visual loss associated with, 28f, 29b, 30t

Children
developmental milestones in, 176t
occurrence of seizures in, 103, 104, 104f
See also Pediatric neurology

Cholinergic crisis, as differential dx for myasthenic crisis, 167

Chorea
causes of, 114, 114b
as movement disorder, 114, 114b

Choriocarcinoma, 130b

Choroid-plexus carcinoma, 130b

Choroid-plexus papilloma, 130b

Chromosomal abnormalities
dementia associated with, **184, 194**
mental retardation syndromes associated with, 177, 178t

Chromosomal translocations, mental retardation associated with, 177

Chronic daily headaches, as primary headache disorder, 70, 70t

Chronic inflammatory demyelinating polyradiculopathy (CIDP), 125, 125b, 156b, 157, 157t, 159b, 160, 165t

Chronic progressive distal symmetric diabetic polyneuropathy, 161t

Chronic subdural hematoma, dementia associated with, 82b

Churg-Strauss disease, 123t

Cingulate herniation, 121

Circle of Willis
arteries of, 95f
as common site of aneurysms, 100, 100f
MRA findings of, 14, 14f

Cisplatinum toxicity, PN associated with, 157t, 159b, 164

Classic migraine, 69, 70t

Clonic phase of seizures, 103

Clonus
associated with MS, 138t
reflexes associated with, 8

Cluster headaches
characteristics of, 68, 69, **192, 200**
lacrimation and rhinorrhea associated with, 68, 69
pain associated with, 68, 69

as primary headache disorder, 68, 69–70, 70t
triggers of, 68, 69

CNS lymphoma, CSF findings associated with, 11t

Cocaine eyedrops test, 29–30

Coccidioides immitis, in CNS fungal infections, 148

Color vision, 28

Coma
associated with thyroid disease, 128t
clinical approach to, 20, 20f, 21, 22, 22f/t
defined, 20, 119t
differential dx for, 22–23
diffuse causes of, 23, 24b
Glasgow Coma Scale of, 20, 119t
noxious stimuli in assessment of, 20, 21, 22
structural causes of, 23b

Common migraine headache, 69, 70t

Complete spinal cord transection, 152

Complex partial seizures
as differential dx for acute confusion, 26
features and automatisms with, 102

Compound muscle action potential (CMAP), 16, 17t

Compressive mononeuropathy, 157t

Compressive neuropathy, 159b, 163

Computed tomography (CT)
contraindication for, 10
contrast-enhanced, 12–13
indications for, 12–13, **188, 197**
technical abilities of, 11–12

Concomitant eye misalignment, 33t

Concussion, labyrinthine, 52, 53b

Conduction aphasia, 76–77

Confusion
acute state of, 25–26, 81
associated with vitamin deficiencies, 126, 127, 127t

Congenital malformations of the spine, 154

Congenital muscle disorders, 169

Congenital nystagmus, 36t

Conjugate gaze deviation, 37

Consciousness
altered/depressed, 20, 20f, 21–22, 22f/t
in neurologic examinations, 3–4

Continuous positive airway pressure (CPAP), 91, **189, 198**

Contralateral homonymous hemianopia, associated with pure alexia, 77

Contrast agents, in imaging studies, 12

Contrecoup contusions, 120

Contusions, 120

Conus medullaris, 150, 154

Coprolalia, as vocal tic, 116

Corneal reflex
brainstem function of, 21, 22t
performing test for, 22t

Corpus callosum, lesions in, 77

Cortex, sensory changes with disorders of, 50t, 51

Corticobasal ganglionic degeneration, 110t

Corticospinal tract
effects of MS on, 138, 138t
motor pathways in, 150, 151f
signs of dysfunction in, 150, 152, 154, **189, 198**

Cover test, 34

Coxsackievirus, in viral meningitis or encephalitis, 146

Cranial nerves (CN)
CN I (olfactory), 4, 5t
CN II (optic nerve), 4, 5t
CN III (oculomotor), 4, 5t, 30, 32–33, 68
CN IV (trochlear), 4, 5t, 32–33
CN V (trigeminal), 4–5, 5t, 67, 67f, 152, **188, 197**
CN V1 (forehead), 5, 5t
CN V2 (cheek), 5, 5t
CN V3 (jaw), 5, 5t
CN VI (abducens), 4, 5t, 32–33
CN VII (facial), 5, 5t, **183, 194**
CN VIII (vestibulocochlear), 5, 5t, **183, 194**
CN IX (glossopharyngeal), 5, 5t
CN X (vagus), 5, 5t
CN XI (accessory), 5, 5t
CN XII (hypoglossal), 5, 5t
areas in the brain of, 94f
diabetic neuropathies of, 125, 125b
effects of MS on, 138, 138t
effects of thyroid disease on, 128t
involvement in brainstem reflexes, 21–22, 22f/t
in neurologic examinations, 3t, 4–5, 5t
as pain-sensitive structures, 67, 67f

Craniopharyngioma, 29b, 130b

Creatine kinase (CK), serum levels of, 39

Creutzfeldt-Jakob disease (CJD)
ataxia associated with, 57b/t
as cause of myoclonus, 115b

dementia associated with, 82b, 87
14,3,3-protein associated with, 10
Cri-du-chat syndrome, mental retardation associated with, 177
Critical care neuropathy, 159b, 162
Critical illness myopathy, 174t
Crohn's disease, inflammatory myopathies associated with, 172
Crossed signs, 43, **190, 198**
Cryoglobulinemia, neurologic symptoms associated with, 123t
Cryptococcus neoformans, in CNS fungal infections, 148
Cryptogenic sensory polyneuropathy, 157t, 158
CT. See Computed tomography (CT)
Cushing's disease, related to pituitary tumors, 136
Cyanide poisoning, PN associated with, 159b
Cysticercosis, 149
Cystometry, 61–62
Cystourethroscopy, 62
Cytomegalovirus (CMV)
    congenital infection as cause of mental retardation, 177
    incidence of GBS related to, 159
    PN associated with, 159b, **187, 197**
    in viral meningitis, 146
    visual changes associated with, 29b

Dawson's fingers, 139
Deafness, as differential dx for autism, 179
Decerebrate posturing, 21–22, 22f
Decorticate posturing, 21–22, 22f
Deep tendon reflexes (DTRs)
    delayed relaxation of, 128t
    in fatigable muscles, 167
    in neurologic examination, 7, 7f, 8
Dejerine-Sottas disease, peripheral neuropathy associated with, 165t
Delirium, defined, 25, 26, 81
Delta waves, in EEG, 15, 15f
Deltoid muscle, shoulder abduction associated with, 6f
Dementia
    associated with extrapyramidal features, 85–87
    associated with neurosyphilis, 145
    associated with PD, 111
    ataxia associated with, 57b/t
    causes of, 82–88
    epidemiology of, 81
    evaluating and diagnosing of, 81, 82b
    imaging studies of, 15

impaired functions associated with, 81
infectious causes of, 87–88
morbidity and mortality associated with, 81
normal aging vs., 81
personality changes with, **184, 194**
related to progressive multifocal leukoencephalopathy, 147
signs/symptoms of, 81, **184, 195**
therapies for, 83–84, 84t
thyroid disease associated with, 128, 128t
urinary incontinence associated with, 62f
vitamin deficiencies related to, 127, 127t
Dementia with Lewy bodies
    features of, 82b, 85, **183, 193**
    management and therapy for, 85
Demyelinating diseases
    multiple sclerosis (MS) in, 137–138, 138t, 139, 139f, 140, 140f, 141, 141t
    NCS and EMG findings with, 16, 16t, 17, 17t
Demyelination
    CSF findings associated with, 11t
    INO associated with, 33
Dental abscess, 68
Denver Developmental Screening test, 175, 177
Depressed consciousness, associated with cerebellar ataxia, 57b/t
Depression
    associated with MS, 138t
    pseudodementia associated with, 81
    sleep disorders with, 92
Dermatomal map, 8, 49f, 152
Dermatomyositis (DM), 169, 172–173
Detrusor hyperreflexia (DH), 63, 64
Detrusor instability (DI), 63
Detrusor-sphincter dyssynergia (DSD), 63, 65t
Developmental delay, 177–178, 179
Developmental milestones, 176t
Developmental regression disorders, 179, 179t, 180
Developmental venous anomaly, 101
Diabetes mellitus
    autonomic neuropathies associated with, 163
    neurologic symptoms associated with, 125–126
    neuropathies associated with, 161, 161t, 165t

peripheral neuropathies associated with, 125, 157, 157t, 158, 159b, 165t
    as risk factor for cerebrovascular diseases, 126
    as risk factor for vascular dementia, 85
    urinary incontinence associated with, 62f, 64, **184, 195**
Diabetic amyotrophy, 43, 125, 125b, 161t, **191, 199**
    cystopathy, 62f, 64
    ketoacidosis, 24b
    mononeuropathy, 161t
    neuropathies, 125, 125b, 126
    proximal motor neuropathy, 161t
    radiculopathy, 161t
Diffuse axonal injuries, 120
Diffuse encephalitis, 24b
Diffuse Lewy body disease, 110t
Diffusion-weighted imaging (DWI), 12, 13f
Diparetic cerebral palsy, 175
Diphtheria, peripheral neuropathy associated with, 165t
Diplopia
    associated with vertigo, 52, 53
    evaluation of, 31–32, 32t, 33, 33t, 34, 34f, 35
Direction-changing nystagmus, 52
Disseminated intravascular coagulation, neurologic symptoms associated with, 123t
Dissociated sensory loss, 49
Distal myopathies, 172
Distal sensory polyneuropathy
    associated with SLE, 127
    related to HIV, 163
Distal symmetric predominantly sensory neuropathy, 125b
Dix-Hallpike test, 53, 54f
Dizziness, defined, 52
Doll's eyes
    brainstem reflex of, 22t
    testing for, 34–35
Doppler studies
    extracranial Doppler sonography, 14
    transcranial Doppler (TCD), 14
Dorsal columns
    fiber arrangement in, 46, 48f
    signs of dysfunction of, 151, 154
Dorsal interossei, 6f
Double simultaneous stimulation, 4
Downbeat nystagmus, 36t, 57t

Down syndrome
     mental retardation associated with, 177
     as risk factor for AD, 82
Doxorubicin toxicity, peripheral neuropathy associated with, 165t
Dropped reflex, 2
Drowsiness, 20
Drug-induced myopathies, 173, 174t
Drug-induced neuropathy, 157t, 159b, 164
Drug-induced tremor, 113b
Drugs/medications, as differential dx
     for altered consciousness, 24b
     for ataxia, 57b
     for chorea, 114b
     for dystonia, 115
     for movement disorders, 111
     for syncope, 55
     See also specific condition or diagnosis
Drusen bodies, optic disc abnormality associated with, 32t
Duchenne's muscular dystrophy (DMD), 167t, 169–170, **189, 198**
Duret hemorrhages, 120
Dysesthesias, 48
Dysarthria
     associated with aphasia, 74
     associated with MS, 138t
     associated with thyroid disorders, 128t
     associated with vertigo, 52, 53
     in cerebellar disease, 56b
Dysdiadochokinesia, 56b, **189–190, 198**
Dysdiadochokinesis, 8
Dysequilibrium, 52
Dysmetria, 8, 56b
Dysphagia
     associated with inflammatory myopathies, 172
     associated with vertigo, 52
Dyssomnias, 90–91
Dystonia
     causes of, 115
     geste antagoniste in, 114
     as idiopathic or symptomatic, 114–115
Dystrophia myotonia protein-kinase (DMPK), 170
Dystrophic muscle changes, 169

Eastern equine encephalitis, 146
Echolalia, 178
Echovirus, in viral meningitis or encephalitis, 146
Edinger-Westphal nuclei (EWN), 29

Elderly population, incidence of seizures in, 104, 104f
Electroencephalogram (EEG)
     bipolar or referential montages in, 15
     clinical indications for, 15, 15f, 16
     in diagnosing seizure disorders, 106
     frequency patterns in, 15, 15f
     interictal, 15
     limitations of, 15
     montage of electrodes in, 15
     technical ability of, 15, 15f, 16
Electromyography (EMG)
     activation and/or recruitment in, 16
     identifying primary muscle disorders with, 39
     indications for, 16, 16t, 17, 17t
     insertional and spontaneous activities in, 16
     volitional motor unit potentials in, 16
Embolic retina, 29b
Embolus
     as cause of ischemic stroke, 95–96
     paradoxical, 96
     as risk factor for vascular dementia, 85
     sources of, 95–96
Embryonal tumors, 130b
Emerin gene, mutations of, 171
Emery-Dreifuss muscular dystrophy, 167t, 171, 172
Encephalitis
     associated with neurosyphilis, 145
     CSF findings associated with, 11t
     hemorrhagic, 11t
     from viral infections, 146
Encephalopathy
     associated with vitamin deficiencies, 126, 127, 127t
     as cause of altered consciousness, 24b
     defined, 25, 26
     EEG findings with, 15
Encephalopathy, progressive, 179t
Endocrine disorders
     associated with pituitary tumors, 136
     myopathies associated with, 173
Endpoint nystagmus, 36t
Enterovirus, in viral meningitis or encephalitis, 146
Entrapment neuropathy, 125, 125b, 159b, 163, 164t, 165t
     as differential dx for peripheral nerve disorders, 41
     related to thyroid disease on, 128t
Enzymatic disorders, as cause of progressive encephalopathy, 179t
Ependymoma, 130b

Epidural blood patch, 11, 72
Epidural hematoma, 119–120, 120f, 122, **186, 190, 191, 196, 199**
Epilepsy
     antiepileptic drugs (AEDs) for, 106, 107t
     first aid for seizures, 108
     licensing for drivers with, 108
     regional brain metabolism with, 14–15
     risks for, 104
     sleep disorders with, 92
     status epilepticus (SE) in, 107–108, 108f, **185–186, 195**
     surgical procedures for, 107
     syndromes of, 105t
     vagus nerve stimulation as treatment of, 107
Epileptic cry, 102
Epileptic myoclonus, 115, 115b
Episodic ataxia, inherited, 57b, 58
Epley maneuver, 53, 54f
Epstein-Barr virus (EBV)
     CSF findings associated with, 10, 11t
     incidence of GBS related to, 159
     in viral meningitis, 146
Epstein-Barr virus polymerase chain reaction (EBV PCR), 11t
Erectile dysfunction (ED)
     anatomy/physiology of, 64–65
     causes of, 65–66
     evaluation and treatment of, 66
Erythema chronicum migrans, 146
Erythrocyte sedimentation rate (ESR), 71
Escherichia coli, in bacterial meningitis, 144t
Esotropia, 33, 34
Essential myoclonus, 115, 115b
Essential tremors (ET), 113, 113b, 114
Ethylene poisoning, peripheral neuropathy associated with, 159b
Examination, neurologic. See Neurologic examination
Exercise, as cause of myoclonus, 115b
Exocytosis, 166
Exotropia, 34
Extensor digitorum, 6f
Extensors carpi radialis, 6f
Extinction, with neglect, 79, 79f
Extracranial Doppler sonography, 14
Extraocular movements, cranial nerves of, 4, 5t
Extrapyramidal disorders, 8
Extrapyramidal signs

associated with cerebellar ataxia, 57t
dementia associated with, 85–87
Eye deviation, 33
Eye misalignment, 33, 33t
Eye movements
anatomy of, 32–33
disorders of, 138, 138t
rapid eye movements in, 35
supranuclear, 35

Fabry's disease, peripheral neuropathy associated with, 165t
Facial droop, focal sign of, 23
Facial expression (CN VII), 5, 5t, **183, 194**
Facial pain syndrome, 71
Facial palsy, associated with thyroid disorders, 128t
Facial sensation, testing for, 4–5, 5t
Fasciculations, in motor examinations, 6
Fasciculus cuneatus, 151
Fascioscapulohumeral muscular dystrophy, 172
Fat, on MRI imaging, 12
Fatal familial insomnia, 87
Fatigue
associated with MS, 138t
fatigable muscles in weakness, 166, **188, 197**
Febrile seizures, 104
Femoral nerve, testing of, 40t
Femoral neuropathy, 159b, 164t
Fever
associated with cerebellar ataxia, 57t
seizures associated with, 104
Filum terminale, 150
Fine motor adaptive skills, 175, 176t
Finger agnosia, 78
Finger flexor, testing reflex of, 41t
Finger tapping, 3t, 8
Finger-to-nose testing, 3t, 8
First-order Horner's syndrome, 31b
First-order neurons, 29, 46
Fistula, perilymph, 52, 53b
Flapping, associated with autism, 178
Flexors carpi radialis, 6f
Flexors digitorum profundus, 6f
Flexors digitorum superficialis, 6f
Fluid-attenuated inversion recovery (FLAIR), 12, 13f, 139
Fluorescent treponemal antibody (FTA), 145
Focal compression neuropathy, 125, 125b, 161t
Focal signs, in coma or altered

consciousness, 21–22, 22f/t, 23, 23b, 24, 24b
Foramen magnum, 150
Foramen magnum compression, 57b/t
Forced expiratory volume (FEV), 167
Forced vital capacity (FVC), 160
Forehead (CN V₁), 5
Foster-Kennedy syndrome, 31
Fourth ventricle, closure of, 10
Fragile-X syndrome, mental retardation associated with, 177
Friedreich's ataxia, 57t, 58, 125
Frontal gait, 59, 59t
Frontal lobe
gait associated with dysfunction of, 9
mental status assessments of, 3t, 4
urinary incontinence related to dysfunction of, 62f
Frontotemporal dementia (FTD)
associated with chromosome 17 (FTD-17), 82b
features of, 87
Fungal infections
CSF findings associated with, 11t
in meningitis, 24b
neurologic, 146t, 148

Gadolinium, 12
Gag reflex
brainstem function of, 21, 22t
performing test for, 22t
related to CN IX, 5, 5t
Gait apraxia, 9
Gait ataxia, 56b
Gait disorders
differential dx for, 59, 59t, 60
etiologies of, 59t
types of, 58–59, 59t, 60
Galactorrhea, related to pituitary tumors, 136
Galactosemia, mental retardation associated with, 177
Ganglionopathy, peripheral neuropathy associated with, 157t, 159b
Gangliosidosis, as cause progressive encephalopathy, 179t
Gaucher's disease, as cause of progressive encephalopathy, 179t, 180, 181t
Gaze, disorders in, 33, 34f, 35, 36t, 37, 52, **195**
Gaze-evoked nystagmus, 36t, 52
Generalized epilepsy, as cause of myoclonus, 115b
Generalized tonic-clonic seizures (GTC), 102–103, 104

Genetic defects
associated with AD, 83
in SCAs, 58
Germ-cell tumors, 130b
Germinoma, 130b
Gerstmann-Sträussler-Scheinker syndrome, dementia associated with, 87
Gerstmann's syndrome, 78–79, 78f
Giant cell arteritis, 71, 123t
Gigantism, related to pituitary tumors, 136
Gilles de la Tourette's syndrome, 116
Glasgow Coma Scale (GCS), 20, 118, 119t, **188, 197**
Glaucoma, 29b
Glial tumors
astrocytic and oligodendroglial, 131
low-grade astrocytomas in, 131
ring-enhancing lesions of, 131, 131f, 132
treatments of, 132
Glioblastoma multiforme, 130b/t, 131, 131f
Gliomas
clinical presentation of, 129
vision loss associated with, 29b
Global aphasia, 77
Glossopharyngeal neuralgia, 68
Glue inhalation, peripheral neuropathy associated with, 159b
Glutamic acid decarboxylase (GAD), 112
Glycogen storage disease type II, as cause of progressive encephalopathy, 180
Grotton patch, 172
Gower's sign, 169
Grand mal seizure. See Generalized tonic-clonic seizures (GTC)
Granulomatosis meningoencephalitis, fungal infections as cause of, 148
Gray matter, disorders as cause of progressive encephalopathy, 179t
Gross motor skills, 175, 176t
Guillain-Barré syndrome (GBS)
acute ascending weakness associated with, 158–159, **187, 197**
autonomic neuropathy associated with, 163
CSF findings associated with, 11t, **187, 197**
diagnostic evaluation of, 159–160
differential dx for, 159
as differential dx for peripheral nerve disorders, 41
as immune-mediated neuropathy, 158–159, 159b, 160, 165t
Miller-Fisher variant of, 58, 159, 165t

Guillain-Barré syndrome (GBS) (*continued*)
pathogenesis and presentation of, 158–159, **187, 197**
PN associated with, 156*b*, 157*t*
treatment of, 160
urinary incontinence associated with, 64
Gustatory sweating, 125

Haemophilus influenzae, in bacterial meningitis, 143, 144*t*
Hallucinations, hypnagogic, 90, **191, 200**
Headaches
associated with brain tumors, 129, 132, 133, 136
associated with thyroid disease, 128*t*
classification of, 68–70, 70*t*, 71–72
cluster headaches in, 68, 69, **192, 200**
history and physical examination for, 68, **189, 198**
imaging studies for, **189, 198**
migraine headaches in, 68, 69, 70*t*, **184, 194**
pathogenesis of, 67, 67*f*
primary headache disorders in, 68, 69–70, 70*t*
related to lumbar puncture (LP), 10–11
secondary headache disorders in, 70–72
tension headaches in, 68
trigeminal neuralgia in, 68
triggers of, 68
Head injury
as cause of dystonia, 115
seizures related to, 104
skull fractures in, 119
See also Head trauma
Head trauma
acute subdural hematoma in, 119, 119*f*
central (transtentorial) herniation in, 121
cingulate herniation in, 121
classification of, 118, 119*t*
contusions in, 120
dementia associated with, 82*b*
diffuse axonal injuries in, 120
epidural hematoma in, 119–120, 120*f*, **186, 190, 191, 196, 199**
herniation syndromes in, 121, **188, 197–198**
management of, 118, 121–122, **188, 197**
mortality and morbidity associated with, 118
as risk factor for AD, 82
skull fractures in, 119

subarachnoid hemorrhage (SAH) in, 11*t*, 21, 24*b*, 71, 100, 100*f*, 120, 120*f*, **183, 190, 194, 199**
tonsillar herniation in, 121
treating increased ICP of, 121–122, **183–184, 194**
types of, 118–119, 119*f*/*t*, 120, 120*f*, 121
uncal (tentorial) herniation, 121, **188, 197–198**
Hearing
as cranial nerve III, 5, 5*t*, **183, 194**
sense of, 46
Hearing loss
associated with acoustic neuroma, 135
associated with thyroid disorders, 128*t*
associated with vertigo, 52, 53
Heavy metal poisoning, altered consciousness associated with, 24*b*, 159*b*
Heel tapping, 3*t*, 8
Heel-to-shin testing, 3*t*, 8
Heliotrope rash, 172
Hemangioblastoma, 130*b*
Hematomyelia, 153
Hemiballismus, 114
Hemibody anesthesia, 50*t*
Hemidystonia, 115
Hemigait, 60
Hemiparesis
associated with brain tumors, 130
examination of, 21
focal sign of, 23
Hemiparetic cerebral palsy, 175
Hemiparetic gait, 59, 59*t*
Hemorrhage
cerebellar, 56, 57*b*/*t*, **189, 198**
epidural, 119–120, 120*f*, 122, **186, 190, 191, 196, 199**
intracranial, 23, 23*b*, **188, 189, 197, 198**
intraparenchymal, 98*f*, 100, 101
intrathecal, 10, 11
pontine, 22
subarachnoid (SAH), 11*t*, 21, 24*b*, 71, 100, 100*f*, 120, 120*f*, **183, 190, 194, 199**
Hemorrhagic encephalitis, CSF findings of, 11*t*
Hemotympanum, 118
Hepatic encephalopathy, 123–124
Hepatic failure, 24*b*, 104
Hepatitis, PN associated with, 159*b*
Hepatocerebral degeneration, as cause of chorea, 114*b*

Hereditary autonomic neuropathy, 159*b*
Hereditary neuropathies, 157*t*, 158, 162
Hereditary neuropathy with liability to pressure palsy (HNPP), 157*t*, 159*b*, 165*t*
Hereditary peripheral neuropathies, 159*b*
Hereditary sensory and autonomic neuropathy (HSAN), 162, 165*t*
Hereditary sensory neuropathies, 159*b*
Herniated disc, as differential dx for radiculopathy, 42
Herniation syndromes, 121, **188, 197–198**
Herpes simplex virus (HSV), in viral meningitis, 146, 147, **190, 199**
Herpes virus, incidence of GBS related to, 159
Herpes zoster, urinary incontinence associated with, 62*f*
Hexacarbon poisoning, peripheral neuropathy associated with, 159*b*
Hiccups, as cause of myoclonus, 115*b*
Higher cortical function, disorders of
agnosia in, 78
anosognosia in, 80
aphasia in, 74–75, 75*f*/*t*, 76, 76*t*, 77
apraxia in, 77–79, 79*f*, 80, **192, 200**
Gerstmann syndrome in, 78–79, 79*f*, 80
neglect as, 79, **185, 195**
nondominant hemispheric syndromes in, 80
Hip adductor muscle, testing reflex of, 41*t*
Histoplasma capsulatum, in CNS fungal infections, 148
Hoffmann's sign, 8
Homocystinuria, as cause of progressive encephalopathy, 179*t*
Homunculus of the motor strip, 43, 45, 45*f*
Horner's syndrome (HS)
causes of, 29–30, 31*b*
characteristics of, 29, 31*b*, **187, 196–197**
ipsilateral, 96–97
Human immunodeficiency virus (HIV)
congenital infection as cause of mental retardation, 177
dementia associated with, 87–88
neurologic complications associated with, 147
neuropathies associated with, 157*t*, 159*b*, 163, 165*t*, **187, 197**
Hunter's syndrome, as inherited neurodegenerative disorder, 181*t*
Huntingtin protein, 86, **194**

Huntington's disease (HD)
as cause of dystonia, 115
as cause of progressive
encephalopathy, 179*t*
dementia associated with, 82*b*
features of, 86
as hereditary chorea, 114, 114*b*, **194**
Hurler's syndrome, as inherited
neurodegenerative disorder, 181*t*
Hydrocephalus
associated with type II Chiari
malformation, 153
ataxia related to, 57*b*
as complication of basilar
meningitis, 144
dementia associated with, 82*b*
gait disorders associated with, 9
Hypercalcemia
as cause of altered consciousness,
24*b*
dementia associated with, 82*b*
Hyperesthesia, 48, 50*t*
Hyperglycemia
as cause of chorea, 114*b*
neurologic effects of, 125, 125*b*
neuropathy associated with, 125*b*
Hyperkalemic periodic paralysis, 167*t*,
171
Hypermagnesemia, as cause of altered
consciousness, 24*b*
Hypermetric saccades, 35
Hypernatremia, as cause of altered
consciousness, 24*b*
Hypertension
as cause of intraparenchymal
hemorrhage, 100–101, **188, 198**
as risk factor for vascular dementia,
85
Hypertensive leukoencephalopathy, 142
Hyperthyroidism
as cause of chorea, 114*b*
paralysis and proximal myopathy
related to, 128
Hypertropia, 34
Hyperventilation, as trigger of absence
seizures, 103
Hypesthesia, 48
Hypnic jerks, 115*b*
Hypocalcemia, as cause of altered
consciousness, 24*b*
Hypoglossal nerve (CN XII), 5, 5*t*
Hypoglycemia
as cause of altered consciousness,
24*b*
as cause of chorea, 114*b*
effect on cerebral functioning, 22
neurologic effects of, 126

Hypokalemic periodic paralysis, 167*t*, 171
Hypomagnesemia, as cause of altered
consciousness, 24*b*
Hypometric saccades, 35
Hyponatremia, as cause of altered
consciousness, 24*b*
Hypophosphatemia, as cause of altered
consciousness, 24*b*
Hypopituitarism, related to pituitary
tumors, 136
Hyporeflexia, associated with cerebellar
ataxia, 57*t*
Hypotension, orthostatic, 125
Hypothyroidism
ataxia associated with, 57*b/t*
as cause of progressive
encephalopathy, 179*t*
dementia associated with, 82*b*
mental retardation associated with,
177
neurologic manifestations of, 128*t*
Hypothyroid myopathy, 173
Hypothyroid neuropathy, 157, 159*b*
Hypotonic infant, 180
Hypotropia, 34
Hypoxic-anoxic encephalopathy, as cause
of mental retardation, 177
Hypoxic brain injury, as cause of
myoclonus, 115*b*

Idiopathic intracranial hypertension
(IIH), 71–72
Idiopathic Parkinson's disease (PD)
as cause of tremor, 113, 113*b*, **191,
200**
presentation and clinical course of,
110, 110*t*, 111, **189, 191, 198,
200**
Idiopathic sensory ganglionitis, 159*b*
Idiopathic torsion dystonia, 115
IgM paraproteinemia, peripheral
neuropathy associated with, 165*t*
Iliopsoas, nerve to, 40*t*
Ill-defined dizziness, 52
Imaging studies. See
Investigations/studies
Immune-mediated ataxic neuropathy,
159*b*
Immune-mediated inflammatory
myopathies, 172–173
Immune-mediated neuropathy, 159*b*
Immune-mediating agents, in treatment
of MS, 140–141, 141*t*
Inclusion body myositis (IBM),
172–173

Incontinence. See Bladder incontinence;
Bowel incontinence; Urinary
incontinence
Incoordination, 8
Increased intracranial pressure (ICP)
altered consciousness associated
with, 24, **183–184, 194**
associated with cysticercosis, 149
causes of, 129, 132
headache disorder of, 68, 70*t*
in herniation syndromes, 121
ODS associated with, 31
treatment of, 24
Infantile ceroid lipofuscinosis, 179*t*
Infants
causes of seizures in, 104
See also Pediatric neurology
Infections
acute confusion associated with, 26
as cause of altered consciousness, 24*b*
as cause of dementia, 87–88
congenital infections as cause of
mental retardation, 177
CSF findings associated with, 11*t*
dementia associated with, 82*b*
of the nervous system, 143–144,
144*t*, 145, 145*f*, 146, 146*t*,
147–149
neuropathies associated with, 159*b*,
162–163, 165*t*
See also *specific organism*
Inflammatory conditions
CSF findings associated with, 11*t*
myopathies in, 172–173, 174*t*
neuropathies in, 165*t*
Inherited episodic ataxias, 57*b*, 58
Inherited neurodegenerative diseases,
179, 179*t*, 180, 181*t*
Insertional activity, 16
Insomnia, fatal familial, 87
Intelligence, testing for, 177
Intention tremor, 8, 56*b*, 113, 113*b*, 138*t*
Internal carotid artery aneurysm, vision
loss associated with, 29*b*
Internal cerebral artery (ICA), 95*f*
International normalized ratio (INR), 128
Internuclear ophthalmoplegia (INO), 33,
34*f*, 35, 138, 138*t*, **186, 195**
Interstitial lung disease, associated with
inflammatory myopathies, 172
Intoxication, acute alcohol, 126*t*
Intracerebral hemorrhage
as cause of mental retardation, 177
hypertension as cause of, 100–101,
188, 198
Intracranial hemorrhage, 23, **188, 189,
197, 198**

Intraparenchymal hemorrhage
  causes and locations of, 100–101
  as form of cerebral hemorrhage, 98f, 100–101
  presentation of, 98f, 101
Intrathecal hemorrhage, 10, 11
Investigations/studies
  cerebral angiography in, 13, 13f, 14
  cerebrospinal fluid (CSF) analysis, 10–11, 11t
  computed tomography (CT) in, 11–13
  electroencephalogram (EEG) in, 15, 15f, 16
  electromyography (EMG) in, 16, 16t, 17
  magnetic resonance angiography (MRA) in, 14, 14f
  magnetic resonance imaging (MRI) in, 11–12, 12f, 13, 13f
  nerve conduction studies (NCS) in, 16, 17, 17t
  positron emission tomography (PET) in, 14–15
  vascular imaging studies, 13, 13f, 14, 14f
  See also Neurologic examination
Ion channel dysfunction, 167t, 171
Ionizing radiation, as risk factor for brain tumors, 130
Ipsilateral gaze, 33, **195**
Ipsilateral limb ataxia, 56
Iris, sphincter and dilator muscles of, 29
Ischemic stroke
  diagnosis and treatment of, 97–98, 98f, 99, 99f
  embolic, 96
  findings on imaging of, 97, 98f, 99f
  of lesion in left PCA, 96
  medical and surgical treatments of, 98–99
  pure motor stroke as, 97
  pure sensory stroke as, 97, **186, 196**
  by right hemispheric lesion, 96
Ishihara plates, 28
Isoniazid, PN associated with, 165t
Ixodes, tick species of, 146

Jacksonian march, 102
Jaw claudication, 71
JC virus, 142, 147–148
Jerk nystagmus, 35
Joint position
  effects of MS on, 138t
  sense of, 3t, 8
Juvenile myoclonic epilepsy, 105t

Kayser-Fleischer ring, 116, **195–196**
Kearns-Sayre syndrome, 171
Kennedy's disease, 155
Knee, reflexes associated with, 7, 7f, 8
Knee jerk, testing of, 41t
Korsakoff's syndrome, 126, 126t
Krabbe's disease
  as cause of progressive encephalopathy, 179t, 180, 181t
  PN associated with, 159b
Kugelberg-Welander disease, 155

L3, reflexes associated with, 7, 7f, 8
L4, reflexes associated with, 7, 7f, 8
Laboratory studies. See Investigations/studies
Labyrinth, infarct of, 52, 53b
Labyrinthine artery, 95f
Labyrinthine concussion, 52, 53b
Lactate, metabolic disorders of, 57b
Lambert-Eaton myasthenic syndrome (LEMS)
  autonomic neuropathy associated with, 163
  as differential dx for NMJ disorders, 40
  fatigable muscle weakness as feature of, 166, 167t
Lamin A, mutations of, 171
Lamin C, mutations of, 171
Landau-Kleffner syndrome, 179
Language
  abilities to repeat in, 4
  aphasia and acquired abnormalities of, 74–75, 75f/t, 76, 76t, 77
  comprehension of, 4, 75, 76t
  fluency of spontaneous speech in, 4
  functions of, 76t
  naming common/less common objects in, 4
  in neurologic examinations, 3t, 4
  pediatric developmental milestones in, 175, 176t
  prosody of, 80
  reading abilities in, 4, 76t
  repetition skills of, 76t
  semantic elements of, 80
  testing fluency of, 76t
  "tip-of-the-tongue" phenomenon in, 74
  word salad of, 76
  word substitution errors (paraphasias) in, 74, 76t
  writing of, 74, 76t, 77
Lateral corticospinal tract, 151, 151f
Lateral geniculate nuclei (LGN), 28, 30t
Lead neuropathy, 159b

Left hemispheric lesion, 96
Leigh disease, as inherited neurodegenerative disorder, 181t
Lennox-Gastaut syndrome, 105t
Lenticulostriate arteries, 95f
Leprosy, PN associated with, 157t, 159b, 163, 165t
Leptomeningeal metastases, 129
Lethargy, 20
Leukemia, PN associated with, 161
Leukodystrophy
  dementia associated with, 82b
  PN associated with, 159b
Leukoencephalopathies, 142
Levodopa-responsive dystonia, as differential dx for CP, 177
Lewy body dementia, 82b, 85, **183, 193**
Lewy body disease, 92, 110t
Lhermitte's sign, associated with MS, 138, 138t
Licking, associated with autism, 178
Light-headedness, 52
Light-near dissociation (LND), 30, 31
Limb-girdle muscular dystrophy, 167t, 170
Lipid storage diseases, dementia associated with, 82b
Listeria monocytogenes, in bacterial meningitis, 144t
Locked-in syndrome, 25
Lou Gehrig's disease, 155
Lower motor neuron (LMN)
  anatomy of, 44f
  disorders of, 44f, **186, 196**
Low-grade astrocytoma, 130b
Low-pressure headache, 72
Lumbar puncture (LP)
  contraindication for, 10–11, 144, **183–184, 194**
  CSF findings of neurologic infections, 146t
  indications for, 10–11, 42, 43, 100, 130, 134, 143
  low pressure headaches associated with, 72
  traumatic tap of, 10
Lumbosacral plexus
  diabetic amyotrophy in, 43
  disorders of, 40t, 42, 42f, 43
Lumbosacral polyradiculopathy, related to HIV, 163
Lyme disease
  CSF findings associated with, 11t, **189, 198**
  neurologic manifestations and treatment of, 145–146, **189, 198**

peripheral neuropathy associated with, 157, 157t, 159b, 165t

Lymphocytic meningitis, **196**

Lymphoid granulomatosis, peripheral neuropathy associated with, 165t

Lymphoma, peripheral neuropathy associated with, 161

Lymphomatosis, peripheral neuropathy associated with, 157t

Macroglobulinemia, peripheral neuropathy associated with, 161

Macrovascular dementia, 85

Macular degeneration, 29b

Magnetic resonance angiography (MRA) fat-suppressed, 14
of vascular anatomy, 14, 14f

Magnetic resonance imaging (MRI) contrast-enhanced, 12
fluid-attenuated inversion recovery (FLAIR) sequence of, 12, 13f
indications for, 12–13
susceptibility- and diffusion-weighted sequences of, 12, 13f
T1- and T2-weighted images with, 12, 12f, 13f
technical abilities of, 12, 12f
time to echo (TE) of, 12
time to repetition (TR) of, 12

Magnetic resonance spectroscopy, 15

Magnetic resonance venography (MRV), 14

Malnutrition, associated with cerebellar ataxia, 57t

Maple syrup urine disease, as cause of progressive encephalopathy, 179t

Marchiafava-Bignami syndrome, associated with alcohol use/abuse, 126t

Marcus-Gunn pupil, 28

Medial lemniscal system, 46, 48f

Medial longitudinal fasciculus (MLF), 33, 34f, 35, **186, 195**

Median nerve, 6f

Median neuropathy, 159b, 164t

Medical Research Council (MRC), muscle power scale of, 7, 7t

Medications. See Drugs/medications, as differential dx; *specific condition or diagnosis*

Medulloblastoma, 130b/t, 132, 133f

Memory
in mental status assessment, 3t, 4
visual memory in, 4

Ménière's disease, 52, 53b

Meningeal carcinomatosis, PN associated with, 157t

Meningeal irritation, 68

Meningeal tumors, 130b/t

Meninges, as pain-sensitive structures, 67

Meningioma
clinical presentation of, 129, 132–134, 134f, **190, 199**
CSF findings associated with, 11t
as primary brain tumor, 130b/t
treatment of, 133–134
vision loss associated with, 29b

Meningismus, 33

Meningitis
aseptic, 147, **185, 195**
associated with cysticercosis, 149
carcinomatous, 24b
as cause of altered consciousness, 24b
CSF findings associated with, 11t
fungal infections as cause of, 148
lymphocytic, **196**
radiologic contraindications for, 10
seizures associated with, 104

Meningoencephalitis, 124, 146

Menstruation, headaches associated with, 68

Mental retardation
causes of, 178
chromosomal abnormality syndromes associated with, 177, 178t
classification of, 178
developmental delay in, 177–178
as differential dx for autism, 179

Mental status
attention in, 3t, 4
frontal lobe function studies in, 4
language in, 3t, 4
level of consciousness in, 3–4, 21
memory testing in, 3t, 4
neglect findings in, 3t, 4
in neurologic examinations, 3, 3t, 4, 4f
visuospatial function in, 3t, 4, 4f

Meralgia paresthetica, 164t

Mercury neuropathy, 159b

Metabolic disorders
acute confusion associated with, 26
as cause of altered consciousness, 24b
as cause of chorea, 114b
as cause of dystonia, 115
as cause of seizures in elderly population, 104
in childhood, 57b/t
dementia associated with, 82b
diabetes mellitus in, 125, 125b, 126
mental retardation associated with inherited forms of, 177
thyroid disorders in, 128, 128b

Metabolic encephalopathy, as cause of myoclonus, 115, 115b

Metabolic neuropathies, 157t, 159b, 161, 161t, 162

Metabolism
of the brain, 14–15
See also Metabolic disorders

Metachromatic leukodystrophy
as cause of progressive encephalopathy, 179t, 180, 181t
as differential dx for CP, 177
peripheral neuropathy associated with, 159b

Metastatic brain tumors, 129, 129f, 130, 130b

Microvascular dementia, 85

Micturition
neuroanatomic connections of, 61–62, 62f
syncope with, 54t, **190, 199**

Middle cerebral artery (MCA), 75, 76, 95f, 100, 100f

Migraine headaches
characteristics of, 68, 105t, **184, 194**
focal neurological deficits associated with, 69
prodromal symptoms of, 68
triggers of, 68
vertigo with, 53, 53b
visual disturbances with, 27
with/without aura, 69

Milkmaid grip, 114

Miller Fisher syndrome (MFS), 57t, 58, 159, 165t, **192, 200**

Mitochondrial, Myopathy, Encephalopathy, Lactoacidosis, and Stroke (MELAS), 174

Mitochondrial disorders, 125
ataxias associated with, 57b
as cause of progressive encephalopathy, 179t
diabetes associated with, 125
myopathies associated with, 171–172, 174

Mitochondrial encephalomyelopathy, 57b

Mixed connective tissue disease, inflammatory myopathies associated with, 172

Mixed incontinence, 63

Mnemonics
DANG THE RAPIST (Diabetes, Alcohol, Nutritional, Guillain-Barré, Trauma, Hereditary, Environmental, Rheumatic, Amyloid, Paraneoplastic, Infections, Systemic diseases, Tumors), 158
DR GATT (Demyelinating, Resolving hematoma, Granuloma, Abscess, Tumors, Toxoplasmosis), 132

Mnemonics (*continued*)
TORCH (Toxoplasmosis, Other agents, Rubella, Cytomegalovirus, Herpes simplex), 148
Monoclonal gammopathy (M protein), PN associated with, 161
Mononeuropathies, 40–41, 158, 163
Mononeuropathy multiplex, 41, 125*b*, 158, **185, 195**
Monotherapy in AEDs, 106
Moro reflex, 177*t*
Motor examination
muscle bulk in, 3*t*, 6
muscle power in, 3*t*, 6, 6*f*, 7, 7*t*
in neurologic examinations, 3*t*, 6, 6*f*, 7, 7*t*
Motor function, 94*f*
Motor neuron diseases (MNDs), 155, 157*t*
Movement, pathways for voluntary movement, 150, 151*f*
Movement disorders
akathisia in, 111
ballism in, 114
chorea as, 114, 114*b*
as differential dx for CP, 177
drug-induced, 111
dystonia in, 114–115
idiopathic Parkinson's disease (PD) as, 110, 110*t*, 111, **189, 191, 198, 200**
myoclonus in, 115, 115*b*
neuroleptic malignant syndrome (NMS) in, 111
paroxysmal dyskinesias in, 116–117
stiff-person syndrome in, 112–113
tardive dyskinesia in, 111
tic as, 115–116
Mucolipidoses, as cause of progressive encephalopathy, 180
Mucopolysaccharidosis, as cause of progressive encephalopathy, 179*t*, 180
Multifocal motor neuropathy (MMN), PN associated with, 157*t*, 158, 159*b*, 160–161, 165*t*
Multi-infarct dementia. See Vascular dementia
Multiple myeloma, PN associated with, 161
Multiple sclerosis (MS)
ataxia associated with, 57*b/t*
"black hole" and Dawson's fingers of, 139
as cause of dystonia, 115
chronic therapies for, 140–141, 141*t*
clinical course and prognosis of, 139, 139*f*, 140
CSF findings associated with, 11*t*
as demyelinating disease of CNS, 137–138, 140

diagnostic evaluation of, 139–140, 140*f*
as differential dx for trigeminal neuralgia, 71
environmental and genetic influences in, 137
as immune-mediated process, 10
lesions associated with, 12, 140*f*, **199**
oligoclonal bands in CSF of, 140, **199**
relapses and flares of, 139, 139*f*, 140
symptoms/manifestations of, 137–138, 138*t*, **186, 195**
treatment of, 140–141, 141*t*, **186, 195**
tremor associated with, 113*b*
urinary incontinence associated with, 62*f*, 64
Multiple sleep latency test (MSLT), 90, 91
Multiple system atrophy (MSA)
autonomic neuropathy associated with, 163
as cause of dystonia, 115
as parkinsonian syndrome, 110*t*
Muscle endplate, 166
Muscles
bulk and tone in motor exams of, 3*t*, 6, 6*f*, 7, 7*t*, 21–22, 22*f/t*
effects of thyroid disease on, 128*t*
of facial expression, 5, 5*t*, **183, 194**
of mastication, 4–5, 5*t*, **188, 197**
primary disorders as cause of weakness, 39, **184, 194**
testing for power of, 3*t*, 6, 6*f*, 7, 7*t*
See also Muscle stretch reflexes
See also Skeletal muscle disorders
Muscle-specific kinase (MUSK), 168
Muscle stretch reflexes
findings with coma/altered consciousness, 22
in neurologic examination, 7, 7*f*, 8
testing of, 41*t*
Muscular dystrophy, 169
Musculocutaneous nerve
elbow flexion associated with, 6*f*
testing of, 40*t*
Myalgia, 169
Myasthenia gravis (MG)
fatigable muscle weakness as feature of, 166, **188, 197**
as immunologic disorder, 166, **188, 197**
inflammatory myopathies associated with, 172
INO associated with, 33
thyroid disease associated with, 128
Myasthenia gravis (MG), as differential dx
for GBS, 159
for NMJ disorders, 40
for thyrotoxic myopathy, 173

Myasthenic crisis, 167, 168
Mycobacterial infections, CSF findings associated with, 11*t*
Mydriasis, 33
Myelin-associated glycoprotein (MAG), 161
Myelitis, 147
Myeloma, PN associated with, 161
Myelomeningocele, 153, 154
Myoclonic epilepsy with ragged red fibers (MERRF), 171, 179*t*
Myoclonic seizures, 16, 104
Myoclonus
forms of, 115*b*
in motor examinations, 6
as movement disorder, 115
Myopathies, 16, 16*t*, 17, 17*t*, 159, 169
Myositis, 147, 169
Myotonic dystrophy, 125, 167*t*, 169, 170, **185, 195**
Myxedema coma, 24*b*

Nailbed pressure, 20, 21
Naming, problems with (anomia), 74, 76*t*
Narcolepsy, 90, 91, **191, 200**
Nasal tickle, 20
Necrotizing myopathy, 174*t*
Negative inspiratory force (NIF), 167
Negative visual phenomena, 27
Neglect
diagnosis of, 79, 79*f*
etiology of, 79
extinction of double simultaneous stimulation, 79
in mental status assessments, 3*t*, 4
signs of, 79, 79*f*, **185, 195**
Neisseria meningitidis, in bacterial meningitis, 143, 144*t*
Neonatal adrenoleukodystrophy, as cause of progressive encephalopathy, 179*t*, 181*t*
Neoplastic disease, dementia associated with, 82*b*
Nerve conduction studies (NCS)
compound muscle action potential (CMAP) in, 16, 17*t*
indications for, 16, 16*t*, 17, 17*t*
Nerve root disorders
patterns of weakness in, 41, 41*t*, 42
polyradiculopathies in, 41, **187, 197**
radiculopathies in, 41
Nerve roots
dermatomal sensory loss of, 49*f*, 50
muscles innervated by, 40*t*
root syndromes in peripheral neuropathy, 158, 158*t*
sensory modalities in, 50*t*

Neural tube defects, 154

Neuritis, 147

Neuroacanthosis, as hereditary chorea, 114*b*

Neurocardiogenic syncope, 54*t*

Neurocutaneous syndrome, 179*t*, 180

Neurofibrillary tangles (NFTs), 83, 86

Neurofibromatosis
as cause of progressive encephalopathy, 179*t*
peripheral neuropathy associated with, 165*t*
type 1 and 2 as neurocutaneous syndrome, 182*t*

Neurogenic bladder
anatomy and physiology of, 61–62, 62*f*
associated with diabetes, 125
atonic, 63, 63*t*, 65*t*, **184, 195**
spastic, 63*t*
urodynamic findings of, 61–62, 63*t*

Neurogenic disorders, EMG findings with, 16, 16*t*, 17, 17*t*

Neurogenic syncope, 54–55

Neuroleptic malignant syndrome (NMS), 111, 173–174

Neurologic examination
of coordination, 3*t*, 8
cranial nerve testing in, 3*t*, 4–5, 5*t*
gait evaluation in, 3*t*, 8–9
localizing with, 2
mental status in, 3, 3*t*, 4, 4*f*
mild vs. hard findings in, 2
motor examinations in, 3*t*, 6, 6*f*, 7, 7*f/t*
observation vs. confrontation, 2
principles of, 2, 3
reflexes in, 3*t*, 7, 7*f*, 8
sensory exams in, 3*t*, 8, 49*f*

Neurologic infections
bacterial, 143–144, 144*t*, 145, 145*f*, 146, 146*t*
CSF findings of, 146*t*, **187, 197**
fungal, 146*t*, 148
parasitic, 148–149
viral infections in, 146, 146*t*, 147–148

Neuromuscular junction (NMJ)
effects of thyroid disease on, 128*t*
NCS evaluation of, 16
pattern of weakness in problems of, 39–40

Neuromuscular junction (NMJ) disorders
as cause of hypotonic infant, 180
as differential dx for GBS, 159
Lambert-Eaton myasthenic syndrome (LEMS) in, 167*t*, 168
myasthenia gravis (MG) in, 166–167, 167*t*, 168

Neuronal ceroid lipofuscinosis, as cause of progressive encephalopathy, 180

Neuronitis, 52

Neurons
first-order, 29, 46
second-order, 29, 46
third-order, 29, 46

Neuro-ophthalmologic disturbances
anatomy of visual pathway, 27, 28*f*
diplopia in, 27, 31–32, 32*t*, 33, 33*t*, 34, 34*f*, 35
visual loss in, 27–28, 29*b*, 30*t*

Neurosarcoidosis, 124

Neurosyphilis, 145

Nicotinic acetylcholine receptor (nAChR), 166, 167

Niemann-Pick disease, as autosomal recessive disorder, 180, 181*t*, **183, 193**

Nightmares, 91

Nitrous oxide inhalation, peripheral neuropathy associated with, 159*b*

N-methyl-D-aspartate (NMDA) receptor antagonist, 84, 88

Noninfectious immune-mediated inflammatory myopathies, 172–173

Nonketotic hyperosmolar coma, 24*b*

Non-REM sleep, 89, 89*f*, 90, 91, 92

Nonvasculitic AION, 29*b*

Noxious stimuli, 21, 22

Nucleus of Cajal, 35

Nutritional cerebellar degeneration, 57*b/t*

Nutritional disorders, neurologic effects of, 126–127, 127*t*, 177

Nystagmus
associated with cerebellar disease, 56*b*
associated with MS, 138, 138*t*
associated with thyroid disorders, 128*t*
types of, 35, 36*t*
vertigo associated with, 52

Obesity, as risk factor for obstructive sleep apnea, 91

Oblique diplopia, 33

Obsessive-compulsive disorder (OCD), 116

Obstructive sleep apnea, 90–91, 128*t*, **188, 189, 197, 198**

Obtundation, 20

Obturator nerve, 40*t*

Occipital cortex, visual loss with disturbances of, 28*f*, 30*t*

Occipitoparietotemporal junction, 35

Ocular flutter, 35

Oculocephalic maneuver, 34–35

Oculocephalic reflex
brainstem reflex of, 21, 22*t*
performing test for, 22*t*

Oculomotor apraxia, 35

Oculomotor nerve (CN III), 4, 5*t*, 32–33, 68

Olfactory nerve (CN I), 4, 5*t*

Oligoclonal bands, 10, 11*t*, 140

Oligodendroglial tumors, 131, 132

Oligodendroglioma, 130*b/t*, 132

Olivopontocerebellar atrophy
ataxia associated with, 57*b/t*
as cause of dementia, 82*b*

"One-and-a-half syndrome," 33, 34*f*, **195**

Ophthalmic artery, 95*f*

Ophthalmoparesis, 33

Ophthalmoplegia, associated with cerebellar ataxia, 57*t*

Opsoclonus, 35

Optic atrophy, 28

Optic disc
abnormalities of, 27, 28, 31, 32*t*
pallor associated with MS, 138, 138*t*
visual loss associated with disturbances in, 29*b*

Optic disc swelling, 31

Optic nerve
as CN II, 4, 5*t*
pupillary light reflex in, 4, 5*t*
visual acuity in, 4, 5*t*
visual fields in, 4, 5*t*
visual loss associated with disturbances in, 28, 28*f*, 29*b*, 30*t*, **183, 193**

Optic neuritis (ON)
associated with cerebellar ataxia, 57*t*
optic disc abnormality with, 29*b*, 31, 32*t*
as symptom of MS, 138, 138*t*

Optic radiations, visual loss with disturbances of, 28*f*, 30*t*

Optic tract, 28*f*

Optokinetic nystagmus, 36*t*

Orbital compressive lesions, optic disc abnormality with, 31

Organophosphorous poisoning, peripheral neuropathy associated with, 159*b*

Orolingumasticatory dyskinesia, 111

Orthodromic study, 16

Orthostatic hypotension, 54–55, 125

Overflow incontinence, 63

Pain
in different types of headaches, 68
sense of, 46
sensory pathways for, 151
sleep disorders associated with, 92
Pain-sensitive structures
cranial, 67, 67f
outside of the cranium, 67, 67f
Palate, movement related to CN IX, 5, 5t
Pandysautonomia, PN associated with, 157t, 163
Papilledema
associated with MS, 138, 138t
associated with thyroid disorders, 128t
as cause of visual loss, 29b, 31
Parachute reflex, 177t
Paradoxical emboli, 96
Paramedian pontine reticular formation (PPRF), 33, 35
Paraneoplastic cerebellar degeneration (PCD), 57, 57b/t, 58, **184, 194**
Paraneoplastic disorders
anti-Hu antibodies with, 157, **183, 194**
associated with small cell lung cancer, 157, **194**
dementia associated with, 82b
PN associated with, 157, 157t, 164, 165t
Paraparetic gait, 59
Paraphasias, 74, 76
Paraplegic gait, 59t
Parasitic infections, neurologic effects of, 148–149
Parasomnias, 91
Parenchymal hemorrhage, 122
Paresthesias, 48, 138t
Parietal lobe, visual loss with disturbances in, 30t
Parinaud's syndrome, 33
Parkinson's disease (PD)
as cause of dystonia, 115
clinical features of, 110, 110t, 111
cogwheel movement associated with, 111
corticobasal ganglionic degeneration syndrome of, 110t
dementia associated with, 82b, 86–87, 111
epidemiology and pathology of, 110
gait associated with, 8
Lewy body disease of, 110t
multiple system atrophy with, 110t
pill rolling motion associated with, 111
progressive supranuclear palsy (PSP) syndrome of, 110t

pursuit disorder associated with, 35
rigidity associated with, 111
sleep disorders with, 92
treatments for, 111, 112t, 113t
tremors associated with, 111
urinary incontinence associated with, 62f, 64
vascular parkinsonism of, 110t
Parkinsonism, syndromes of, 110, 110t, 113b
Park's three-step test, 34
Paroxysmal dyskinesias, 116–117
Paroxysmal dystonic choreoathetosis (PDC), 117
Paroxysmal exercise-induced dystonia, 117
Paroxysmal hemicrania
pain associated with, 70, **192, 200**
as primary headache disorder, 70, 70t
Paroxysmal kinesogenic choreoathetosis (PKC), 117
Paroxysmal neurologic events, 105t
Paroxysmal nocturnal dyspnea, 92
Partial seizures, 102, 104, 105t
Partial thromboplastin time (PTT), 124
Patellar reflexes, 8, 41t
Pathologic nystagmus, 36t
Pediatric autoimmune neurologic disorders associated with streptococcal infection (PANDAS), 116
Pediatric neurology
autistic spectrum disorders in, 178–179
cerebral palsy (CP) in, 175, 177
developmental assessments of, 175, 176t
developmental regression disorders in, 179, 179t, 180
febrile seizures in, 104
hypotonic infant in, 180
inherited neurodegenerative diseases in, 179, 179t, 180, 181t
mental retardation in, 177–178, 178t
Moro reflex in, 177t
parachute reflex in, 177t
pervasive developmental disorders in, 178–179
seizures in, 104, 175, **187, 196**
special reflexes in, 177t
tonic neck reflex in, 177t
traction response in, 177t
Pelizaeus-Merzbacher disease, 179t, 180, 181t
Pellagra, peripheral neuropathy associated with, 165t
Perilymph fistula, 52, 53b
Periodic alternating nystagmus, 36t
Periodic paralysis (PP), 167t

Periosteum, as pain-sensitive structure, 67
Peripheral nerve disorders
commonly tested movements in, 40t
differential dx for, 41
mononeuropathies in, 40–41
pattern of weakness in, 40, 40t, 41
polyneuropathy in, 41
Peripheral nervous system (PNS)
anatomy of, 156
classification of disorders in, 156, 156b
demyelination of, 156, 156b
neuronal/axonal degeneration of, 156, 156b
reflexes associated with, 7, 7f, 8
sensory modalities in, 50t
Wallerian degeneration of, 156, 156b
Peripheral neuropathy
anatomic distribution of, 156, 156b
associated with alcohol use/abuse, 126, 126t
associated with infections, 159b, 162–163, 165t
associated with mitochondrial myopathies, 172
associated with vitamin deficiencies, 127, 127t
autonomic forms of, 163, 165
classification of, 156, 156b
compressive form of, 159b, 163
entrapment forms of, 159b, 163, 164t, 165t
evaluating and testing symptoms of, 156, 156b, 157, 157t
forms of, 125, 125b, 126
functional involvement of, 156, 156b
hereditary, 159b, 162
immune-mediated, 158–159, 159b, 160
metabolic neuropathies in, 159b, 161, 161t, 162
mnemonic for causes of, 158
mononeuropathy in, 158
mononeuropathy multiplex in, 41, 158, **185, 195**
pathologic mechanism of, 156, 156b
polyneuropathy in, 158
radiculopathy in, 158, 158t
recognizing patterns of, 156, 157t
remembering forms of, 165t
root syndromes in, 158, 158t
temporal course of, 156, 156b
vasculitis, 159b
Peripheral nystagmus, 36t
Perisylvian aphasia, 77
Peroneal nerve, 40t
Peroneal neuropathy, 159b, 164t
Peroxisomal disorder, as cause of progressive encephalopathy, 179t, 180

Persistent vegetative state, 25

Personal/social developmental milestones, 175, 176t

Pervasive developmental disorders, 178–179

Phakomatoses, syndromes associated with, 180, 182t

Phenylketonuria, as cause of progressive encephalopathy, 179t

Phonophobia, 68, 69

Phoria, 34

Phoria eye misalignment, 33t

Photophobia, 68, 69

Physiological tremor, 113b

Physiologic myoclonus, 115, 115b

Physiologic nystagmus, 36t

Pick's disease, dementia associated with, 82b, 87

Pilocytic astrocytoma, 130b

Pinprick sensation, 8, **191, 200**

Pituitary adenoma, 130b, 135, 135f, 136, **189, 198**

Pituitary dysfunction, associated with pituitary tumors, 136

Plasmapheresis, 160, 168, 173

Plexopathy, peripheral neuropathy associated with, 157t

Plexus disorders
    pattern of weakness in, 42, 42f, 43
    sensory changes in, 50t
    sensory findings and dropped reflexes with, 42

Poisoning, peripheral neuropathy associated with, 159b

Poliomyelitis, 62f, 155

Polyarteritis nodosa
    neurologic symptoms associated with, 123t
    peripheral neuropathy associated with, 165t

Polymerase chain reaction (PCR), 147, 148

Polymyalgia rheumatica, 71

Polymyositis (PM), 172–173

Polyneuropathy, 41, 158

Polyradiculopathy
    nerve root disorders associated with, 41, **187, 197**
    peripheral neuropathy associated with, 157t

Polysomnography, 89

Pons
    intracerebral hemorrhages in, 100–101, **188, 198**
    lesions in, 43, 44f, 45, 45f, **190, 198**
    M-region of, 61, 62f

Pontine hemorrhage, 22

Pork tapeworm, infection of, 149

Porphyria, peripheral neuropathy associated with, 157t, 159b, 162, 165t

Positional vertigo, 52–53, 53b

Positive visual phenomena, 27

Positron emission tomography (PET), 14–15

Posterior cerebral artery (PCA), 30t, 77, 95f, 96

Posterior columns, 151, 151f

Posterior communicating artery, 95f

Posterior fossa mass, ataxia related to, 57b/t

Posterior inferior artery (PICA), 94, 95f, 100, 100f

Posterior spinal artery, 95f

Postganglionic Horner's syndrome, 31b

Postictal hemiparesis, 106

Postictal state, as cause of altered consciousness, 24b

Post-lumbar puncture headache, 72

Post-organ transplant leukoencephalopathy, 142

Poststreptococcal chorea, 114b

Postural orthostatic tachycardia syndrome (POTS), 163

Postural tremor, 113, 113b

Postvoid residual (PVR), 61–62, 63, **192, 200**

Pott's disease, 144

Prader-Willi syndrome, mental retardation associated with, 177

Preganglionic Horner's syndrome, 31b

Pregnancy
    as cause of chorea, 114b
    risks with AED therapies and, 108

Presenilin 1 (PS1), 83

Presenilin 2 (PS2), 83

Presyncope, 53–54

Pretectal midbrain nuclei, 29

Primary CNS lymphoma (PCNSL), 130b, 134

Primary headache disorders
    chronic daily headaches in, 70, 70t
    cluster headaches in, 69–70, 70t
    migraine headaches in, 68, 69, 70t, **184, 194**
    paroxysmal hemicrania in, 70, 70t, **192, 200**
    rebound headaches in, 70, 70t
    tension-type headaches in, 69, 70t

Primary muscle disorders, 39, **184, 194**

Primitive neuroectodermal tumors, 130b

Prion-related diseases, dementia caused by, 87–88

Progressive aphasia, dementia associated with, 87

Progressive encephalopathy, causes of, 179t

Progressive external ophthalmoplegia (PEO), 171

Progressive multifocal leukoencephalopathy (PML), 142, 147–148

Progressive supranuclear palsy (PSP)
    as cause of dystonia, 115
    dementia associated with, 82b, 86
    eye movement and gaze disorders with, **191, 200**
    pursuit disorder associated with, 35
    syndrome of, 110t

Prolonged prothrombin time (PT), 124

Pronator drift, 6f

Proprioception, sense of, 8, 46–47, 151

Prosody, 80

Prosopagnosia, 78

Proximal diabetic neuropathy, 125, 125b, **191, 199**

Pseudomotor cerebri, 128t

Pseudopapilledema, 32t

Pseudotumor cerebri, 71–72

Psychogenic disorders, 50t

Psychogenic gait, 60

Psychogenic nonepileptic seizures, 109

Psychosis
    associated with thyroid disease, 128t
    as differential dx for acute confusion, 26

Ptosis
    associated with thyroid disorders, 128t
    bilateral, 33

Pupillary reflex, 21, 22t

Pupilloconstrictor, 29

Pupillodilator, 29

Pupils
    Adie/tonic, 30, 31
    anatomy of, 29
    Argyll Robertson, 31
    disorders of, 28, 29–31, 31b
    examination of, 29–31
    testing of, 28, 35
    unequal, 27, 29–31, 31b

Pure alexia, 77

Pure motor stroke, 97

Pure sensory stroke, 97, **186, 196**

Purified protein derivative (PPD), 144

Pursuit, in extraocular movements, 4

Pursuit movements, 35

Pyridoxine toxicity, PN associated with, 165*t*

Pyruvate, metabolic disorders of, 57*b*

Quadrigeminal cistern, 10

Quantitative sudomotor axon reflex test (QSART), 163

Raccoon eyes, 118

Radial nerve, 6*f*, 40*t*

Radial neuropathy, 159*b*, 164*t*

Radiculitis, 147

Radiculopathy, 41
    NCS and EMG studies of, 16, 16*t*, 17, 17*t*
    PN associated with, 157*t*, 158, 158*t*

Radiofrequency (RF), 12

Ramsay Hunt syndrome, 147

Rapid alternating movements, 3*t*, 8

Rapid-eye movement (REM)
    erections with episodes of, 66
    in normal sleep, 89, 89*f*, 90

Rapid plasma reagin (RPR), 145

Reactive CSF-VDRL, 145

Reading, area in the brain, 94*f*

Rebound headaches, as primary headache disorder, 70, 70*t*

Rebound nystagmus, 36*t*

Recombinant tissue-type plasminogen activator (rt-PA), 98, 99

Recurrent vertigo, 52–53, 53*b*

Red desaturation, 28, 138, 138*t*, **186, 195**

Reflexes
    abnormalities associated with MS, 138, 138*t*
    of brainstem function, 21, 22, 22*f/t*
    delayed relaxation of DTRs, 128*t*
    muscle stretch ("deep tendon"), 7, 7*f*, 8, 41, 41*t*
    pediatric reflexes in, 177*t*
    symmetry/asymmetry findings of, 23

Reflex syncope, 54, 54*t*

Refsum disease, peripheral neuropathy associated with, 165*t*

Relative afferent pupillary defect (RAPD)
    associated with MS, 138, 138*t*
    visual changes associated with, 28, 30*t*, **183, 193**

REM sleep behavior disorder, 91

Renal failure, seizures associated with, 104

Repetitive nerve-stimulation studies, 16, 17

Respiratory failure, as cause of altered consciousness, 24*b*

Resting tremor, 113, 113*b*, **191, 200**

Restless leg syndrome, 91

Retina, visual loss associated with disturbances in, 29*b*, 30*t*

Retinal detachment, 29*b*

Retinal nerve fiber, 28

Retinitis pigmentosa, 29*b*

Retrochiasmal, disturbances causing visual loss in, 29*b*

Retrograde urethrography, 62

Rett's syndrome
    as cause of progressive encephalopathy, 179*t*, 181*t*
    mental retardation associated with, 178*t*

Rheumatoid arthritis, neurologic symptoms associated with, 123*t*, 159*b*

Rheumatologic disease, as differential dx for peripheral nerve disorders, 41

Right hemispheric lesion, 96

Right-left confusion, 78

Rigidity, evaluating in motor examinations, 6

Rinne test, 5

Rocking, associated with autism, 178

Romberg sign, 8, 145

Rostral interstitial nucleus of the MLF (riMLF), 33, 35

Rubella, congenital, as cause of mental retardation, 177

Rubrospinal tract, 150

S1, reflexes associated with, 7, 7*f*, 8

S2, reflexes associated with, 7, 7*f*, 8

Saccades
    abnormalities of, 35, 37
    in extraocular movements, 4, 35

Saccadic intrusions, 35

Sandhoff's disease, 180

Sarcoidosis
    inflammatory myopathies associated with, 172
    neurologic effects of, 124–125, **186, 196**
    PN associated with, 157*t*, 165*t*
    visual loss associated with, 29*b*

Scapuloperoneal muscular dystrophy, 172

Sciatic nerve, 40*t*

Scissoring gait, 59

Second-order Horner's syndrome, 31*b*

Second-order neurons, 29, 46

See-saw nystagmus, 36*t*

Seizure(s)
    absence seizures in, 103, 103*f*, **184, 194**

antiepileptic drugs (AEDs) for, 106, 107*t*, **190, 199**
associated with brain tumors, 129–130, 131, 133
associated with cysticercosis, 149
associated with thyroid disease, 128, 128*t*
associated with vitamin deficiencies, 127, 127*t*
atonic, 104
as cause of altered consciousness, 24*b*
classification of, 102–103, 103*f*, 104
clonic phase of, 103
complex partial, 102
defined, 102, 104
diagnosis and evaluation of, 105–106
as differential dx for autism, 179
EEG findings with, 15–16, **185, 195**
epidemiology and etiology of, 102, 104, 104*f*
epilepsy syndromes with, 105*t*
febrile seizures in, 104
first aid for, 108
generalized, 102, 104
jacksonian march in, 102
licensing for drivers with, 108
myoclonic, 104
partial, 102, 104, 105*t*
postictal state with, 103
pregnancy and AED therapies for, 108
psychogenic nonepileptic forms of, 109
regional brain metabolism with, 14
simple partial seizures in, 102
surgical procedures for, 107
tonic phase of, 102, 104
vagus nerve stimulation as treatment of, 107
visual disturbances with, 27
See also Status epilepticus

Sellar region, tumors of, 130*b*

Semantic dementia, 87

Sensation
    in neurologic examinations, 3*t*, 8
    pinprick, 8, **191, 200**
    of temperature, 8

Sensory ataxia, 56, 60

Sensory nerve action potential (SNAP), 16

Sensory pathways
    dorsal columns of, 151, 151*f*
    of the spinal cord, 151, 151*f*
    spinothalamic tract of, 151, 151*f*

Sensory system
    allodynia in, 49, **187, 196**
    anatomy of, 46, 47*f*
    anterolateral system in, 46, 47*f*
    dermatome map of, 49*f*
    dissociated sensory loss in, 49

dorsal columns in, 46, 48f
dysesthesias in, 48
examination of, 46–49
hyperesthesia in, 48
hypesthesia in, 48
localizing dysfunction in, 49, 50, 50t, 51
medial lemniscal system in, 46, 48f
negative and positive symptoms of, 49
paresthesias in, 48–49
primary modalities of, 46–49
somatosensory and special senses in, 46
spinothalamic tract (STT) in, 46, 47f
symptoms associated with MS, 138, 138t
terms for abnormalities in, 48–49
Serpentine tongue, 114
Sexual dysfunction, causes of, 65–66
Shingles, 147
Short-stepped gait, 8
Shuffling gait, 8, 59
Shy-Drager syndrome, 62f
Sialidoses, as cause of progressive encephalopathy, 180
Simple partial seizure, features and sensory phenomena with, 102
Single-fiber EMG studies, 16, 17
Single-photon emission computed tomography (SPECT), 15
Sinusitis, 68
Sjögren's syndrome
    neurologic symptoms associated with, 123t
    PN associated with, 157t, 159b, 165t
Skeletal muscle disorders
    Becker's muscular dystrophy (BMD) in, 167t, 169–170
    congenital, 169
    Duchenne's muscular dystrophy (DMD) in, 167t, 169–170, **189, 198**
    Emery-Dreifuss muscular dystrophy in, 167t, 171, 172
    focal patterned weakness in, 169
    hyperkalemic periodic paralysis in, 167t
    hypokalemic periodic paralysis in, 167t
    inherited vs. acquired, 169
    limb-girdle muscular dystrophy in, 167t, 170
    mitochondrial myopathies in, 171–172, 174t
    muscular dystrophies in, 169
    myopathies in, 169
    myositis in, 169

myotonia in, 169
myotonic dystrophy, 125, 167t, 169, 170, **185, 195**
Skew deviation, 33–34
Skull fractures, 119
Slapping gait, 59t, 60
Sleep
    dreaming during, 89–90
    EEG findings with, 15, 15f
    as interdisciplinary specialty, 89
    REM and non-REM sleep stages in, 66, 89, 89f, 90, 91, 92
    stages of, 15, 89, 89f, 90
Sleep apnea
    associated with thyroid disorders, 128t
    obstructive, 90–91, **188, 189, 197, 198**
Sleep bruxism, 91
Sleep disorders
    dyssomnias in, 90–91
    as interdisciplinary specialty, 89, 89f, 90–92
    with medical conditions, 92
    narcolepsy in, 90, 91, **191, 200**
    neurologic conditions with, 92
    nightmares in, 91
    obstructive sleep apnea in, 90–91, **188, 189, 197, 198**
    parasomnias in, 91
    with psychiatric conditions, 92
    REM sleep behavior disorders in, 91
    restless leg syndrome in, 91
    sleep bruxism in, 91
    sleep paralysis in, 91
    sleep terrors in, 91
    sleepwalking in, 91
Sleep spindles, 89
Slurring (dysarthria), 52, 53, 56b, 74, 128t, 138t
Small cell lung cancer
    LEMS associated with, 168
    paraneoplastic disorders associated with, 157, **194**
Small-fiber neuropathy, 8, **191, 200**
Smell, sense of, 46
Snellen chart, 28
Social/personal developmental milestones, 175, 176t
Somatosensory system, abnormalities in, 46
Sonography, Doppler studies with, 14
Spastic bladder, 63, 63t, 65t
Spastic gait, 59
Spasticity
    evaluating in motor examinations, 6
    related to subacute combined degeneration, 154
    as sign of MS, 138, 138t

as symptom of UMN dysfunction, 43, 44f, **189, 198**
Spastic quadriplegic cerebral palsy, 175
Speech
    area in the brain for, 94f
    See also Language
Sphenoid mucocele, vision loss associated with, 29b
Sphincter dyssynergia, 62, 63, 65t
Sphingolipidoses, as cause of progressive encephalopathy, 180
Spina bifida occulta, 154
Spinal arteries, 150
Spinal bifida cystica, 154
Spinal cord
    anatomy of, 150
    cauda equina of, 150
    cerebrospinal fluid (CSF) of, 10–11, 11t
    congenital malformations of, 154
    conus medullaris of, 150
    corticospinal tract in, 150, 151f, 152
    filum terminale of, 150
    foramen magnum of, 150
    gray and white matter in, 150
    motor neuron diseases (MNDs) of, 155
    motor pathways in, 150, 151f
    sensory pathways in, 151, 151f
    subacute combined degeneration of, 126–127, 127t
    syndromes of, 152–153, 153f, 154–155
    vascular supply of, 150
Spinal cord compression, 152–153
Spinal cord disorders
    as cause of hypotonic infant, 180
    differential dx for, 43
    pattern of weakness in, 43
    sensory changes with, 50t, 51
    UMN weakness in, 43, 44f
    urinary incontinence associated with, 62f, 64
Spinal cord injuries, 62f, 64, 152
Spinal cord transection, 152
Spinal muscular atrophy (SMA), 155
"Spinal shock," 152
Spinal stenosis, 62f
Spinocerebellar ataxias (SCAs), 58
Spinocerebellar degeneration
    autosomal dominant ataxia associated with, 57b
    as cause of dementia, 82b
Spinothalamic tract (STT)
    fiber arrangement in, 46, 47f
    signs of dysfunction of, 151, 151f, 154
    somatotopic organization of, 154

Spongiform encephalopathy, dementia associated with, 87

Spontaneous activity, 16

Spontaneous vertigo, 52–53, 53*b*

Square wave jerks, 35

St. Louis encephalitis, 146

Stance, normal/abnormal forms of, 8

Stanford-Binet IQ test, 177

Staphylococcus, in bacterial meningitis, 144

Status epilepticus (SE)
  emergency treatment of, 108, 108*f*, **185–186, 195**
  etiologies of, 107–108
  types and forms of, 107

Status migranosus, 69

Steele-Richardson-Olszewski syndrome, 86

Stereotactic biopsy, 134

Stereotyped speech, associated with autism, 178

Sternal rub, 20, 21

Sternocleidomastoid, strength related to CN XI, 5, 5*t*

Steroid myopathy, 173

Stiff-person syndrome, 112–113, 125

Strabismus, 33*t*

Streptococcus. See also Group A Streptococcus; Group B Streptococcus

Streptococcus pneumoniae, in bacterial meningitis, 143, 144*t*

Stress incontinence, 63, 65*t*

Striate cortex, 27

Stride, normal/abnormal forms of, 8

Stroke
  aphasia associated with, 75
  in brainstem, 33
  as cause of seizures in elderly population, 104
  as differential dx for cerebral palsy, 177
  DWI findings associated with, 12
  focal neurologic deficits associated with, 69
  incidence in diabetic patients, 126
  as risk factor for dystonia, 115
  unilateral, 23
  urinary incontinence associated with, 62*f*, 63
  visual disturbances with, 27, 29*b*
  See also Ischemic stroke

Studies/investigations. See Investigations/studies; Neurologic examination

Stupor, 20

Sturge Weber syndrome, as neurocutaneous syndrome, 182*t*

Subacute combined degeneration, 154

Subacute sclerosing panencephalitis
  as cause of progressive encephalitis, 179*t*
  post-measles dementia associated with, 82*b*

Subarachnoid hemorrhage (SAH)
  altered consciousness with, 21, 24*b*
  CSF findings associated with, 11*t*, **183, 194**
  as form of cerebral hemorrhage, 11*t*, 21, 24*b*, 71, 100, 100*f*, 120, 120*f*, **183, 194**
  as secondary headache disorder, 71, **190, 199**

Subclavian artery, 94

Subcortical aphasia, 77

Substance abuse, PN associated with, 159*b*

"Sundowning," 83

Superior gluteal nerve, 40*t*

Supinator muscles, reflexes associated with, 7, 7*f*, 8

Supranuclear eye movements, 35

Supraspinal disorders
  DH associated with, 63
  urinary incontinence associated with, 62*f*, 63–64

Susceptibility-weighted imaging, 12, 13*f*

Sydenham's chorea, 114*b*

Symptomatic myoclonus, 115, 115*b*

Syncope
  autonomic failure as cause of, 54–55
  cardiac causes of, 53–54
  evaluating patients with, 53–54, 54*t*, 55, **190, 199**
  micturition syncope in, 54*t*, **190, 199**
  neurogenic, 54, 55

Syphilis
  Argyll Robertson pupil associated with, 31
  congenital infection as cause of mental retardation, 177
  congenital infection as cause of progressive encephalopathy, 179*t*
  dementia associated with, 82*b*
  neurologic effects of, 145, 154
  peripheral neuropathy associated with, 165*t*

Syringomyelia, 153, 153*f*

Systemic diseases, neurologic effects of, 123*t*
  alcohol-related disorders, 126, 126*t*, 127
  antiphospholipid syndrome in, 128

central pontine myelinolysis in, 128
  diabetes mellitus in, 125, 125*b*, 126
  hepatic encephalopathy in, 123–124
  neurosarcoidosis in, 124–125
  nutritional disorders in, 126–127, 127*t*
  thyroid disease in, 128, 128*b*

Systemic lupus erythematosus (SLE)
  as cause of chorea, 114*b*
  CSF findings associated with, 11*t*
  neuropsychiatric manifestations of, 127
  PN associated with, 127, **185, 195**

Systemic vasculitis, as differential dx for peripheral neuropathy, 41

T1, finger and thumb abduction with, 6*f*

Tabes dorsalis, 145, 154

Taenia solium, 149

Tandem gait, 8

Tangier disease, PN associated with, 165*t*

Tapeworm, pork, 149

Tardive dyskinesia, 111

Taste, sense of, 5, 5*t*, 46

Tau protein, 83, 87

Tay-Sachs disease
  as inherited neurodegenerative disorder, 180, 181*t*
  mental retardation associated with, 177

Teeth
  abscess of, 68, 143
  grinding/clenching during sleep of, 91

Temperature, sensation of, 8, 46–47, 151

Temporal arteritis, 68, 71, **188, 197**

Temporal lobe, visual loss with disturbances in, 30*t*

Temporomandibular joint dysfunction, 68

Tension-type headaches
  pain associated with, 68
  as primary headache, 69, 70*t*

Tentorial edge compression, 33

Tentorial herniation, 121, **188, 197–198**

Teratoma, 130*b*

Thalamus
  sensory stroke related to, 97–98, 98*f*, **186, 196**
  in sensory system, 46, 47*f*, 48*f*, 50*t*, 51

Thallium neuropathy, 159*b*

Theta waves, in EEG, 15, 15*f*

Third-order Horner's syndrome, 31*b*

Third-order neurons, 29, 46

Thoracolumbar radiculopathy, 125, 125*b*

Thrombotic thrombocytopenic purpura (TTP), 123t

Thrombus
as cause of ischemic stroke, 95
causes of, 95

Thyroid disorders
as cause of altered consciousness, 24b
neurologic signs/symptoms of, 128

Thyroid ophthalmopathy, vision loss associated with, 29b

Thyrotoxic myopathy, 173

Thyrotoxicosis, as cause of altered consciousness, 24b

Tibial nerve, 40t

Tic douloureux, 68, 71

Tick-borne disease, 145–146

Tics
as idiopathic or secondary, 116
as motor or vocal, 115–116
as movement disorder, 115–116

Tilt-table testing, 55

Tinnitus
associated with thyroid disorders, 128t
associated with vertigo, 52, 53

"Tip-of-the-tongue" phenomenon, 74

Tobacco-alcohol amblyopia, 126t

Todd's paralysis, 106, 130

Toe-walking, associated with autism, 178

Tolosa-Hunt syndrome, 31b

Tongue, movement of, 5, 5t

Tonic neck reflex, 177t

Tonic phase of seizures, 102, 104

Tonic pupil, associated with thyroid disorders, 128t

Tonsillar herniation, 121

Torsin A protein, 115

Touch
sensing light touch in, 46
sensory pathways for, 151
testing in neurologic examinations, 3t, 8

Tourette's syndrome, 116

Toxins/toxic exposure
as cause of altered consciousness, 24b
chorea associated with, 114b
dementia associated with, 82b
mental retardation associated with, 177
myopathies associated with, 173, 174t
neuropathy associated with, 159b
peripheral neuropathy associated with, 157t
vision loss associated with, 29b

Toxoplasma gondii, 148

Toxoplasmosis
congenital infection as cause of mental retardation, 177
as parasitic infection, 148
visual changes associated with, 29b

Toxoplasmosis, other agents, rubella, cytomegalovirus, herpes simplex (TORCH), 148

Traction response, 177t

Transcortical aphasia, 77

Transcranial Doppler (TCD), 14

Transient ischemic attack (TIA)
features/characteristics of, 105t
visual disturbances with, 27

Transtentorial herniation, 121

Transverse myelitis
as differential dx for GBS, 159
as differential dx for spinal cord disorders, 43
as symptom of MS, 138, 138t
urinary incontinence associated with, 62f

Trapezius, movement related to CN X, 5, 5t

Tremor(s)
action, 113, 113b
alcohol-related, 113b
associated with PD, 111
cerebellar outflow tract type of, 113b
defined, 113
drug-induced, 113b
essential tremor (ET) in, 113, 113b, 114
intention tremors in, 8
in motor examinations, 6
physiological, 113b
postural, 113, 113b
resting, 113, 113b
types of, 113, 113b

Treponema pallidum, neurologic manifestations of, 145

Triceps muscles
elbow extension associated with, 6f
testing reflexes of, 7, 7f, 8, 41t

Trichloroethylene, peripheral neuropathy associated with, 159b

Trigeminal nerve
CN V, 4–5, 5t, 67, 67f, 188, 197
dermatomal innervation of, 67, 67f, 188, 197
facial sensation of, 46, 49f

Trigeminal neuralgia
associated with thyroid disorders, 128t
pain characteristics of, 68
as secondary headache disorder, 71

Trigeminal palsy, 159b

Trinucleotide (CTG), defect of, 170

Trochlear nerve (CN IV), 4, 5t, 32–33

Tropia eye misalignment, 33t

Truncal ataxia, 56b

Tuberculosis meningitis, 11t, 144

Tuberous sclerosis, as neurocutaneous syndrome, 182t

Tuberous sclerosis complex (TSC), as cause of progressive encephalopathy, 179t, 187, 196

Tumors
CSF findings associated with, 11t
edema associated with, 24
visual loss associated with, 29b
See also Brain tumors

Tuning forks
Rinne, 5
sensation of, 8
Weber, 5

T1-weighted MRI, 12, 13f

T2-weighted MRI, 12, 12f, 13f

Uhthoff's phenomenon, 138, 138t

Ulnar nerve, 6f

Ulnar neuropathy, 159b, 164t, 190, 199

Uncal herniation, 121, 188, 197–198

Unequal pupils, 27

Unidirectional nystagmus, 52

Unwanted saccades, 35

Upbeating nystagmus, 36t

Upper motor neuron (UMN), 150
anatomy of, 44f
disorders of, 43, 44f, 184, 189, 194, 198

Uremia
as cause of altered consciousness, 24b
neuropathy associated with, 159b, 162

Urge incontinence, 63, 65t

Urinary bladder dysfunction, 61–62, 62f, 63, 63t, 64, 65t

Urinary incontinence
anatomy and physiology of, 61
associated with spinal disorders, 43, 184, 194
classification of, 63, 184, 194
diagnostic evaluation of, 61–62, 63t, 192, 200
level of lesion causing, 62f, 63–64
mixed incontinence of, 63
neuroanatomic connections in, 61–62, 62f
overflow incontinence of, 63
related to UMN (spastic) bladder, 63t, 184, 194
stress incontinence of, 63, 65t
treatment/therapy for, 64, 65t
urge incontinence in, 63, 65t

Vagus nerve (CN X), 5, 5*t*, 107

Varicella zoster virus
as differential dx for radiculopathy, 42
in viral meningitis, 146

Vascular dementia
macrovascular and microvascular
forms of, 85
as multi-infarct dementia, 82*b*, 85
risk factors for, 85
therapies for, 84*t*, 85

Vascular parkinsonism, 110*t*

Vascular system
EEG findings of dysfunction in, 15
imaging studies, 13, 13*f*, 14, 14*f*

Vasculitic AION, 29*b*

Vasculitis
dementia associated with, 82*b*
inflammatory myopathies associated
with, 172
neuropathies associated with, 157,
157*t*, 159*b*, 165*t*

Vasovagal syncope, 54*t*

Venereal Disease Research Laboratory
(VDRL), 145

Venezuelan equine encephalitis, 146

Venous sinus thrombosis, imaging of, 14

Vermal lesions, ataxia associated with, 56

Vertebral arteries, 14, 93–94, 94*f*, 95, 95*f*,
150

Vertebrobasilar artery, 96

Vertical nystagmus, 52

Vertical saccades, 35, 37

Vertigo
associated with migraine headaches,
53, 53*b*
BPPV in, 53, 53*b*, **187–188**
etiologies of, 52–53
evaluating acute onset of, 37
examining patients with, 52–53,
53*b*, **187–188, 197**
labyrinthine concussion in, 52, 53*b*
Ménière's disease in, 52, 53*b*
as spontaneous, recurrent or
positional, 52–53, 53*b*
types of, 52–53, 53*b*
vestibular neuronitis in, 52, 53*b*

Vestibular function (CN VIII), 5, 5*t*, **183,
194**

Vestibular neuronitis, 52, 53*b*

Vestibular nystagmus, 35, 36*t*, 37

Vestibular schwannoma, 135

Vestibular sensation, 46

Vestibulo-ocular movement, 4, 34–35

Vestibulo-ocular nystagmus, 36*t*

Vestibulo-ocular reflex (VOR), 35

Vestibulospinal tract, 150

Vibration
loss associated with MS, 138*t*
sensation of, 3*t*, 8, 46
sensory pathways for, 151

Vincristine, PN associated with, 157*t*,
159*b*, 164

Viral infections
CSF findings associated with, 11*t*
neurologic, 146, 146*t*, 147–148
postinfectious cerebellitis associated
with, 57, 57*b/t*

Viral meningitis
as cause of altered consciousness, 24*b*
causes of, 146, **190, 199**
CSF findings associated with, 11*t*,
185, 190, 195, 199

Vision
anatomy of, 27, 28*f*
area in the brain for, 94*f*
changes with MS, 137–138, 138*t*,
186, 195
color vision in, 28
evaluating/localizing loss of, 27–28,
29*b*, 30*t*
monocular or binocular loss of, 27, 29
positive or negative phenomena of, 27
red desaturation in, 28, **186, 195**
sensory system of, 46
visual association of, 78
See also Neuro-ophthalmologic
disturbances

Visual acuity (VA), 28, 138, 138*t*

Visual agnosia, 78

Visual area 1 (V1), 27

Visual field, testing of, 28, 30*t*

Visual memory, in mental status
assessments, 4

Visuospatial function, in mental status
assessments, 3*t*, 4, 4*f*

Vitamin B$_{12}$ deficiency
dementia associated with, 82*b*, 88
subacute combined degeneration
related to, 154

Vitamin B$_6$ toxicity, peripheral
neuropathy associated with, 157*t*, 159*b*

Vitamin deficiencies
associated with alcohol use/abuse,
126, 126*t*, 127, 127*t*
subacute combined degeneration of
spinal cord associated with,
126–127, 127*t*
syndromes associated with,
126–127, 127*t*

Vitamin E deficiency
peripheral neuropathy associated
with, 165*t*
symptoms of, 57*b/t*

Voice, palatal movement with, 5, 5*t*

Volitional motor unit potentials, 16

Vomiting, associated with cerebellar
ataxia, 57*t*

von Hippel Lindau syndrome, as
neurocutaneous syndrome, 182*t*

Waddling gait, 59, 59*t*

Wakefulness, EEG findings with, 15, 15*f*

Walking
gait evaluation in, 3*t*, 8–9
See also Ambulation; Neurologic
examination

Wallenberg's syndrome
as cause of HS, 31*b*
as vertebrobasilar stroke, 96–97

Water, on MRI imaging, 12

Weakness
associated with ALS, 155, **191, 200**
associated with GBS, 159, **187, 197**
associated with skeletal muscle
disorders, 167, 169
defined, 38
differential dx for, 39–40, 40*t*, 41,
41*t*, 42, 42*f*, 43, 44*f*, 45, 45*f*
patterns of, 40, 40*t*, 41, 41*t*, 42, 42*f*,
43
principles in diagnosis of, 38–39, 39*f*
as sign of MS, 138, 138*t*

Weber test, 5

Wegener's granulomatosis
neurologic symptoms associated
with, 123*t*
PN associated with, 157

Werdnig-Hoffmann disease, 155

Wernicke's aphasia
as differential dx for acute
confusion, 26
features of, 75, 75*t*, 76, 76*t*

Wernicke's area, 65*f*, 66

Wernicke's encephalopathy
associated with alcohol and
nutritional disorders, 126, 126*t*,
127
ataxia associated with, 57, 57*t*
INO associated with, 33
precipitation of, 21

Wechsler Preschool and Primary Scale of
Intelligence-Revised, 177

Western equine encephalitis, 146

West Nile virus, 146

Whipple's disease, 123*t*

White matter, disorders as cause of
progressive encephalopathy, 179*t*

Wilson's disease (WD)
ataxias associated with, 57*b/t*
as cause of dystonia, 115
as cause of myoclonus, 115, 115*b*

chorea associated with, 114*b*
dementia associated with, 82*b*
features/characteristics of, 116, **186, 195**
as genetic movement disorder, 116
Kayser-Fleischer ring associated with, 116, **195–196**
neuropsychiatric symptoms with, 116, **185, 195**

related to copper dysfunction, 116, **185, 195**
tremor associated with, 113*b*, **185, 195**
Withdrawal, acute alcohol, 126*t*
Word salad, 76
Writing, aphasia and problems with, 74, 76*t*, 77

Xanthochromia, 10, 11, 100
X-linked adrenoleukodystrophy, as cause of progressive encephalopathy, 180
X-ray, attenuation of, 11

Zellweger's syndrome, as cause of progressive encephalopathy, 180